PEDIATRICS
for the Physical Therapist Assistant

SECOND EDITION

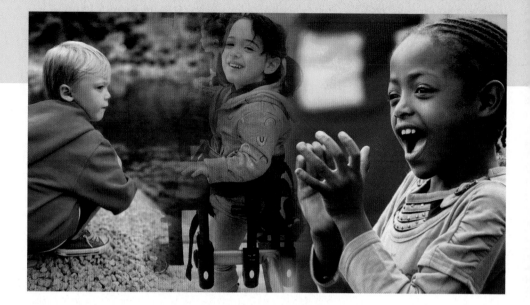

PEDIATRICS
for the Physical Therapist Assistant
SECOND EDITION

Roberta Kuchler O'Shea, PT, DPT, PhD
Professor
Physical Therapy
Governors State University
University Park, IL
Countryside

ELSEVIER

Elsevier
3251 Riverport Lane
St. Louis, Missouri 63043

PEDIATRICS FOR THE PHYSICAL THERAPIST ASSISTANT, SECOND EDITION   ISBN: 978-0-323-88142-5

Notices

Knowledge and best practice in this field are constantly changing. As new research and experience broaden our understanding, changes in research methods, professional practices, or medical treatment may become necessary.

Practitioners and researchers must always rely on their own experience and knowledge in evaluating and using any information, methods, compounds, or experiments described herein. In using such information or methods they should be mindful of their own safety and the safety of others, including parties for whom they have a professional responsibility.

With respect to any drug or pharmaceutical products identified, readers are advised to check the most current information provided (i) on procedures featured or (ii) by the manufacturer of each product to be administered, to verify the recommended dose or formula, the method and duration of administration, and contraindications. It is the responsibility of practitioners, relying on their own experience and knowledge of their patients, to make diagnoses, to determine dosages and the best treatment for each individual patient, and to take all appropriate safety precautions.

To the fullest extent of the law, neither the Publisher nor the authors, contributors, or editors, assume any liability for any injury and/or damage to persons or property as a matter of products liability, negligence or otherwise, or from any use or operation of any methods, products, instructions, or ideas contained in the material herein.

Previous edition copyrighted 2009.

Senior Content Strategist: Lauren Willis
Content Development Manager: Ranjana Sharma
Senior Content Development Specialist: Rishabh Gupta
Publishing Service Manager: Deepthi Unni
Senior Project Manager: Manchu Mohan
Senior Book Designer: Brain Salisbury

Printed in India

Last digit is the print number: 9   8   7   6   5   4   3   2   1

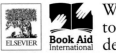

This book is dedicated to my parents, Bob and Joy Kuchler.
Although they died during the last year and before this text went to press,
I hope they are as proud of my work now as they were previously. Their belief
in me propels me forward, and their expectation for best effort, despite the
eventual result, is deeply engrained. I love you and miss you. In addition, my
family, supportive girlfriends, and numerous colleagues never fail when I am all
consumed with a writing project. I appreciate all the cups of tea, back rubs, and
space they provide. Without them I am nothing.

"I can do things you cannot, you can do things I cannot; together we can do great things."

—Mother Teresa

CONTRIBUTORS

Catherine Bookser-Feister, PT, DPT
Board-Certified Specialist in Pediatric Physical Therapy
Adjunct Associate Professor
Doctor of Physical Therapy Program
Department of Rehabilitation
Exercise and Nutrition Sciences
College of Allied Health Sciences
University of Cincinnati
Physical Therapist II
Division of Occupational and Physical Therapy
Cincinnati Children's Hospital Medical Center
Cincinnati, Ohio

Maureen (Mo) Connelly Boyle
Clinician
Prosthetist/Orthotist
Hanger Clinic
Northwestern University
Evanston, Illinois

Kara Boynewicz, PT, DPT, PHD, PCS, ATC
Associate Professor
Department of Rehabilitative Science
East Tennessee State University
Physical Therapist
Department of Rehabilitation
Niswonger Children's Hospital
Johnson City, Tennessee

Kristine (Tina) Chase, PT, DPT, PCS
Clinical Assistant Professor
Department of Physical Therapy
University of Illinois at Chicago
Chicago, Illinois

David Diers, EdD, PT, MHS, ATC
Department Chair
Physical Therapy
Governors State University
University Park, Illinois

Maryleen K. Jones, PT, DHSc, CLT, NCS, CSRS
Physical Therapist
Governors State University
University Park, Illinois

Shruti V. Joshi, PT DPT PCS
Physical Therapy Specialist
Department of Rehabilitation Services
University of Illinois at Chicago
Chicago, Illinois

Leann Kerr, PT, DHS, CBIS
Associate Professor
School of Movement and Rehabilitation Science
Bellarmine University
Louisville, Kentucky

Howe Liu, PhD, MS, MD
Professor
Physical Therapy
Director of Collaborative Research
School of Health Science
Allen College
Waterloo, Iowa
Adjunct Professor
Anatomy
University of North Texas Health Science Center
Fort Worth, Texas

Margaret Mizera, PT, DPT, PCS
Adjunct Faculty
Physical Therapy
Governors State University
University Park, Illinois

Roberta Kuchler O'Shea, PT, DPT, PhD
Professor Emeritus
Physical Therapy
Governors State University
Countryside, Illinois

Matthew Okon, CPO
Clinic Manager
Prosthetist Orthotist in Hanger Clinics
Northwestern University Fienberg School of Medicine
Chicago, Illinois

Susan Ronan, DPT, PT
Board-Certified Clinical Specialist in Pediatric Physical
    Therapy
Clinical Associate Professor
Physical Therapy
Sacred Heart University
Fairfield, Connecticut

Yasser Salem, PT, PhD, MS, NCS, PCS
Professor and Program Director
Allied Health and Kinesiolgy
Hofstra University
Hempstead, New York

Erin Simpson, DrOT, MOT, OTR/L
Assistant Professor
Department of Occupational Therapy
Governors State University
University Park, Illinois

Alison Garlock Small
Pediatric Occupational Therapist
La Rabida Children's Hospital
Chicago, Illinois

Renee Theiss, PhD
Associate Professor
Physical Therapy
Governors State University
University Park, Illinois

Nia Mensah, PT, DPT, PhD, PCS, C/NDT
Associate Professor
Physical Therapy
Long Island University
Brooklyn, New York
President
Kusudi International Incorporated
New York, New York

Jessica Trenkle, PT, DPT, PCS
Physical Therapist
Jessica Trenkle, LLC
Associated Faculty
Physical Therapy & Human Movement Sciences
Northwestern University Feinberg School of Medicine
Chicago, Illinois

PREFACE

This book is the long overdue second edition of *Pediatrics for the Physical Therapy Assistant* written more than 10 years ago. I was so pleased when the editors at Elsevier recognized the need to update this text. The current text includes many new features and topics such as the addition of the Movement Systems Assessment for certain chapters. The chapter authors have worked hard to bring the most current knowledge and evidenced-based PT practice to these pages. In the past 10 years much has changed, and the world has weathered a pandemic that will impact the health care and the development of children for many years and in ways yet untold.

Although this book is designed to be an integral text in PTA education, I also see novice PTs and PTs new to the field of pediatrics using this book as a reference. In the next 10 years I hope the stark line between adult medicine and PT and pediatric rehab and PT will blur, and our profession will realize that children with lifelong disabilities do indeed grow up to live fruitful adult lives. However, they do not shed the impact of their childhood impairments as they venture into adulthood. These young to middle-age adults require, and are currently demanding, rehab teams that understand the impact of their impairments on their aging bodies. Therapists who treat adults will see clients who have lifelong impairments, not just adult-onset issues. Therapists must recognize that the child with CP, for example, may have shoulder impingement syndrome not from being a weekend warrior but from being an everyday warrior who injured their shoulder from overuse of mobility that includes upper extremity use as the norm. The examples and realities are many.

ACKNOWLEDGMENTS

I would like to take this opportunity to thank all the chapter authors who dedicated countless hours to the formation of their chapters. Each has sacrificed many other priorities and opportunities to create a superior educational product that will guide novice, and on occasion veteran, therapists in their clinical decision making. I would also like to give a huge heap of thanks and gratitude to the professionals at Elsevier. Without their foresight, patience, and gentle prodding this second edition would still be a thought. These people include Lauren Willis and Rishabh Gupta in particular. I cherish that the chapter authors and Lauren and Rishabh joined me on this project and as a team we created a respectable product that hopefully will influence many. However, the most important people in all of our clinical lives are the children and families we serve. Their guidance and teachings give us depth and allow us to humbly serve and help to make their world a better place. Without them we are nothing.

CONTENTS

1

Development

Susan Ronan, PT, DPT

LEARNING OBJECTIVES

At the end of the chapter, the reader should be able to do the following:
1. Trace the development of the nervous system.
2. Identify the levels of the central nervous system.
3. Identify stages of development.
4. Recognize primitive reflexes and their impact on development.
5. Understand the issues of how tone can impact development.
6. Recognize the effects of poverty on child development.

CHAPTER OUTLINE

KEY TERMS

Atypical development
Blastocyte
Central nervous system (CNS)
Embryonic stage
Fetal stage
Germinal stage

Homunculus
Nervous system development
Nervous system function
Peripheral nervous system (PNS)
Postnatal
Poverty

Prenatal
Primitive reflexes
Rigidity
Tone
Typical physical development
Zygote

A complete discussion of development should include a general understanding of how the brain, spinal cord, and nervous system develop. Disease or injury to the developing central nervous system (CNS) or peripheral nervous system (PNS) can result in disruption in development.

NERVOUS SYSTEM DEVELOPMENT

Nervous system development encompasses fascinating processes. The brain develops from a few dozen cells of the primitive ectoderm and weighs 800 grams at birth, approximately 1200 grams at age 6 years, and approximately 1400 grams in adulthood. By the sixth week of gestation, the basic form of the human CNS is completed. Peak myelination of the nerves occurs during the third trimester of pregnancy, and development continues as life experiences contribute to functional maturity.[1]

The neural tube in the fetus develops into the brain and spinal cord, or the CNS. The rostral end becomes the brain, and the remainder of the tube closes to become the spinal cord. A condition called *spina bifida* results when the posterior tube does not properly close.

The spinal nerves, or the PNS, can be described as *afferent, efferent, general,* or *special.* Afferent fibers carry sensory messages; efferent fibers carry motor messages; and general fibers innervate the skin, muscles, bones, and viscera. Special fibers innervate sensory organs in the head, such as taste buds, olfactory epithelium, retina, and the cochlear and vestibular apparatus.[1]

Afferent fibers begin in the dorsal root ganglia and exit the spinal cord. Messages coming into the CNS regarding sensory information travel along these pathways. Conversely, efferent fibers originate in the ventral horn of the spinal cord and carry motor messages to the appropriate targets.[2]

NERVOUS SYSTEM FUNCTION

The human nervous system comprises three systems: CNS, PNS, and visceromotor nervous system. We will discuss the CNS and PNS in this section.

Central Nervous System

The CNS consists of the brain and spinal cord. It begins in utero as the neural tube, and in a short time, it folds on itself and differentiates into sections. At the basic level, the nervous system is composed of neurons and glial cells. Neurons synapse with each other, allowing incoming sensory information and outgoing motor responses to pass between the periphery and the CNS. The CNS may be referred to as *gray matter* and *white matter.* This nomenclature indicates which structures are myelinated and which are not. Myelinated structures are considered white matter, whereas nonmyelinated structures are considered gray matter.

The CNS consists of the spinal cord, brainstem, and two cerebral hemispheres (Fig. 1.1). The spinal cord has five levels: cervical, thoracic, lumbar, sacral, and coccygeal. Descending pathways (efferent) originate in the motor cortex and travel to the periphery carrying messages that control voluntary movement. Descending pathways will influence neuronal activity in the spinal cord gray matter. Specific parts of the motor cortex control specific areas of the body. As evident in the homunculus (Fig. 1.2), the lower extremities are controlled in an area close to the central sulcus and midline, whereas upper extremities are controlled more laterally in the motor cortex. Ascending pathways (afferent) carry sensory information from the periphery to the cortex. There are several pathways that carry different sensations from the limbs to the cortex.

Similarly, the lobes of the cerebral hemispheres are diversified to control different functions. The frontal lobe controls cognition and impulse control and contains the motor cortex; the occipital lobe controls visual stimuli; and the temporal lobe controls the language centers, including receptive and expressive language skills. The parietal lobe receives messages from all sensory neurons except those involved with vision and hearing.[3]

The brainstem consists of the medulla oblongata, pons, cerebellum, midbrain, and thalamus. The medulla contains ascending and descending pathways and some nuclei of the cranial nerves. It is also an important relay center for the regulation of respiration, heart rate, and various visceral functions. Embryologically, the pons and the cerebellum originate from the same part of the neural tube. The pons contains nuclei of several cranial nerves and acts as the relay station between the cortex, cerebellum, and descending motor fibers. The cerebellum controls coordination and helps the body produce smooth, purposeful movements. The midbrain houses the descending pathways and nuclei for several cranial nerves; midbrain centers are concerned with vision and auditory pathways, pain transmission, and motor function. The thalamus is surrounded almost completely by the cerebral hemispheres. Except for smell, all sensory

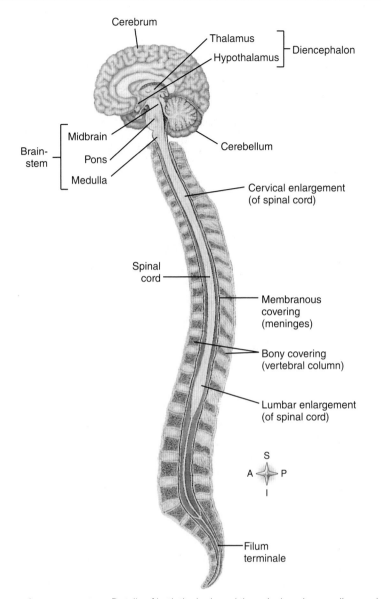

Cerebrum

Thalamus

Hypothalamus

Diencephalon

Brain-stem

Midbrain

Pons

Medulla

Cerebellum

Cervical enlargement
(of spinal cord)

Spinal
cord

Membranous
covering
(meninges)

Bony covering
(vertebral column)

Lumbar enlargement
(of spinal cord)

S
A — P
I

Filum
terminale

Fig. 1.1 The central nervous system. Details of both the brain and the spinal cord are easily seen in this figure. (From Thibodeau GA, Patton KT. *Anatomy & Physiology*. 6th ed. St Louis: Mosby; 2007.)

information reaching the cortex passes through the thalamus. The thalamus conveys information regarding muscle tension and limb position sense to the cortex. This information allows for smooth, coordinated movements to take place. The relatively smaller hypothalamus influences sexual behavior, feeding, hormone output of the pituitary gland, and body temperature regulation.

There are two cerebral hemispheres. Each hemisphere has three subdivisions: the cortex, subcortical white matter, and the basal ganglia. The cortex covers the entire surface of each hemisphere. It is divided into sulci (the indentations in the brain surface) and gyri (the raised areas of the brain surface). The sulci and gyri formations of the brain allow an incredible amount of information to be stored; if the brain had a smooth surface, it would be limited in the amount of information it could process and store. The subcortical white matter is made up of myelinated axons carrying information to and from the

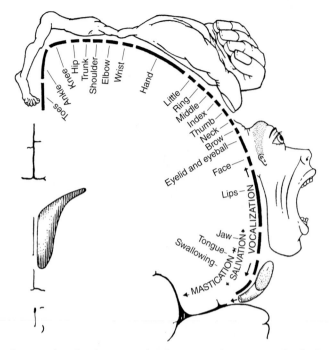

Fig. 1.2 The motor homunculus showing proportional somatotopic representation in the main motor area. (From Standring S. *Gray's Anatomy: The Anatomical Basis of Clinical Practice*. 39th ed. London: Churchill Livingstone; 2005.)

cortex. The most organized portion of this white matter is known as the *internal capsule*. The basal ganglia contain a prominent group of cell bodies involved with motor function. Basal ganglia damage is implicated in disease processes such as Parkinson disease.

Peripheral Nervous System

The PNS is made up of the nerves and nerve pathways that allow signals to travel between the cortex, the spinal cord, and the peripheral muscles of the body (Fig. 1.3). The PNS has sensory fibers and motor fibers that innervate glands and skeletal, cardiac, and smooth muscle. It can regenerate after an injury, whereas the CNS cannot. It is vital to human development that the nervous system form new pathways in the event of injury or damage. This ability to adapt is known as *neuroplasticity*.

TYPICAL PHYSICAL DEVELOPMENT

Human physical development has been well documented and researched. This chapter will provide an overview of typical motor development in infants, toddlers, and children. Motor development can be influenced by individual social, emotional, and cognitive factors, as well as environmental and cultural factors. These influences are beyond the scope of this text and will not be discussed, but several chapters in addition to this one address atypical development secondary to risk factors and physical disabilities.

Typical physical development is based on an uncomplicated pregnancy lasting for a gestational period of approximately 37 to 40 weeks. During gestation, the fetus undergoes significant changes. These changes continue after the child is born, with some occurring well into adolescence and young adulthood.

At conception, fertilization occurs when the sperm and the ovum combine to form a new cell called a zygote. The zygote duplicates itself multiple times by cell division to eventually form a fetus. This duplication process is known as *mitosis* and includes the duplication of all the genes and chromosomes. If there is a disruption in the duplication process—for instance, if there are too many or not enough chromosomes or the chromosomes are improperly located—typical development is compromised.

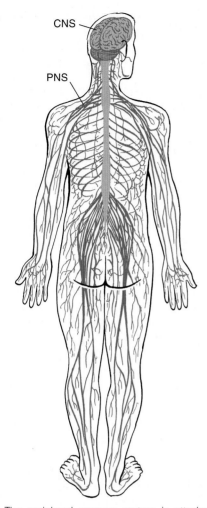

CNS

PNS

Fig. 1.3 The peripheral nervous system is attached to the central nervous system, but its nerve fibers are distributed throughout the body. (From Nolte J. *The Human Brain: An Introduction to Its Functional Anatomy.* 5th ed. St Louis: Mosby; 2002. Redrawn from Krstić RV. *General Histology of the Mammal.* Berlin: Springer-Verlag; 1985.)

Each cell in the human body contains approximately 60,000 to 100,000 genes. Genes carry developmental instructions to form a human being from a zygote. The genes are located in specific locations on the chromosomes. Each human cell, except the sex cells, should contain 23 pairs of chromosomes, totaling 46 chromosomes in all. The sex cells contain 23 single chromosomes, and when they combine at fertilization, the zygote has 46 chromosomes.

Prenatal

There are three major stages in prenatal (before birth) development: germinal, embryonic, and fetal. The germinal stage occurs from fertilization until roughly 2 weeks' gestational age. During this stage, the zygote implants in the uterine wall and divides. When the cell divides, it is no longer a zygote, but instead is referred to as a blastocyte. The blastocyte cells will begin to differentiate into several areas. A thickened area will evolve into two layers, the ectoderm and endoderm. The ectoderm will eventually become the outer layer of skin, nails, teeth, sensory organs, and nervous system, including the brain and spinal cord. The endoderm will transform into the digestive system, liver, pancreas, salivary glands, and respiratory system. In due time, a middle layer, the mesoderm, will differentiate and become the inner layer of skin, muscles, skeleton, and excretory and circulatory systems. Other areas of the blastocyte will evolve into protective components for the fetus, specifically the placenta, umbilical cord, and amniotic sac.

The embryonic stage occurs during weeks 2 to 8 of gestation. During this time, there is continued rapid growth and development of the major body systems, including the respiratory, digestive, and nervous systems. This stage is considered a high-risk time because the developing embryo can sustain significant damage from a host of factors. Most severely defective embryos will not survive past this stage.

The fetal stage constitutes the period between 8 weeks after conception and birth. During this stage, rapid growth continues, and organs and body systems become more refined (Table 1.1). Fingernails, toenails, and eyelashes develop. The fetus actively moves within the uterus, and these movements can be tracked by means of ultrasonography. Motor patterns arise spontaneously and are not reflexive.[4] Other aspects of fetal development, including heart rate and cardiac activity and sleep/wake states, can also be monitored. Beginning at approximately 26 weeks' gestation, fetuses also begin to respond to familiar voices, sounds (mother's heartbeat), and external environmental stimuli (vibration). The fetus's brain is highly vascularized between 28 and 32 weeks' gestation.[2] If a fetus experiences aggressive movements (such as birth or transfer via ambulance to a neonatal intensive care unit [NICU]) during this time, there is great potential for injury to the motor cortex.

TABLE 1.1	Motor Development of the Fetus		
	10–15 Weeks	**17–18 Weeks**	**20 Weeks**
Upper extremity	Isolated extremity movements; hands to face; thumb sucking		Wide arcs of arm movement
Locomotion	Full body rotation around the umbilicus; climbing on the uterine wall	Vigorous extensor thrusts against uterine wall repositions fetus	Period of greatest mobility; creeping/crawling movement
Atypical behaviors	Fetal akinesia	Symmetric, stereotypic movements lacking dissociation	

From Long T, Toscano K. *Handbook of Pediatric Physical Therapy.* 2nd ed. Philadelphia: Lippincott Williams & Wilkins; 2002.

Postnatal

Following birth (postnatal), the stages of human development continue. They include infant and toddler (0–3 years); early (3–6 years) and middle (6–12 years) childhood; adolescence (12–20 years); and young (20–40 years), middle (40–65 years), and late (older than 65 years) adulthood. Similar to prenatal development, childhood motor development is affected by several factors, including social-emotional and cognitive development, as well as the environment and culture (see Box 1.1).

THEORIES OF GROSS MOTOR DEVELOPMENT

Motor development is the outcome of many systems working together. This includes neural, environmental, kinesiological, and musculoskeletal. Development can be viewed through several lenses and theories. This section will address several theories of development. Motor development in neonates and infants typically occurs in three directions: cephalocaudal, proximal-distal, and flexion into extension. The infant's

BOX 1.1	Key Facts About American Children
Every 2 seconds a public-school student is suspended	Every 2 hours and 36 minutes a child or teen is injured with a gun
Every 9 seconds a high school student drops out	Every 3 hours and 11 minutes a child or teen dies by suicide
Every 45 seconds a child is arrested	Every 5 hours a child is killed by abuse or neglect
Every 48 seconds a child is confirmed abused or neglected	Every 11 hours and 40 minutes a mother dies from complications of childbirth or pregnancy
Every 49 seconds a public-school student is corporally punished	More than 1 in 3 children live in households burdened by housing costs
Every 1 minute a baby is born into poverty	1 in 3 youth in the juvenile justice system has a condition qualifying them for special education
Every 2 minutes a baby is born without health insurance	1 in 4 children are children of immigrants
Every 2 minutes a baby is born into extreme poverty	1 in 5 children of color are poor
Every 2 minutes a baby is born at low birthweight	Nearly 1 in 6 children under six years of age were poor in 2019 and almost half lived in extreme poverty
Every 2 minutes a child is removed from their home and placed in foster care	1 in 7 children lived in food-insecure households before the COVID-19 Pandemic
Every 6.5 minutes a child is arrested for a drug offense	1 in 15 children eligible for after school suppers received them
Every 12 minutes a child is arrested for a violent offense	
Every 25 minutes a baby dies before their first birthday	
Every hour and 11 minutes a child or teen dies from an accident	

From the Children's Defense Fund (website): https://www.childrensdefense.org/wp-content/uploads/2021/04/The-State-of-Americas-Children-2021.pdf. Accessed June 21, 2023.

movement must also be observed in several positions, including prone, supine, sitting, suspended prone, and standing. At birth, the neonate is dominated by primitive reflexes and a flexion posture but should be able to breathe and suck independently. Over the next few months, head and neck control and visual and auditory acuity are acquired. The baby will bat at objects, kick (randomly at first), and begin to prop up on forearms and later hands as the shoulder and hip/pelvis musculature become stronger. The baby learns to roll and differentiate the upper half of the body from the lower half.[5]

Neural Maturational Theory was pioneered by Arnold Gesell. Gesell viewed development as an intrinsic property of the child, with development occurring in predetermined patterns caused by the brain and nervous system.[6] Examples of this view of development include developmental reflexes and milestones that occur in a set sequence. These reflexes and milestones will be discussed later in this chapter. Cognitive theories of development include work by Piaget and Skinner.

Cognitive Theories: Piaget's work focused on maturation of cognition as children understand their environment by interpreting their experiences through interaction. Examples of Piaget's theory include developmental periods such as the sensorimotor, representational thought, concrete operations, and formal operations periods.[7] As a child develops, their understanding becomes more complex and logical. B. F. Skinner's work is identified with behavioral psychology. Skinner viewed behavior as being shaped and developed through experiences and outcomes.[8] The outcomes can be reinforced, which makes them more likely to occur, or discouraged, making them less likely to occur. The Dynamic Systems Theory regards development as the sum of multiple influences. Esther Thelen is the pioneer of this theory. Dynamic Systems Theory recognizes the complexity of development. A child's development can be influenced by factors such as environmental affordances that make one behavior more likely than another. Self-organizing patterns of behavior emerge and over time move from simpler to more complex.[9,10] The Neuronal Group Selection Theory was developed by Edelman and Hadders-Algra.[11] This theory uses knowledge about the nervous system, which is viewed as having primary and secondary variability. "In primary variability, development is occurring through the variability of motor experiences and output, which are minimally adapted. In secondary variability, trial and error is one learning strategy used by the child to refine their movements and responses. This theory recognizes the impact of genetic information on development as well as motor development and the environment."[11] This theory does not view nervous system development or genetic factors as the sole determinants of movement. Rather, the interplay of the child's experiences and the ability to learn from the environment and motor outcomes will result in movement development.

It is also important to consider the role of genes and genomics. Each person has their own unique genetic code, but the expression of some genes can be altered by influences in the environment, such as diet and stress.[12] "Genomics is the study of all of a person's genes (the genome), including interactions of those genes with each other and with the person's environment."[13] A child's development can be affected by their parent's experiences and genetic code. For example, lower socioeconomic status has been an influence on worse birth outcomes.[14] Poverty and poor air quality are related to children having asthma.[15] Research has demonstrated that parents', and even grandparents', exposures to poverty influence child outcomes in subsequent generations.[14]

Reflexes

During the first year of life, children learn to roll, sit, crawl, and move into and out of those positions safely. Although primitive reflexes dominate the movement of young infants, as the child matures and develops control, the once obligatory reflexes become inhibited, and volitional control is available. Many of the postural reflexes, such as the Landau response, will assist the child in developing upright antigravity control. One may see a resurgence of reflexes when the child/adult is involved in high-stress situations. For example, clonus is the rapid beating of the foot in response to a quick stretch of the gastrocnemius tendon. If this reflex fails to be integrated, ambulation proves difficult. Picture a group of young adults experiencing a high ropes course for the first time. At 40 feet in the air, while standing on a 2-inch-diameter rope, the clonus may reoccur in the novice climber. Uncontrolled foot tapping during an important exam, or even during an intense job interview, may also be observed. These uncontrolled foot-tapping behaviors, although very inhibited in normal situations, may be an indication of clonus.

Primitive reflexes are dominant when a child is born and often reappear in the presence of an upper motor neuron lesion. Reflexes are important to the infant as they learn to move against gravity and develop postural control. In infancy, as development proceeds, primitive reflexes become integrated as motor skills, and postural/balance reactions emerge.[16]

The following reflexes will be described in more detail: suck/swallow, rooting, Galant, flexor withdrawal, Landau, plantar and palmar grasp, and asymmetric tonic neck reflex (ATNR).

Suck/swallow reflex. Most babies are born with a strong suck/swallow reflex. This reflex allows the child to obtain and maintain oral nutrition. It is usually integrated at age 2 to 5 months. In response to a stimulus in the mouth, the baby begins to suck and swallow and learns how to feed and control flow from a breast or bottle. Some infants born with medical risks, especially prematurity, may lack the suck/swallow reflex. Early therapeutic intervention works to rectify the deficit and help the baby develop strong suck/swallow skills.

Rooting reflex. The rooting reflex is related to the suck/swallow reflex and is integrated at 3 months. Stroking either side of the mouth will cause the baby to turn toward the ipsilateral (same) side. This reflex allows babies to locate their food source. When they feel the breast or bottle brush up against their cheek, they automatically turn toward the source. If it is a food source, the baby may find a nipple in their mouth, the suck/swallow reflex is activated, and the baby is feeding. If the rooting reflex is not appropriately integrated, the baby may be obligated to turn the head toward any stimulus that touches the cheek area. In a severe circumstance, if a child has a dominant rooting reflex, the child's wheelchair head rest/neck rest or even a strong breeze could elicit the rooting response, and the child may turn toward the stimulus even when it is not appropriate to do so.

Galant reflex. The Galant reflex occurs in response to stroking the paraspinals. The body's involuntary response is to bend to the stimulated side. This side bending helps a baby to develop rolling and controlled trunk movements. If not appropriately integrated bilaterally, the child may develop musculoskeletal deformities in response to repeated side-bending postures when stimulated by a back cushion or may be at risk for ipsilateral hip dislocation.[3]

Flexor withdrawal reflex. Flexor withdrawal is a reflex that causes the baby to pull the lower extremity into flexion after a sudden stimulus to the bottom of the foot. This reflex is helpful for safety reasons. For example, if you were walking along barefoot on a rug and stepped on a sharp tack, the flexor withdrawal reflex would cause you to pull your foot away immediately, thus keeping you safe. However, if you could not control this reflex, it stands to reason that every time you took a step, your lower extremities would go into an exaggerated lower extremity flexor movement pattern.

Landau response. The Landau response is an extension response to being in the prone position. When prone, the child plays in the "airplane position": extension of the hips, shoulders, and trunk. While prone, the child will also move into and out of flexion and extension patterns. This response helps the infant develop co-contraction of the proximal joints and coordination of movement between flexion and extension. The Landau response is usually integrated by 6 months, as the child learns to push up into a four-point position, requiring flexion of the hips and shoulders while maintaining trunk extension.

Grasp reflexes. Plantar grasp is the curling of the toes in response to pressure at the ball of the foot; palmar grasp is the curling of the hand and fingers in response to pressure in the palm. The plantar reflex makes it difficult to put on an infant's shoes. Dominant plantar reflexes may inhibit children from walking with a typical gait pattern.

The palmar grasp indirectly assists in bonding. Some infant-parent dyads have difficulty bonding for a myriad of reasons (such as social-emotional issues and medical frailty). The palmar grasp results in a child automatically grasping and not releasing an object put into the hand. While the baby is feeding, the caregiver can massage the baby's palm, and that hand will immediately assume the grasping position and maintain a hold on the person's fingers for a bit. The best outcome will be that the caregiver feels the child is expressing love, and the upward cycle begins: caregiver plays with child, child inadvertently grasps, caregiver finds this cute and encourages the behavior. This behavior works well for an infant, but the obligatory grasp inhibits development if not integrated. Imagine the toddler or preschooler who cannot release an object. If this child grabs something hot and holds on, the child will be injured. Both the palmar and plantar grasps should be integrated by 9 months.

Asymmetric tonic neck reflex. The ATNR is often referred to as the *fencing reflex* and is normally seen in infants 3 to 5 months old. As they turn to look to the left or right, the ipsilateral upper extremity goes into extension, and the contralateral upper extremity comes up into horizontal flexion. Similarly, the ipsilateral lower extremity extends, and the contralateral lower extremity flexes; hence, the baby appears to be "fencing." This reflex is helpful when the child is developing hand-eye coordination and learning about cause and effect. For example, a noise on the left might attract a baby's attention. The baby looks left, causing the left upper extremity to extend, and while extending, this arm inadvertently hits the baby's overhead mobile and causes the toy to move and make noise; the baby notices the mobile (cause-and-effect knowledge develops). Although the ATNR is useful to the developing infant, a person with an inappropriately dominant ATNR will have difficulty completing midline, two-handed activities and difficulty mastering independent living skills such as self-feeding and dressing.

Motor Development

Typical motor milestones for infants are as follows: head control develops at 4 months, rolling begins between 6 and 8 months, sitting develops between 5 and 7 months, creeping usually appears at 9 to 10 months, competent in cruising furniture begins at 10 to 11 months, and ambulation skills are mastered between 12 and 15 months (Table 1.2). Some children will walk as early as 10 months or as late as 18 months. Children who have not begun ambulating by 16 to 18 months should be assessed by a developmental professional. Infants gain the status of toddler after mastering ambulation. As a child becomes a toddler and masters upright mobility, developmental fine-tuning emerges.

As children learn to roll, they begin to differentiate segments of their bodies. The head and trunk and legs learn to move independently of one another. Similarly, children learn to differentiate between moving the left

TABLE 1.2 Motor Milestones for Infants	
Skill	Typical Acquisition Age
Head control	4 months
Rolling	6–8 months
Sitting	5–7 months
Creeping	9–10 months
Cruising	10–11 months
Ambulation	12–15 months
Steps and higher level skills	18 months

side of the body and the right side of the body. This allows for reciprocal movements between the arms and legs when crawling, walking, and riding a bike.

As the child grows and develops, typical gait parameters (step and stride length, base of support, cadence) change. These changes happen in response to overall changes occurring system-wide and include changes in the neuromuscular system, the musculoskeletal system, and the sensory system.[17] Children begin to ambulate with a wide base of support, upper extremities in a high- or low-guard position, and lower extremities in slight flexion. At this phase, the child tends to posture with the upper extremities in high-guard or arms-in-the-air position, where the shoulders are horizontally flexed to approximately 90 degrees, the elbows are flexed to 90 degrees, the wrist and hands are extended, and the hands are at about the level of the child's ears. As balance develops, the toddler will assume a low-guard position of the upper extremities. In this posture, the shoulders tend to be more in a neutral position, with the elbows in flexion and the hands/fingers in extension. Thus, the child's arms are closer to waist level, but the child is prepared for a stumble or fall, using upper extremity extension as needed.

As the child gains confidence and experience in ambulating, the base of support narrows, the step length and stride length increase, and the child moves with a slower cadence. The overall gait cycle becomes smoother and more fluid. Near 17 months, or after a few months of mobility practice, the child will begin to demonstrate a more heel-toe gait pattern, lateral weight shift, and reciprocal arm swing. After 18 months, a typically developing child begins to ascend and descend steps, kick, and catch a ball and try to jump, hop, and run well. The child masters the three latter skills at about 3 years of age. Between 6 and 10 years, the child should have mastered the adult forms of running, hopping, jumping, and throwing.[18]

ATYPICAL DEVELOPMENT

Several factors may affect a child's development. There are hallmark methods to describe delays or differences in development, including increases and decreases in tone, delayed motor development, delayed cognitive and communicative development, and inappropriately dominant primitive reflexes. Some of the delays may be significant at birth but diminish over time. Other delays will influence the child's growth and development over the entire life span. Atypical development may be caused by upper motor neuron disease, lower motor neuron disease, muscle disease, or genetic malformation and toxin exposure.

Upper motor neuron diseases affect the upper motor neuron systems in the CNS: the cortex, cranial nerve nuclei in the brainstem, and spinal cord. Cerebral palsy and spinal cord injury are examples of upper motor neuron pathologies. Lower motor neurons include the PNS and cranial nerves. Erb's palsy is an example of a lower motor neuron disease. Muscle disease, such as muscular dystrophy, will also cause disruptions in development.

Tone

Tone is the normal tension found in muscles. It can be described as the slight resistance felt when a joint is moving in its total range of motion.[19] Atypical tone becomes an issue when it affects the child's ability to move and be independent. Tone is often a relative term when the total population is considered, and the range of normal is quite variable. As clinicians become more experienced with the feeling of tone, they can discriminate when variances may cause developmental complications.

Atypical tone includes hypertonia, mixed or fluctuating tone, rigidity, and hypotonia. The Modified Ashworth Scale of spasticity (Table 1.3) can be used to quantitatively describe tone. The Modified Ashworth Scale represents a grading scale for degree of spasticity. The patient receives a grade of 0 for no tone; 1 for slight increase in tone, with minimal resistance during flexion and extension; 1+ for slight increase in tone, with minimal resistance in remainder of range of motion; 2 for marked increased tone, but the limb can be easily flexed; 3 for considerable increase in tone, making passive range of motion (PROM) difficult; and 4 for rigidity in flexion and extension.[3]

Increased tone is also known as *hypertonia*. Hypertonia is commonly seen in individuals with upper motor neuron disease and is described as an increase in stiffness in muscles of the limb or trunk; it may also be called *spasticity*. Resistance to movement increases in response to rapid movement of the joint or limb, as if the joint were "catching." Hypertonia can often be reduced with the use of handling techniques and orthotics.

TABLE 1.3   Modified Ashworth Scale

Grade	Description
0	No increase in muscle tone
1	Slight increase in muscle tone, manifested by a catch and release or by minimal resistance at the end of the range of motions (ROM) when the affected part(s) is moved in flexion or extension
1+	Slight increase in muscle tone, manifested by a catch, followed by minimal resistance throughout the remainder (less than half) of the ROM
2	More marked increase in muscle tone through most of the ROM, but affected parts move easily
3	Considerable increase in muscle tone; passive movement difficult
4	Affected part(s) rigid in flexion or extension

Athetoid tone involves writhing, uncontrolled movements. Athetoid tone is a result of damage to the extrapyramidal region near the basal ganglia, not damage in the motor cortex. Fluctuating tone indicates fluctuations between hypertonia and near-normal tone. Children with spastic cerebral palsy often have underlying athetoid movements of the extremities and may exhibit fluctuating tone. Orthotic intervention techniques to normalize tone will be described in later chapters in detail.

Rigidity is also a significant resistance to movement; however, the typical causes are extrapyramidal syndromes (dystonias) and damage such as that from Parkinson disease or after an anoxic event. Rigidity differs from spasticity because it is present through the entire range of motion. It is described as "lead pipe" or "cogwheel rigidity." In the first type, the individual's extreme tone does not break and feels as if you are trying to bend a lead pipe. Cogwheel rigidity is described as intermittent breaks in increased tone throughout range of motion, so the limb moves in a cogwheel pattern.[3]

Hypotonia, on the other hand, is "floppiness" or lack of resistance to movement. Marked hypotonia is referred to as *flaccidity*. Hypotonia may be associated with lower motor neuron involvement and would be present in association with polio, spinal cord injury, or brachial plexus injuries. Additionally, some genetic diseases, such as Down syndrome, are often characterized by increased hypotonia.

Other Developmental Issues

Other developmental issues will also affect typical development. If a child is born blind or with visual impairments, acquisition of gross motor movements will be delayed. As the child learns about the environment and begins to explore, motor skills rapidly improve. Typically, by the time the child is a toddler, motor skills are age appropriate.[17]

Conversely, children with hearing impairments appear to develop typically as infants, but as they age, it becomes apparent that they may have cognitive and language delays. With intervention, many of these delays can be minimized.

Children with peripheral nerve damage or missing limbs may also experience early motor delays. As children cognitively advance and learn how to adapt their movements using intact body segments or prosthetics or orthotics, motor skills and independent activities-of-daily-living skills develop. Often, by the time the children are nearing early childhood (ages 3–5), they have adapted their movement patterns, and their skills are independent and age appropriate. Several developmental sequelae and relevant interventions are discussed in depth in the following chapters.

Social Determinants of Health

The Centers for Disease Control and Prevention has organized social determinants of health into five areas: healthcare access and quality, economic stability, social and community context, neighborhood and built environment, and education access and quality.[20] Poverty seriously affects health and human development, and it has a significant and detrimental effect on child development. According to the United States 2019 census, nearly 1 in 7 children live in poverty, with 71% being members of minority racial groups.[21] Poverty has been linked to higher rates of infant mortality, asthma, overweight or obesity, and increased risk factors for lack of learning readiness and mental health conditions for children.[22] Each of these conditions has significant health implications, and some are discussed elsewhere in the text.

Living in poverty often results in suboptimal and infrequent healthcare, exacerbation of chronic conditions, and risky environments. Children are less likely to see a healthcare professional and receive recommended care when affected by poverty.[23] Poverty directly affects a society's health issues by increasing the number of premature births or infants with low birth weight resulting from inadequate maternal prenatal care. "In United States in 2020, preterm birth affected 1 in 10 infants born, with the rate of preterm birth for African-American women (14.4%) 50% higher than the rate of preterm birth among White or Hispanic women (9.1% and 9.8% respectively)."[24] Stress, racism, and poverty contribute to rates of preterm birth. The phenomenon of "weathering" also contributes to worse birth and maternal outcomes.[25] Weathering is the cumulative effect of stressors such as poverty.

SUMMARY

Knowledge of typical and atypical child development is important because it forms a basis for physical therapy practice. Each child is unique, and recognizing the skills and abilities of each child enables the physical therapist assistant to manage successful interventions.

CHAPTER DISCUSSION QUESTIONS

1. Identify three ways poverty may impact a child's development.
2. Conceptualize one community-based strategy to help address environmental deficit.
3. Identify the three components of the human nervous system.
4. Describe motor development progression and how that progression affects the developmental sequence.
5. What is the developmental impact on a child if the following are not integrated?
   a. Rooting reflex
   b. ATNR
   c. Galant reflex
6. Define hypotonia.
7. Choose a type of atypical tone and describe how this tonal influence can affect a 6-year-old child's ability to function in an inclusive classroom setting.
8. List the components of the CNS.

9. How does the CNS differ from the PNS?
10. At what week of gestation is the basic CNS developed?

REFERENCES

1. Haines DE, Mihailoff GA. *Fundamental Neuroscience.* 5th ed. New York: Elsevier; 2018.
2. Gilman S, Newman SW. *Essentials of Clinical Neuroanatomy and Neurophysiology.* 10th ed. Philadelphia: FA Davis; 2003.
3. Accardo PJ, Whitman BY. *Dictionary of Developmental Disabilities Terminology.* 3rd ed. Baltimore: Paul H. Brookes; 2011.
4. Long T, Battaile B, Toscano K. *Handbook of Pediatric Physical Therapy.* 3rd ed. Philadelphia: Lippincott Williams & Wilkins; 2018.
5. Kobayashi Y, Yozu A, Watanabe H, Taga G. Multiple patterns of infant rolling in limb coordination and ground contact pressure. *Exp Brain Res.* 2021;239(9):2887–2904.
6. Gessell at Yale Program in Early Childhood: Gesell theory. Accessed June 18, 2022. https://www.gesell-yale.org/pages/gesell-theory.
7. Houdé O. Ethical views and considerations. *Handb Clin Neurol.* 2020;173:15–21. doi:10.1016/B978-0-444-6410-2.00003-4.
8. Gewirtz JL, Pelaez-Nogueras M. B. F. Skinner's legacy to human infant behavior and development. *Am Psychol.* 1992;47(11):1411–1422.
9. Thelen E, Ulrich BD. Hidden skills: a dynamic systems analysis of treadmill stepping during the first year. *Monog Soc Res Child Dev.* 1991;56(1):1–98.
10. Rahlin M, Barnett J, Becker E, Fregosi CM. Development through the lens of a perception-action-cognition connection: recognizing the need for a paradigm shift in clinical reasoning. *Phys Ther.* 2019;99(6):748.
11. Hadders-Algra M. Early human motor development: from variation to the ability to vary and adapt. *Neurosci Biobehav Rev.* 2018;90:411–427.
12. Armstrong-Carter E, Wertz J, Domingue BW. Genetics and child development: recent advances and their implications for developmental research. *Child Dev Perspect.* 2021;15(1):57.
13. National Institutes of Health. National Human Genome Research Institute: A brief guide to genomics. Accessed November 5, 2021. https://www.genome.gov/about-genomics/fact-sheets/A-Brief-Guide-to-Genomics.
14. Weightman AL, Morgan HE, Shepherd MA, Kitcher H, Roberts C, Dunstan FD. Social inequality and infant health in the UK: systematic review and meta-analyses. *BMJ OPEN.* 2012;2(3):e000964.
15. Cook Q, Argenio K, Lovindky-Desir S. The impact of environmental injustice and social determinants of health on the role of air pollution in asthma and allergic disease in the United States. *J Allergy Clin Immunol.* 2021;148(5):1089–1101.e5.
16. Modrell AK, Tadi P: Primitive reflexes. In Abai A, et al, editors: *StatPearls,* Treasure Island, FL, 2022, StatPearls Publishing. Updated March 9, 2022.
17. Bierman JC. Developing ambulation skills. In: Connolly BH, Montgomery PC, eds. *Therapeutic Exercise in Developmental Disabilities.* 3rd ed. Thorofare, NJ: Slack; 2005.
18. Cech D, Martin S. *Functional Movement Development Across the Life Span.* 2nd ed. Philadelphia: Saunders; 2002.
19. Fuller G. *Neurological exam made easy.* 2nd ed. Edinburgh: Churchill Livingstone; 2002.
20. Centers for Disease Control and Prevention: Social determinants of health at CDC. Accessed on April 11, 2022. https://wwwcdcgov/socialdeterminants/indexhtm, https://www.cdc.gov/socialdeterminants/index.htm.
21. Children's Defense Fund. The state of America's children 2021. Child poverty. (website). Accessed April 11, 2022. https://www.childrensdefense.org/state-of-americas-children/soac-2021-child-poverty/.
22. Gupta RP, de Wit ML, McKeown D. The impact of poverty on the current and future health status of children. *Paediatr Child Health.* 2007;12(8):667–672.
23. Cree RA, Bitsko RH, Robinson LR, others. Health care, family, and community factors associated with mental, behavioral, and developmental disorders and poverty among children aged 2–8 years—United States, 2016. *MMWR Morb Mortal Wkly Rep.* 2018;67:1377–1383.
24. Centers for Disease Control and Prevention. Reproductive health: preterm birth. Accessed April 11, 2022. https://www.cdc.gov/reproductivehealth/maternalinfant-health/pretermbirth.htm.
25. Love C, David RJ, Rankin KM, Collins JW Jr. Exploring weathering: effects of lifelong economic environment and maternal age on low birth weight, small for gestational age, and preterm birth in African-American and white women. *Am J Epidemiol.* 2010;172(2):127–134.

RESOURCES

National Institute of Child Health and Human Development
www.nichd.nih.gov
Society for Research and Child Development
University of Michigan
3131 S. State Street, #302
Ann Arbor, MI 48108-1623
734-998-6578
www.srcd.org

National Association for Child Development
International Headquarters, 5492 S 500 E
Washington Terrace, Utah 84405
Phone: +1 (801) 621-8606
www.nacd.org

Foundation for Child Development
475 Riverside Drive, Suite 248
New York, NY 10115
www.fcd-us.org
Children's Defense Fund
www.childrensdefense.org

Assessments

Roberta Kuchler O'Shea, PT, DPT, PhD
Shruti V. Joshi, PT, DPT, PCS

LEARNING OBJECTIVES

At the end of the chapter, the reader will be able to do the following:

1. Differentiate between norm- and criterion-referenced assessments.
2. Discuss psychometric properties of different assessments.
3. Determine the purpose and design of each assessment tool.
4. Appreciate that one assessment is not appropriate for all testing purposes and all children.

CHAPTER OUTLINE

KEY TERMS

Criterion-referenced assessment tools

Norm-referenced assessment tools

Qualitative assessment

Quantitative assessment

This chapter introduces several assessment tools used in pediatric settings. Although the physical therapist assistant (PTA) does not evaluate children directly, it is helpful to be familiar with the types of assessment tools commonly used in pediatric physical therapy examination and diagnosis. Familiarity with this component of the record gives a PTA background knowledge essential to being able to read assessment reports and understand their content. Data describing motor development (Fig. 2.1) are typically divided into three areas: gross motor skills, fine motor skills, and oral motor skills. Since physical therapy traditionally focuses on gross motor and fine motor development, only these two areas will be discussed in this chapter. Oral motor skills are outside the scope of this text.

PURPOSE

The purpose of assessment is to screen for delays or abnormalities, provide a diagnosis and/or prognosis, evaluate outcomes and progress, develop goals, collect data, and ultimately help direct the plan of care. When an assessment is used to determine a diagnosis, it is attempting to distinguish individual characteristics based on some feature of interest. Data can also be used to classify children for program placement. When

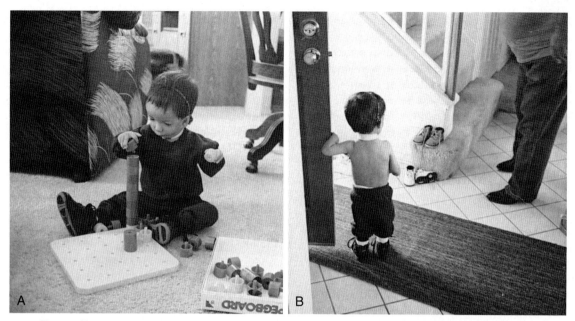

Fig. 2.1 Physical therapists and physical therapist assistants help children with their fine motor skills **(A)** and gross motor skills **(B)**. (From Parham LD, Fazio LS. *Play in Occupational Therapy for Children.* 2nd ed. St Louis: Mosby; 2008.)

making determinations or diagnosis decisions, it is best to use a standardized and norm-referenced assessment tool designed to be demographically representative of a given population as a whole. The reference group used in developing such tests is called a *norming sample*.

If an assessment tool is being used to evaluate outcomes and progress, the tool should document change over a period of time or evaluate the effectiveness of a program or intervention. The tool should be standardized and sensitive enough to measure change in performance over time.

To develop goals and outcomes, the preferred assessment tool should measure individual competencies and needs, be standardized, and document validity of the intervention for program planning. Some definitions and descriptions you may find useful are as follows[1]:

- Age-equivalent score: the mean chronological age represented by a certain score. This score is useful when assessing and describing developmentally delayed children who cannot achieve a developmental index score. Parents and caregivers may understand the age-equivalent scores more easily than other statistical data. However, these data are not necessarily statistically sound. It is better to use percentile or standard scores for data reporting.

- Percentile score: the percentage of children at the same age or grade level who should perform at a lower level. For example, if a boy is in the 60th percentile, he performed better than 60% of children in the norm group or reference group population. The average range of scores is between the 16th and 84th percentiles.

- Percentage score: expresses the percent of items passed on a scale.

- Raw score: actual points earned on an assessment or number of items passed on a certain test. Several assessments require the child to achieve a basal (baseline) and a ceiling (cutoff) score. Each tool has particular criteria for establishing a child's basal and ceiling scores.

- Scaled score: provides an estimate of the child's ability level along a continuum of items. Scores range from 0 to 100; 0 is low capacity, and 100 is highly capable.

- Standard scores: describe deviations from the mean, or average, score for the group. Standard deviations are used to describe the divergence.

- Standard tests: tests that include a set of tasks or questions intended to assess a particular type of behavior when presented under standardized conditions.

- Reliability: determines whether the tool is an accurate measure of what it claims to measure. Typically, reliability is measured as the consistency of test item agreement between two or more observers or between two administrations of a test. Error in measurement can occur between two evaluators or because of errors in the test. The standard measure of error demonstrates the range of variability in which the true ability of an individual probably lies. Hence, it expresses test reliability for an individual independent of the variability found in a group.
- Validity: determines whether the assessment tool accomplishes its intended purpose. There are several types of validity. *Face validity* is the concept that the test strongly measures what it claims to measure. (Is the face value of the assessment valid and true?) *Content validity* requires that the assessment sample a reasonable range of target behaviors. (Is the content of the assessment measuring what it claims to measure?) *Concurrent validity* correlates the child's performance on an assessment to another valid assessment. (Will the child achieve the same age or developmental level on two different assessments given in the same time period?) *Construct validity* requires that the test explain the child's achievement within a theoretical framework. *Predictive validity* describes how well the assessment tool predicts the child's performance at a future date.[2]
- Responsiveness: the ability to detect minimally significant clinical change.
- Minimal Clinical Difference (MCD): a determination if the change in performance is based on intervention. A client's performance must exceed MCD value to be considered clinically relevant.

QUALITATIVE ASSESSMENTS

The primary purpose of qualitative assessment is to understand people's perspectives and their interpretation of behaviors and expressions.[3] There are several ways to assess a child and family, and using a combination of methods will provide a richer understanding of the child. Methods include an interview with the child, family, and caregivers; observation in settings familiar to the child (e.g., home, day care, and school); chart reviews of existing medical and educational records; and the assessment tools.

When assessing a young child, it is imperative to discuss the child's progress, or lack thereof, with a person familiar with the child. The reporter may be able to provide necessary history and areas of concern. An older child may provide an understanding of his or her own motor concerns. In either case, identification of family/child priorities is vital to creating a successful plan of care. Existing medical or educational records provide the clinician with a window into the past; without having been there, the clinician gains insight into previous motor assessment performance. This insight can come from previously conducted standardized assessments and provider reports.[1]

QUANTITATIVE ASSESSMENTS

In quantitative assessment, researchers identify an inquiry area within a broad scope that requires investigation. The investigators' questions are narrow and have well-defined boundaries regarding who or what will be investigated. A specific experimental design is employed to answer the defined questions.[3]

STANDARDIZED ASSESSMENT TOOLS

Standardized assessments adhere to a formal administration and scoring protocol. These assessments can be categorized into two types: norm-referenced and criterion-referenced (Table 2.1). The differences between the two are significant and should be recognized prior to choosing an assessment tool.[1]

Norm-referenced assessment tools have been standardized on a demographically representative population and evaluate a child's performance based on comparisons with a normative typical-development sample (i.e., a representative group of the child's peers). Norming samples should mimic the socioeconomic status, racial and ethnic breakdown of the population being studied, typically the census in the United States. Normative assessments are valuable when diagnostic and qualifying information is needed to determine eligibility for services. Normative data allow standard scores, percentiles, and age-equivalent calculations to be made. Examples of norm-referenced assessments include the Bayley Scales of Infant Development, Fourth Edition (BSID-4); the Peabody Developmental Motor Scales, Second Edition (PDMS-2); the Test of Gross Motor Development, Third Edition (TGMD-3); and the Test of Infant Motor Performance (TIMP).

In contrast, criterion-referenced assessment tools are judgment based and compare a child's performance

TABLE 2.1 Pediatric Physical Therapy Assessments

Assessment	Design	Authors/Date	Age Range	Measures
Alberta Infant Motor Scale (AIMS)	Norm-referenced	Piper, Darrah, 1994	Birth to 18 mo	Prone, supine, sit, and stand
Bayley Scales of Infant Development, Third Edition (BSID-3)	Norm-referenced	Bayley, 2005	1 to 42 mo	Cognitive, motor, language, social-emotional, and adaptive behavioral
Bruininks-Oseretsky Test of Motor Proficiency, Second Edition (BOT-2)	Norm-referenced	Bruininks, Bruininks, 2005	4 to 21 yr	Gross and fine motor skills
Gross Motor Function Measure (GMFM)	Criterion-referenced	Russell, Rosenbaum, Hardy, et al., 1994		Motor function in: 1. lying and rolling 2. sitting 3. crawling and kneeling 4. standing 5. walking, running, and jumping
Hawaii Early Learning Profile (HELP)	Criterion-referenced	Parks, 1997	Birth to 6 yr	1. cognition 2. gross motor 3. fine motor 4. social 5. self-help
Home Observation Measurement of the Environment (HOME)	Norm-referenced	Caldwell, Bradley, 1984	Birth to 10 yr	Quantity and quality of stimulation in the home environment
Pediatric Balance Scale	Observational measure	Franjoine, Taylor, et al., 2003	Preschool and school-age children	Balance
Peabody Developmental Motor Scales, Second Edition (PDMS-2)	Norm-referenced	Folio, Fewell, 2002	Birth to 6 yr	Gross and fine motor skills
Pediatric Evaluation of Disability Inventory (PEDI)	Criterion-referenced	Haley, Coster, Ludlow, et al., 1992	6 mo to 7.5 yr	Self-care ability Social function
School Function Assessment (SFA)	Criterion-referenced	Coster, Deeney, Haltiwangar, et al., 1998	Kindergarten to 6th grade	Participation Task support Activity performance Physical tasks Cognitive and behavioral tasks
Test of Gross Motor Development, Second Edition (TGMD-2)	Norm-referenced	Ulrich, 2000	3 to 10 yr	Locomotor and object control skills
Test of Infant Motor Performance (TIMP)	Norm-referenced	Campbell, Kolobe, Osten, et al., 1995	Infants 32 weeks' gestation to 4 mo after term	Functional motor performance
Timed Up and Down Stairs and Timed Up and Go	Reference values available	Zaino, Marchese, et al., 2003	School-age children	Functional mobility, speed, balance
6 Minute-Walk Test (6MWT)	Reference values available	American Thoracic Society, 2002	School-age children	Functional walking capacity

to criteria that have been defined within the test.[4] They are often based on milestones of motor skills performed by typically developing children. Criterion-referenced assessments are more useful when developing a treatment plan or curriculum for a child. Examples of criterion-referenced assessments include the Gross Motor Function Measure (GMFM), the School Function Assessment (SFA), and the Hawaii Early Learning Profile (HELP).

Norm-Referenced Assessments

Bayley Scales of Infant Development, Fourth Edition

The BSID-4[5,6] assesses the development of children from 16 days to 42 months of age. It was standardized on a stratified random sample based on current US Census data in 1999. The BSID-4 consists of five scales: cognitive, language, social-emotional, motor, and adaptive behavior. The scoring is polytomous (2, 1, 0) and includes questions for the caregiver.[5]

The *motor scale* (46 items) evaluates body control and fine and gross motor skills. The scale yields standardized scores with a mean of 100 and a standard deviation of 15.

The BSID-4 norming sample does not include children with diagnosed disabilities. For them, the examiner has two scoring options. Examiners may either adapt the test items and not determine a standardized score or administer the test as directed and risk the child scoring significantly lower than the norm.

The BSID-4 demonstrates concurrent validity with other reputable assessments, including the Motor Developmental Index with the McCarthy Scales of Children's Ability, the General Cognitive Index, and the Wechsler Preschool and Primary Scale of Intelligence, Third Edition.[5]

Peabody Developmental Motor Scales, Second Edition

The PDMS-2[4,7] uses a stratified sample relative to the US Census criteria. The PDMS-2 is designed to assess the gross and fine motor skills of children from birth through 5 years of age. Items are scored on a three-point scale. Age equivalents, motor quotients, percentile rankings, and standard scores can be calculated for each child.

The PDMS-2 gross motor scale assesses skills in four areas: reflexes, stationary, locomotion, and object manipulation. The fine motor scale assesses skills in two areas: grasping and visual-motor integration. Not all test items must be administered to achieve a basal level and a ceiling level.

The PDMS-2 has shown empirical reliability and validity. Features of the PDMS-2 include a software scoring and report system available as an additional option. Strengths include optional awarding of partial credit on items; the ability to determine gross motor quotient, fine motor quotient, and a total motor quotient; and an illustrated administrator's manual. Among its weaknesses are incomplete descriptions of scoring on some items, leading to subjective scoring, and increased administration time when assessing children with delays because more time is needed to establish a basal score.

Test of Gross Motor Development, Third Edition

The TGMD-3[6,8] is appropriate for children aged 3 years to 10 years 11 months. This norm-referenced scale identifies children who may be eligible for special services because of significantly delayed gross motor skills.

The TGMD-3 consists of two scales with six subtests. The locomotor scale includes skills that require coordinated body movements such as run, gallop, hop, leap, horizontal jump, and slide. The ball scale includes striking a stationary ball, stationary dribble, kick, catch, overhand throw, and underhand roll. This assessment can be easily administered in less than 20 minutes.

Test of Infant Motor Performance

The TIMP, version 5, is a comprehensive motor test designed to assess functional motor performance of infants between 32 weeks' gestational age and 16 weeks after term. Initial reports on the TIMP suggest that it yields reliable measurements that are valid for discriminating optimal motor performance from poor motor performance in infants born before term and very young infants.[7] Scoring on the TIMP has been reported to be sensitive to changes related to maturation and medical complications.

The TIMP consists of 42 items divided into 2 sections: elicited and observed. The elicited section items (items 1–13) assess the infant's motor responses to placement in various positions and to visual or auditory stimulation.[10] The observed section (items 14–42) is used to rate spontaneous movement exhibited by the infant. The items on the TIMP have been shown to have ecological validity (i.e., the elicited section items are similar to demands placed on infants in everyday caregiving situations).

Excellent concurrent validity with the Alberta Infant Motor Scale was demonstrated for infants at 3, 6, 9, and 12 months of age.[7,8,8a]

Alberta Infant Motor Scale

The Alberta Infant Motor Scale (AIMS)[8] is an observational tool to be used with infants aged 0 to 18 months. It is a norm-referenced test using a representative infant population sample of Alberta, Canada, compiled between 1990 and 1992. There are four subscales accounting for 58 items: prone, supine, sit, and stand. Each item has descriptors for weight-bearing, posture, and antigravity movements. The manual must be used to accurately score the items. Scores are calculated and plotted as percentiles. The AIMS shows moderate (at 6 months) and excellent (at 12 months) concurrent validity with the Bayley Motor Scale.

The strengths of this test are ease and speed of administering the assessment, its observational format, and its emphasis on quality of movement. Limitations are that therapists must subjectively convert percentile scores and that the number of items for birth to 4 months of age is limited.

Bruininks-Oseretsky Test of Motor Proficiency, Second Edition

The Bruininks-Oseretsky Test of Motor Proficiency, Second Edition (BOT-2),[9] assesses motor control abilities in children and adolescents aged 4 to 21 years. It is a norm-referenced assessment tool. There are eight subtests and a short- and long-scoring form. The long form takes approximately 60 minutes to administer, while the short form takes up to 20 minutes to complete.

The strengths of the BOT-2 are that it covers a wide age range and assesses unique aspects of motor development, including speed, agility, balance, strength, bilateral coordination, and upper-limb coordination. The tasks are child friendly and include photos to accompany the simple instructions. Norms are based on US Census data. The BOT-2 has good concurrent validity with the PDMS-2, the Movement Assessment Battery for Children, Second Edition (MABC-2), and Test of Visual Motor Scales.[9]

Home Observation Measurement of the Environment

The Home Observation Measurement of the Environment-Short Form (HOME-SF)[10] measures the quantity and quality of stimulation in the home environment, thus assessing the home environment from the child's vantage point. The HOME-SF is easy to administer. It can be used with children from birth to age 15 years who live with their mothers. The HOME-SF includes cognitive stimulation and self-help subscores in addition to the total score. The HOME-SF can be administered via interview or observation and usually takes 45 minutes to complete.

The strengths of the HOME-SF are that it is a systematic data-collection system for the home environment, it is easy to administer, it covers a wide age range, and it is used extensively in research.

The Pediatric Evaluation of Disability Inventory

The Pediatric Evaluation of Disability Inventory (PEDI)[11] is a norm-referenced tool that assesses functional skills of children aged 6 months to 7 years, although some selected scales can be used for children older than 7 years. Scoring can be calculated using normative or scaled scoring. The normative scoring allows the child to be measured against same-aged peers, and the scaled scoring is along a scale of 0 to 100. The PEDI allows therapists to measure performance over time. Children with motor delays can be assessed using the PEDI, provided their skills do not exceed those of a typical 7-year-old. The PEDI measures capability and performance of functional activities in three content areas: self-care, ability, and social function. Additionally, the PEDI records the amount of caregiver assistance the child needs to demonstrate a skill and any equipment/object modifications that may be necessary. Scores may be obtained from interviews with parents or primary caregivers or from observation of the child.

The strengths of the PEDI are that it is designed for use with children with disabilities, it can be administered easily, decisions regarding goals and further referrals can be determined from test results, and it has a score range (standard error of measurement) and caregiver-assistance scale. Its limitations are that no composite score can be calculated, and the test was normed on a relatively small regional sample. The PEDI has moderate to high reliability with other developmental tests. The MDC is 3.91 to 9.92 for children without motor delays and 5.19 to 9.38 for children with motor delays. The Minimal Clinically Important Difference (MCID) is 6 to 15 points or 11% on a scale of 0 to 100 for children with disabilities. The PEDI–Computer Adapted Test (PEDI-CAT) uses item response theory. An additional responsibility area and a module specifically for youth with autism spectrum disorder (ASD) are included in the PEDI-CAT.[11]

Hammersmith Infant Neurological Examination

The Hammersmith Infant Neurological Examination (HINE)[12] is a standardized 26-item tool used for infants aged 2 to 24 months at risk for developmental impairments. Some of the items reliably predict future motor impairments. The HINE is easy for clinical staff to administer. It is useful for identifying infants that could benefit from additional rehabilitation services. The HINE can be used over time to document a child's development and motor progress. Chapter 6 further describes the use of the HINE to identify young infants and toddlers that may be at risk for cerebral palsy (CP).

Prechtl's General Movements Assessment

Prechtl's General Movements Assessment (GMA) is unique, as trained assessors view a video of a child from 0 to 20 weeks' adjusted age. The evaluators watch the video and observe the child's spontaneous movements compared with expected age-related standardized movements. A child's movements are predictive of how the child's nervous system is developing.[13,14] More information on how the GMA can be used to identify infants younger than 3 months that are at high risk for CP can be found in Chapter 6.

Criterion-Referenced Assessments

Gross Motor Function Measure-66

The GMFM-66[15] allows a therapist to measure a change in motor function over time in a child aged 0 to 12 years with CP. It is a reliable and valid shorter version of the GMFM-88. It is a criterion-referenced assessment that focuses on how much (the quantity) of an activity the child can accomplish rather than how well (the quality) the child performs the movement. These areas include lying and rolling; sitting; crawling and kneeling; standing; and walking, running, and jumping. The MCID is 0.8 to 1.3.[16,17]

The strengths of the GMFM-66 are that it covers a wide age range, various dimensions can be scored, and it has a goal score. Software is available to help determine the child's performance more accurately. The GMFM-66 has excellent validity with the self-care aspects and mobility portions of the PEDI, the Pediatric Outcomes Data Inventory, and the Child Health Questionnaire.[17,18] Occasionally, the GMFM-66 is used to assess children without

CP, but then this must be considered in the scoring and interpretation of the results. Limitations are that each item must be administered, and only items administered and performed during the testing session can be scored.

School Function Assessment

The purpose of the SFA[3,18] is to assess a child's function and guide program planning for students with disabilities within their educational abilities.[19] This is a criterion-referenced assessment for children in kindergarten through 6th grade. It tests skills in the following areas: participation, task support, activity performance, physical tasks, and cognitive and behavioral tasks.[19]

The strengths of the SFA are that its content is specific to children with physical or sensory impairments and clinical judgment is based on typical performance required in the elementary school setting. A limitation is that it requires collaboration and coordination among team members to obtain valid information.

Hawaii Early Learning Profile

The HELP[20] is a comprehensive and developmentally sequenced, curriculum-based assessment tool that includes six domains: cognitive, language, gross motor, fine motor, social, and self-help. The HELP promotes a cross-disciplinary, integrated approach that focuses on the whole child and includes the importance of supportive environments and interactions, building on strengths, and providing activities for working on specific needs within a curriculum for children from birth to 6 years of age.[20]

Other Standardized Tests Used in Pediatric Physical Therapy

Several measures that were originally designed for use with adults to assess balance, speed of walking, endurance, and functional performance of everyday activities such as navigating stairs have been adapted for use with children. These measures are quick and easy to administer, do not involve complex directions, and need minimal equipment. They can be used for establishing a baseline of the child's performance, to determine goals for a physical therapy plan of care, and to assess change in functional movement because of intervention.

6-Minute Walk Test

The 6-Minute Walk Test (6MWT) involves having an individual walk continuously as fast as they can for 6 minutes. The distance walked over 6 minutes is measured and provides an assessment of cardiopulmonary capacity and functional ambulation.[21] Reference values have been established in several countries for different age groups of children, and the measure has been used to demonstrate changes with age and in health status in boys with Duchenne muscular dystrophy.[22] For children that cannot walk for 6 minutes because of muscle weakness or inability to sustain attention, a modified assessment, the 2-Minute Walk Test has been explored. It has been found to predict values on the 6MWT in children with neuromuscular disorders.[23] It shows promise as a measure of walking speed and endurance and as an outcome measure for younger children or children that are still progressing in their ability to ambulate. It could also be useful in hospitals to assess functional recovery in children having medical or surgical procedures.

Pediatric Balance Scale

Developed as a modification of the Berg Balance Scale for adults, the Pediatric Balance Scale (PBS) is used to evaluate balance in functional movements such as going from sitting to standing, turning to look behind, and picking up an object from the floor. It uses a rating scale of 0 to 4 to score performance of each item. The measure can be used for children 5 to 15 years of age with mild to moderate motor impairments.[24] Recent studies have established its utility in assessing balance impairments in children with visual impairments[25] and adolescents with CP.[26]

Timed Up and Go and Timed Up and Down Stairs

Efficient performance of transitional movements such as standing up from sitting in a chair and standing up from the floor is important for everyday mobility and independence among typically developing children and children with neuromotor disorders. The Timed Up and Go (TUG) assesses how quickly a child can stand up from a chair, walk 3 meters, and return to sitting in the chair. Children with CP and more severe mobility problems take longer than typically developing children, and this test may be useful for measuring change in functional mobility with intervention and with age in children at Gross Motor Function Classification System (GMFCS) levels II and III. Similarly, the Timed Up and Down Stairs (TUGS)[27] measures the time taken by a child to go up a flight of stairs, turn around, and descend the stairs until they land with both feet on the bottom step. Recently, reference values for the TUDS in typically developing school-age children have been developed.[28]

Children with CP between GMFCS levels I and III take two to three times longer to go up the same set of stairs as typically developing children.[27] This measure may be useful for tracking changes in stair navigation in individual children with CP based on age and interventions to improve strength, balance, and functional mobility.

SUMMARY

The assessment tools described in this chapter can be used to complete initial evaluations of a child and to collect data regarding the child's development and performance over time. These measurements can be used to benchmark progress as time goes on and change the plan of care as needed. They can also be used as ongoing assessment strategies for re-evaluating a child's abilities and needs across the spectrum of growth and development. In this way, the assessment tools allow the therapist to measure developmental progress. The assessments featured in this chapter are the most common pediatric assessments currently used. It is by no means an exhaustive list, and there are many other pediatric assessments.

CHAPTER DISCUSSION QUESTIONS

1. Why is reliability important in regard to assessment tools?
2. Should a raw score be used to compare a group of children over time? Why or why not?
3. List at least three purposes of assessment. Describe a setting or environment and why you would use assessment measures in this setting.
4. When and why would you report age-equivalent scores?
5. Why is test validity an important construct?
6. Describe at least two types of test validity. What would be the consequence of violating each of these constructs?
7. Identify one benefit of using qualitative assessment.
8. Compare and contrast criterion-referenced assessments and norm-referenced assessments.
9. Identify and describe one criterion-referenced assessment tool and one norm-referenced assessment tool.
10. Describe a scenario in which you would use quantitative assessment and a scenario in which you would use qualitative assessment.

REFERENCES

1. Long T, Toscano K. *Handbook of Pediatric Physical Therapy*. 3rd ed. Philadelphia: Lippincott Williams & Wilkins; 2018.

2. Accardo PJ, Whitman BY. *Dictionary of Developmental Disabilities Terminology*. 3rd ed. Baltimore: Paul H Brookes; 2011.

3. Balthazar C, Vendrely A. *Rehabilitation Research*. 6th ed. St Louis: Elsevier; 2021.

4. Folio MR, Fewell RR. *Peabody Developmental Motor Scales*. 2nd ed. Austin: PRO-ED; 2002.

5. Aylward GP, Jiajun Zhu. The Bayley Scales: clarification for clinicians and researchers, 2019. Accessed July 9, 2022. https://www.pearsonassessments.com/content/dam/school/global/clinical/us/assets/bayley-4/bayley-4-technical-report.pdf.

6. Ulrich D: Test of Gross Motor Development, 3rd edition. 2019. PRO-ED, inc. Dallas Texas.

7. James D: Alberta Infant Motor Scale (AIMS), 2017. https://www.apta.org/patient-care/evidence-based-practice-resources/test-measures/alberta-infant-motor-scale-aims. Accessed June 25, 2022.

8. Drumm D, Marone J. Test of Infant Motor Performance. https://www.sralab.org/rehabilitation-measures/test-infant-motor-performance. Accessed June 26, 2023.

8a. Campbell SK, Kolobe TH. Concurrent validity of the test of infant motor performance with the Alberta infant motor scale. *Pediatrics PT*. 2002;12:2–9.

9. Dietz L, Mano N, Mazza S and others. *Bruininks-Oseretsky Test of Motor Proficiency*. 2nd ed. (BOT-2); 2019. Accessed June 25, 2022. https://www.apta.org/patient-care/evidence-based-practice-resources/test-measures/bruininks-oseretsky-test-of-motor-proficiency.

10. US Bureau of Labor Statistics. National Longitudinal Surveys. The HOME (Home Observation Measurement of the Environment). Accessed July 7, 2022. https://www.nlsinfo.org/content/cohorts/nlsy79-children/topical-guide/assessments/home-home-observation-measurement.

11. Brew S, Langan E, Link-Dudek A. Pediatric Evaluation of Disability Inventory. Accessed July 7, 2022. https://www.sralab.org/rehabilitation-measures/pediatric-evaluation-disability-inventory.

12. Maitre NL, Chorna O, Romeo DM. Implementation of the Hammersmith Infant Neurological Examination in a high-risk infant follow-up program. *Pediatr Neurol*. 2016;65:31–38.

13. Morgan C, Crowle C, Goyen T-A. GMA and CP in Australia. *J Paediatr Child Health*. 2016;52:54–59.

14. Caesar R, Colditz PB, Cioni G. Clinical tools used in young infants born very preterm to predict motor and cognitive delay (not cerebral palsy): a systematic review. *Dev Med Child Neurol*. 2021;63:387–395.

15. Wei S, Su-Juan W, Yuan-Gui L and others. Reliability and validity of the GMFM-66 in 0- to 3-year-old children with cerebral palsy. *Am J Phys Med Rehabil*. 2006;85:141–147.

16. Oeffinger D, Bagley A, Rogers S. Outcome tools used for ambulatory children with cerebral palsy: responsiveness and minimum clinically important differences. *Dev Med Child Neurol*. 2008;50:918–925.

17. Shah J. Gross Motor Function Measure-66. https://www.sralab.org/rehabilitation-measures/gross-motor-function-measure-66, Accessed July 7, 2022.

18. McCarthy ML, Silberstein CE, Atkins EA. Comparing reliability and validity of pediatric instruments for measuring health and well-being of children with spastic cerebral palsy. Developmental medicine and child neurology. *Dev Med Child Neurol*. 2002;44:468–476.

19. Coster W, Deeney T, Haltiwanger J, Haley S. *School Function Assessment Technical Report*. Pearson Education, Inc; 2008. Accessed July 7, 2022. http://images.pearson-assessments.com/images/tmrs/tmrs_rg/SFA_TR_Web.pdf?WT.mc_id=TMRS_School_Function_Assessment.

20. Li Z, Gooden C, Toland MD. Reliability and validity evidence for the Hawaii Early Learning Profile, birth-3 years. *J Early Interv*. 2019;41:62–83.

21. ATS Committee on Proficiency Standards for Clinical Pulmonary Function Laboratories. ATS statement: guidelines for the six-minute walk test. *Am J Respir Crit Care Med*. 2002;166:111–117.

22. McDonald CM, Henricson EK, Abresch R T. The 6-minute walk test and other endpoints in Duchenne muscular dystrophy: longitudinal natural history observations over 48 weeks from a multicenter study. *Muscle Nerve*. 2013;48:343–356.

23. Witherspoon JW, Vasavada R, Logaraj RH. Two-minute versus 6-minute walk distances during 6-minute walk test in neuromuscular disease: is the 2-minute walk test an effective alternative to a 6-minute walk test? *Eur J Pediatr Neurol*. 2019;23:165–170.

24. Franjoine MR, Gunther JS, Taylor MJ. Pediatric balance scale: a modified version of the Berg balance scale for the school-age child with mild to moderate motor impairment. *Pediatr Phys Ther*. 2003;15:114–128.

25. Zyłka J, Lach U, Rutkowska I. Functional balance assessment with pediatric balance scale in girls with visual impairment. *Pediatr Phys Ther*. 2013;25:460–466.

26. Jantakat C, Ramrit S, Emasithi A. Capacity of adolescents with cerebral palsy on paediatric balance scale and Berg balance scale. *Res Dev Disabil*. 2015;36:72–77.

27. Zaino C, Marchese VG, Westcott SL. Timed up and down stairs test: preliminary reliability and validity of a new measure of functional mobility. *Pediatr Phys Ther*. 2004;16:90–98.

28. Del Corral T, Vivas-Mateos J, Castillo-Pelaz M, Aguilar-Zafra S, López-de-Uralde-Villanueva I. Development of stratified normative data and reference equations for the timed up and down stairs test for healthy children 6–14 years of age. *Physiotherapy*. 2021;112:31–40.

Overview of Physical Therapy Interventions

Nia Mensah, PT, DPT, PhD, PCS, C/NDT
Roberta Kuchler O'Shea, PT, DPT, PhD

LEARNING OBJECTIVES

At the end of the chapter, the reader will be able to do the following:

1. Identify the differences between intervention philosophies.
2. Recognize which interventions would be most appropriate for a given situation.
3. Understand why one intervention may not be appropriate for all situations and all children.

CHAPTER OUTLINE

KEY TERMS

Aquatic therapy
Conductive Education
Constraint-induced movement therapy (CIMT)
International Classification of Functioning, Disability, and Health (ICF)

Motor Learning
Neurodevelopmental treatment (NDT)
Physical Activity
Proprioceptive neuromuscular facilitation (PNF)
Sensory integration

Strengthening
Therapeutic taping
World Health Organization model of enablement

Physical therapy interventions vary, depending on many scenarios. There are standards in the profession that the physical therapist assistant (PTA) will encounter. This chapter is designed to help you become familiar with some of the more common pediatric physical therapy interventions and environments you may encounter. Master clinicians use a wide variety of techniques and interventions that can be modified based on variables including but not limited to the child's pathology, family structure, living situation, age, and history. The following discussion is by no means an all-inclusive discussion of physical therapy interventions; it should be used as an overview and guide.

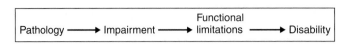

Fig. 3.1 Schematic representation of the four components of health status and the process of disablement in the model developed by Nagi.

TERMINOLOGY

The development of enablement models by the World Health Organization has helped to describe individuals with disabilities. In years past, the Nagi model of disablement (Fig. 3.1) was widely used to describe patients and the effect of their injuries or pathologies on their livelihood. The International Classification of Functioning, Disability, and Health (ICF) (Fig. 3.2) is the current framework utilized to provide theoretical categorization to help to promote proper plans of care for individuals with disability.[1] This model describes how the patient's injury or pathology impacts his or her activities and participation in society. The components of the framework are body structure and function, activity limitations and participation restrictions, and environmental factors. Although the cases in this text generally follow the Guide to Physical Therapy Practice format, the ICF framework and the Movement Systems Analysis have been included following each case (as appropriate) to demonstrate for the reader how patient cases can be analyzed through different lenses. Treatment goals and interventions are then formulated from these perspectives, with the patient and/or family actively participating in the formulation of goals. The prediction of treatment outcomes through research is dependent on homogeneous groups of patients with similar signs and symptoms when movement system analysis is used, and this concept is building traction within the pediatric and neurologic physical therapy setting.[2]

GOALS OF INTERVENTION

Regardless of the age of the child, goals of intervention must be established before treatment begins. Goals should be functional and realistic. A goal becomes meaningful only when it is relevant to the child's lifestyle. For instance, a child and therapist should not be working on increasing active range of motion merely for the sake of increased range. What will the child be able to do differently or more efficiently with increased range of motion? Will the child's gait pattern improve? Will the distance of ambulation increase? Thus, the goal of improving knee extension by 10 degrees is no longer acceptable in pediatric practice. Why does the child need

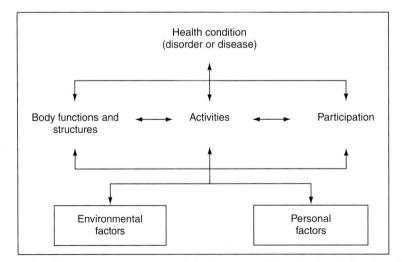

Fig. 3.2 Interactions between the components of the International Classification of Function. (From World Health Organization. *International Classification of Functioning, Disability, and Health (ICF)*, Geneva, 2001, WHO.)

this increased range of motion? The goal should reflect what the child will be accomplishing with improved range of motion. A more appropriate goal would be that the child will ambulate a certain distance to play with peers or will ambulate to class.

Many goals have been written stating that the child will independently hold the head up for a certain amount of time. If the goal is limited to maintaining an upright head position, it can be accomplished with standard head rest/support equipment. The goal is met simply and without extended therapy. A more meaningful statement of the goal might be that the child will be able to maintain an upright head posture in order to drive a power chair safely or participate in dinner. This goal highlights the importance of the child's ability to hold their head up to participate in an activity/program, communicate with family or peers, or navigate through an environment.

Goals are meant to be met, modified, or changed. Reassessment of the goals should occur frequently and vary among settings. The goals will either be met or require revision. Revision or elimination of a goal should occur when it becomes evident that the goal will not be met. Many times, goals must be updated during the intervention timespan to maintain relevancy for the child and the family's functional goal. When this occurs, the goal should be revised to make it more applicable.

INTERVENTION PLAN

After goals have been established, an intervention plan can be devised. The intervention plan should reflect the child's current needs and capabilities. Interventions should be based on what is appropriate for both the child and the family. It is best to first think about intervention based on the age of the child and the pathology. If the injury is acute in nature (flare-up in arthritis, soft tissue shortening secondary to immobilization, torticollis, or an injury/surgery that requires gait training with an assistive device), then service delivery will look very different from therapy given for a chronic pathology (cerebral palsy [CP], traumatic brain injury, Down syndrome, developmental delay).

For children living in the United States ranging in age from birth to 3 years, pediatric physical therapy interventions may take place within the Early Intervention, Part C, system. (Early intervention [EI] is discussed in more depth in Chapter 4.) Services delivered in this way must be family centered. Historically, services for very young children were child centered and mostly focused on the specific needs of the child; however, this model is no longer the best practice. Family-centered care broadens the scope of the interventions and focuses therapy on the family and the child's position in the family. Therapists assume more of a coaching role, working with the child through the family and devising a plan based on the needs of the family.

Interventions should also be embedded in routines that already occur in the home or within the child's day. Much of the practitioner's time and energy will be focused on teaching the family members how to handle, position, and interact with the child to get optimal performance from the child over the span of the day. Therapy goals are worked on throughout the entire day, not just at therapy-designated times. If a child needs to increase strength, then appropriate activities will be designed so that the child works on strength while participating in his or her regularly scheduled activities. Leg strength can be improved with squat-to-stand activities. If a container/toy is placed on a low table surface, and all the pieces are on the floor, the child must repeatedly perform squat-to-stand activities to put all the pieces into the container. Likewise, if therapy is focusing on improved fine motor skills, pulling diaper wipes from a container will work on grasp-and-release movements. These are activities embedded in typically occurring routines. If the child needs to improve a gait pattern, the parent will be taught stretching activities that can occur at every diaper change, for instance. Ambulation can be built into going to check for mail at the mailbox or cruising around the bedroom or kitchen. (A child will be more inclined to cruise if furniture is placed close together to provide ready support.)

Often, the therapist must invest a great deal of effort in slowing down the caregiver to permit time for the child to practice movements/activities. For instance, instead of letting the parent completely dress the child to speed up the process, the therapist should encourage the parent to allow the child to complete some of the activity alone—pulling the shirt over the head, putting the foot into the shoe, using pull-to-sit activities. Thus, the child receives more meaningful practice opportunities and in the long run learns new skills in the context of where they need to be applied.

As the child enters school age, the focus of therapy may switch from a family-centered to an education-centered approach. Therapies delivered within an educational environment must focus on improving school performance. Therapy services outside the educational system continue to be child and family centered. For example, a 6-year-old child with diplegic CP attends school. The child lives on the second floor of a two-story walkup building, which has no elevators. The child has difficulty ambulating up the many steep steps to his or her apartment. The child's school is in a single-story building without steps. If the family wants this child to improve safety on the steps at the apartment, providing practice opportunities would be outside the mandates of the school therapist, since there are no steps in the school building. Thus, the goal is not educationally relevant. However, the astute therapist will think about the child's participation in school activities outside of the building, such as ascending and descending the school bus steps or using playground equipment. In this way, therapy could focus on stair climbing, which is important to the child's ability to be independent and safe both at home and within the educational environment. Additionally, the family may choose to engage the services of a community-based therapist to work on noneducation-based goals.

After the therapist, family, and child (if appropriate) have developed goals, the therapist should decide what intervention technique(s) may be most efficient and effective in helping the child meet the goals. There are several types of interventions and differing philosophies. In this chapter, several of the interventions are discussed. By no means is this an all-inclusive list or a ranking of the "best" interventions. This chapter is designed to give the reader an overview of what is currently practiced, most commonly, in the United States. It should be used as a guide to build on as the therapist accumulates experience and breadth and depth of knowledge.

TYPES OF INTERVENTIONS

Common interventions include the following (Table 3.1):
- Motor learning
- Strengthening and stability
- Constraint-induced therapy
- Physical activity
- Conductive education (Peto)
- Aquatic therapy
- Hippotherapy
- Neurodevelopmental treatment (Bobath)
- Proprioceptive neuromuscular facilitation (Kabat, Knott, Voss)

- Therapeutic taping (Kase)
- Sensory integration (Ayers)

The basis for all treatments must embrace in some form the dynamic systems model of motor control and motor learning. This model explains that all components of a child's world must be considered and will be influenced by all systems working in concert or conflict with each other. The brain is incredibly plastic, and it has great capacity to change as a result of the interaction of genetic, experiential, and environmental factors. There are several physiologic systems, as well as environmental and cultural systems, to consider before determining the optimal intervention. If any component of any of these systems is not on target and not working in concert with the other systems, dysfunction will occur. It is up to the treating therapist to collect all the clues and decipher which component is missing. The treating therapist determines whether the intervention should focus to correct the malfunctioning component or to assist the child and family to adapt and learn new strategies to function as independently and optimally as possible.

The physiologic systems include the *commanding system*, the *regulating and comparing system*, the *sensorimotor system,* and the *musculoskeletal system*. In order to operate functionally, a person's commanding system must integrate and act on stimulation from the sensory system, the cognitive system, and the emotional system. The body also must be able to regulate and compare actions to modify existing skills and learn new ones. The comparing and regulating system includes the predictive central set, accurate knowledge of results, and adequate knowledge of performance. The body must be able to activate an intrinsic error-detection system. An adequately functioning sensorimotor system includes postural orientation made up of a working visual system, a working somatosensory system, and a working vestibular/proprioceptive system; the ability to adapt to the environment; sensory and processing skills; and motor coordination. The typical musculoskeletal system includes postural alignment, appropriate tone, intact primary sensory function, adequate range of motion, appropriate strength, lack of pain, and sufficient coordination.

If a child cannot utilize his or her vestibular/proprioceptive systems efficiently, significant delays in balance and coordination may result. The treating therapist must keep this in mind. A child who appears to fall frequently may do so in response to decreased muscle tone or decreased muscle strength. However, this child may

TABLE 3.1	**Comparison of Common Interventions**	
Intervention	**Philosophy**	**Appropriate Use**
Motor learning	Uses motor control theory and emerges from a complex set of processes, including perception, cognition, and action	Children with cerebral palsy and all developmental disorders
Physical activity and exercise	Use of direct and indirect physical activity measures can provide baseline, intervention, and physiologic information about cardiorespiratory fitness	All children: typical or atypical development
Neurodevelopmental treatment (NDT)	Uses motor control to effect postural control and interactions between many neurologic and physiologic systems. Enhances the individual's capacity to function	Children with cerebral palsy and motor disorders
Proprioceptive neuromuscular facilitation (PNF)	Strengthens muscle groups within diagonal and rotational movement patterns, based on developmental sequence and the sequential mastery of motor milestones	Children with muscle imbalances
Conductive education (CE)	Views child as a whole child, using learning concepts, motor control/motor learning, and the group model to improve function. Learning movements and functional skills requires practice, intention, group motivation, and breaking down skills into task series. Uses specialized equipment to enhance child's orthofunction (ability to be functional and independent)	Children with cerebral palsy, spina bifida, and other motor disorders
Strengthening and stability	Improved function through improved strength, bone density, joint structures, muscle function, and management of obesity	Children with weakness and muscle imbalances
Constraint-induced therapy	Improved use and function of affected arm due to forced use, when strong arm is restricted to complete normal movement (arm sling)	Children with hemiparesis (related to cerebral palsy, brachial plexus injury, stroke, brain injury)
Aquatic therapy	Improved strength, mobility, and activity endurance by use of water therapy that provides special environment with reduced effects of gravity	Children with sensory processing dysfunction, cerebral palsy, developmental disorders
Hippotherapy	Improved mobility of pelvis, postural control and lower-extremity strength from guided horseback riding where movement of pelvis mimics movement of horse	Children with weakness and muscle imbalance, reduced hip and pelvis mobility
Therapeutic taping	Uses rigid or flexible taping to support and influence muscle groups	Children with muscle weakness, joint instability, joint malalignment, and postural asymmetries
Sensory integration (SI)	Provides controlled sensory input to help children with sensory processing	Children with sensory processing dysfunction; children exhibiting dysfunction in ability to take in and process sensory information, organize behaviors and movements, or formulate/plan/and execute motor plans

be just as likely to have delayed balance and vestibular responses that prevent successful efforts to prevent falls; or this child may never see the horizon as straight and the ground as being still. A child with vestibular/processing issues will not benefit significantly from a strengthening program but will benefit greatly from a program that emphasizes linear swinging and vestibular training.

In addition to the physiologic systems, each child is influenced by environmental and cultural systems. Environmental systems include the child's primary living habitat, school or daycare facility, neighborhood, and resources to function in these environments. Cultural systems include the family's traditions and beliefs, the extended family's traditions and beliefs (which may differ somewhat from the immediate family's), and known or perceived expectations of the child from society at large.

For an intervention plan to be successful, all the described systems that influence a child must be continually assessed and monitored. Although a child may have a primary pathology or a functional limitation, various influences from other systems may negatively affect the child and impact the primary impairment.

In the following sections, several common interventions are described. Most require additional training and experience on the part of the therapist. Each intervention has unique principles, but the interventions also have overlapping themes. Often, a combination of different interventions can be employed to provide the child and family with optimal experiences. The master clinician will adapt and modify interventions to meet the child's and family's ever-changing needs.

MOTOR LEARNING

Motor Learning is a set of internal processes associated with practice or experience leading to relatively permanent changes in the capability for skilled behavior.[37] Motor learning principles have been shown to be the most successful method for improving function for children with special needs and specifically for children with CP.[3] There are many theories and options for implementation of motor learning based on the patient population. The most common identifiable features of motor learning principles include set-up and use of the environment to provide optimal acquisition of skills. Motor learning training typically follows a hands-off approach, and manipulation of the task is acquired by practice dosing, feedback, and type of sensory input/cuing that is allowed or given. Aspects of motor learning are sprinkled in almost every intervention option described in this chapter, and understanding the role of motor learning throughout the plan of care is important for successful compliance and carryover of skills into life application.

STRENGTHENING AND STABILITY

Current theories in rehabilitation support the fundamental notion that children with motor impairments must work on strengthening and stability.[4] Many studies have shown the significance of strength training for children with CP and other neuromuscular and developmental disorders, and there are several methods through which this is accomplished.[38] Appropriate weight-bearing through the long bones helps to maintain bone density and joint structure.[5] Exercise and strengthening are mandatory for children with movement disorders to prevent overuse of the strong muscles, atrophy and wasting of weaker muscles, and obesity for children who cannot move as efficiently as their typically developing peers.[6] In each of the following chapters dealing with a specific pathology, strengthening techniques specific to that pathology are addressed. In this chapter, different tools to help a child become stronger and more motorically efficient are discussed. These techniques may be used in addition to any of the other therapeutic techniques when working with a child and/or the child's family.

CONSTRAINT-INDUCED MOVEMENT THERAPY

Constraint-induced movement therapy (CIMT) has been shown to improve strength and mobility to the affected side in persons after a stroke or those with hemiparesis resulting from brain injury.[39] The protocol developed by Drs Ostendorf and Wolf at Emory University included intensive rehabilitation hours with a patient's arm on the strong side restrained in a shoulder sling.[7] The result is forced use of the affected, weaker arm. Since its creation, CIMT has been used with children with hemiplegia during a minimum of 2 weeks of training (6 hours a day) to increase strength to the affected upper extremity (UE) during routine play and functional tasks.[8] Growing research has included use of functional bimanual upper extremity movement training as a successful method to increase use and reduce neglect of the affected arm in children with hemiplegic CP.[9,10]

PHYSICAL ACTIVITY AND FITNESS

Physical activity is defined as any bodily movement produced by skeletal muscle that requires energy expenditure for successful participation in everyday activities.[11] This may include routine walking, cycling, or jogging for children that are able to walk, but this may also include reaching, dressing, manual propulsion of a wheelchair, and use of an adaptive tricycle for children who are not able to walk independently. Energy expenditure is the measure of energy required for daily activities (such as respiration, digestion, circulation) and physical activity. Physical activity encompasses all activities that involve muscle activation that may or may not be related to training principles that involve structured vigor such as exercise prescriptions. Children with CP in adolescence have been shown to participate in less structured and lower intensity physical activity as compared with their age-matched peers.[12] Physical fitness is specific to purposeful tasks related to the perceived vigor of the individual with a corresponding goal of training.[13,14] Physical fitness ascribes to achievable attributes such as the ability to carry out daily tasks with vigor and without undue fatigue. Health-related components of physical fitness are cardiorespiratory endurance, muscular endurance, muscular strength, body composition, and flexibility.[13,15] Cardiorespiratory endurance is typically measured or estimated by VO2 max, which is the maximum oxygen inspired during the most intense level of vigorous exercise. This technique is not always available in a school or clinical setting. Therefore, the use of heart rate (HR) monitoring can provide an objective measure that corresponds to the child's levels of exertion and conditioning based on the therapist's interventions.[16] Other measures to track physical activity may include indirect measures such as surveys and questionaries about the child's and family's activity routine.

Utilization of the Frequency, Intensity, Time, and Type of exercise (FITT) principle to develop exercise programs has been shown to provide highly effective exercise intervention and improvement in cardiorespiratory function for children with CP.[17] Children are encouraged to spend 60 minutes a day within moderate to vigorous physical activity intensity levels per US Department of Health recommendations, and children with special needs are advised to collaborate with a health and wellness specialist to obtain appropriate guidance in dosing as it relates to implementation of physical activity and exercise progression.[11]

CONDUCTIVE EDUCATION

Conductive education was theorized by Andres Peto in 1948 in Budapest, Hungary. It is an integrated system that allows a child with motor dysfunction to learn to move within functional skills. Peto believed that children with motor disorders could learn to move by utilizing their brain's plasticity. He believed that learning movement required practice as well as rhythmic intention, so he based his technique on the educational principles of group learning and motivation.[40]

Conductive education is based on four primary principles: a conductor, the group setting, rhythmic intention, and a specific task series for each functional skill. A conductor or a therapist trained in conductive education leads a session. The children attend in a group setting, with a typical ratio of three children to one adult. Skills are broken down into a series of tasks by the conductor. Children receive individual assistance as needed to complete the task at hand. The group of children practices each task until it is mastered, and then individual tasks are built into mastering skills. Rhythmic intention is the cadence set to time a movement or series of movements. Rhythmic intention allows children to replay the cadence and perform newly learned movements on their own. The cadence helps the children initiate a movement, sequence a movement, and complete the movement. Conductive education focuses on the functional skills a child needs to be optimally independent. This notion is also known as *orthofunction*. Motor learning and motor control principles come into play, and intensive amounts of practice time are part of conductive education programs.

Conductive education programs use specifically designed equipment that assists the child to perform a movement. Slatted plinths and benches allow the child to grasp between the slats for stability. Additionally, horizontal or vertical posts can be attached to tabletops to provide anchors for children to use to stabilize themselves against gravity. Ladder-back standers and ladder-back chairs also provide graspable uprights to use during ambulation practice. Conductive education programs in the United States are typically 3 to 4 hours per session, with sessions occurring three to five times per week. Given that generous amount of treatment time, there is wonderful opportunity to practice and use feedback and feed-forward mechanisms to master a task and eventually master the skill.

In the United States, the trend is to develop transdisciplinary or interdisciplinary teams to provide conductive education programs, with conductors and therapists working together. Some programs also use a hybrid system that allows the child to simultaneously attend his or her educational program (school) and a conductive education program.

In summary, conductive education is an intensive motor training program that uses motor learning and motor control principles, along with educational learning principles, to teach children with movement disorders to master movement to their highest potential. This leads to each child being as functional as possible. Conductive education is not appropriate for all children in its original form. However, many of the principles and tenets of conductive education can be modified, and conductive education has been shown to be as successful as physical therapy intervention for children with CP.[18]

AQUATIC THERAPY

Aquatic therapy has been deemed safe, enjoyable, and effective for children with CP.[19,20] Exercise in water is beneficial to children with CP, movement disorders, and weakness because of the unique quality of buoyancy of water that reduces joint loading and impact and decreases the negative influences of poor balance and poor postural control. Aquatic therapy can also be viewed as a means for learning and participation in activities.[21] Successful implementation in a special education setting may enhance understanding regarding the potential benefits of implementing multidisciplinary aquatic therapy programs in specialist school settings. Aquatic therapy utilizes the effects of water to vary gravitational forces on weight-bearing, strengthening, mobility, and physiologic impact on the child's body.[22]

Three main principles of water are important to emphasize when providing intervention in the hydro-environment. Buoyancy, viscosity, and hydrostatic pressure are to be considered when planning implementation of aquatic therapy. Buoyancy is defined as the upward thrust acting in the opposite direction of gravity. Viscosity can be described as the way the water molecules stick together when you try to move through them. This viscosity means that more muscle fibers are recruited for each movement through water as compared with movement on land. The heart must also work harder in providing blood to the muscles, which results in cardiovascular fitness, as well

as overall toning. Hydrostatic pressure is another property of water that is helpful in decreasing inflammation. Pascal's law states that at any depth in water, the pressure from the water on an immersed object is the same from all directions.[23] Hydrostatic pressure turns down the body's reticular (activating) system (the brain's system of arousal), dampening tactile sensory input to the brain. This is partly why water is such a calming environment for most people. Individuals who are tactilely defensive (having a negative response to touch) are often able to tune out their surroundings and focus on the enjoyment of being in the pool without an adverse response.[23]

HIPPOTHERAPY

There is a growing body of evidence that supports hippotherapy for children with special needs. Both instructor-led horseback riding and licensed therapeutic hippotherapy have shown effectiveness for children with CP: (1) the three-dimensional, reciprocal movement of the walking horse produced normalized pelvic movement in the rider, closely resembling pelvic movement during ambulation in individuals without disability; (2) the sensation of smooth, rhythmical movements made by the horse improved co-contraction, joint stability, and weight shift, as well as postural and equilibrium responses; and (3) both options improved dynamic postural stabilization, recovery from perturbations, and anticipatory and feedback postural control.[24,25] Hippotherapy is provided by a licensed practitioner, and there are certification programs to improve effectiveness of this intervention for children with special needs.

Neurodevelopmental Treatment

Neurodevelopmental treatment (NDT) originally was theorized by Berta and Carl Bobath. Since its inception in the late 1940s, the approach underwent a major shift of focus in the 1990s. Originally, the approach focused on patterns of movement. Dysfunction of the movement patterns was thought to be caused by a loss of control from damaged higher centers in the brain. These lesions unleashed abnormal reflex activity. In the 1990s, a shift from an orthopedic model to a biomechanical and systems model occurred. Current NDT theory embraces knowledge of motor and postural control along with utilization of motor learning principles related to task-specific functional training as a result of interactions between many neurologic and physiologic systems.[26] The overall goal of management and treatment, according to NDT theory and tenets, is to enhance the individual's capacity to function. Intervention may involve a hands-on approach when working with individuals with central nervous system insults that create difficulties in controlling movements; however, the clinical reasoning involved in prioritizing and identifying the optimal system-based impairment is emphasized. The following tenets are consistent with NDT general treatment principles[27]:

- A child with CP must be treated as a whole child with a whole personality.
- A good evaluation or assessment of the child must be completed.
- From the time of initial assessment, treatment programs should be customized to meet the needs of the individual child.
- The child's responses to treatment should be reassessed often.
- Realistic and reachable treatment goals are essential.
- Key points of control are used in treatment. Key points of control are parts of the body, typically in proximal areas, where the therapist can apply light pressure to influence movement through the rest of the body.
- Teamwork is essential and must include the family.

In summary, pediatric NDT is primarily used to treat children with CP and other movement disorders. Unfortunately, minimal evidence supports its use, mainly because of the individualistic approach to treatment and the difficulty in reproducing the results in a research setting.[3] Nonetheless, aspects of NDT theory are currently applicable to many different clinical scenarios, and NDT is internationally recognized as a viable intervention option for individuals with brain-based disorders.[26,28]

Proprioceptive Neuromuscular Facilitation

Proprioceptive neuromuscular facilitation (PNF) was developed in the early 1950s by Dr Herman Kabat and Maggie Knott. The goal of PNF is to strengthen muscles within functional movement patterns rather than straight-plane or anatomic-plane motions. These movement patterns are known as *diagonals*. Physical therapist Dorothy Voss added many clinically relevant techniques to the PNF patterns. The theoretical basis for PNF rests within the hierarchical model of development. Hence, PNF theory is based on the developmental sequence and the sequential mastery of motor milestones.[29]

Diagonal movement patterns are vitally important because they represent mass movements characteristic of normal motor activity. The spiral and diagonal components are directly related to the spiral and rotary characteristics of skeletal muscle. Diagonal patterns can efficiently and effectively address specific problems of musculoskeletal weakness, and PNF is based on the principle that human beings respond in accordance with the demand placed on the neuromusculoskeletal system. Two diagonals of motion exist for each major part of the body, and each diagonal is made up of two patterns that are antagonistic to each other. Each pattern has a component of flexion or extension. Each diagonal involves movement toward and across the midline or movement across and away from the midline and includes rotation with a flexion or extension pattern. When assessing the patient, a therapist using PNF treatment protocols will look first at the patient's functional abilities. The identified stronger areas (agonists) will be used within the treatment session to assist the weaker areas (antagonists). Treatment movement patterns must be specific and directed toward a goal. Additionally, activity that will best develop coordination, strength, and endurance is necessary. Stronger body parts assist in strengthening weaker body parts through cooperation of muscle groups to achieve optimal function. For this reason, PNF places great emphasis on using maximal resistance tolerated throughout the entire range of motion; by resisting stronger muscles, weaker muscles will receive overflow/reinforcement to help them become stronger and more coordinated. To initiate a movement, a PNF technique may call for a stretch of the synergist. This provides the increased proprioceptive stimulation necessary to create a chain of muscle activity from a completely lengthened state to a completely shortened state, where the shortened muscle is the agonist.

In summary, PNF techniques work optimally for individuals with muscle imbalances secondary to spasticity, flaccidity, weakness, or pain. As a patient improves, coordination and balance activities can be added. Treatments tend to be intensive, using the patient's existing capabilities and skills without increasing pain or fatigue. The overall emphasis is on improving the person's function.[30,31]

Therapeutic Taping

Therapeutic taping is used to provide support or input to a muscle group. Flexible taping is also known as *Kinesio taping*, while rigid taping is known as *Leukotaping* or *strapping*.

Kinesio taping helps to support weakened muscles or prevent muscle overuse. Kinesio tape is flexible and has elastic properties. To strengthen a weakened muscle, the tape is applied from origin to insertion. To prevent cramping or overcontraction of a muscle, tape should be applied from insertion to origin.[32,33]

Leukotaping (named after Leuko sports tape) is rigid strapping used to support a joint in normal alignment. Muscle facilitation for appropriate firing can be achieved by laying the tape parallel to the muscle fibers. Similarly, muscles can be inhibited by laying the tape perpendicular to the muscle fibers.[34] Over time, it has been demonstrated that bony remodeling can occur with appropriate and consistent rigid taping.

TheraTogs (www.theratogs.com) is an orthotic product designed to capture the benefits achieved with taping without directly adhering to the skin. The client wears a vest and shorts made of a neoprene-type material. With additional arm and leg cuffs, flexible or rigid straps can be added to the suit to facilitate or inhibit movements. TheraTogs are easy to don and doff, should be worn directly next to the skin, and easily fit under typical street clothes and diapers. TheraTogs provide consistent input, essentially where a therapist would provide manual input for the child, in the absence of handling the child.

Sensory Integration

Sensory integration therapy assists the child by using controlled sensory input to help with sensory processing difficulties through brain-behavior relationships.[35] The theory has three major components: normal sensory function, sensory integration dysfunction, and a programmatic guide for using sensory integration techniques. Ayers felt that learning is dependent on the person's ability to take in and process sensory information from the environment and self-movements, then organize behavior and movements in response to these inputs. If an individual has difficulty integrating and processing, the result will be deficits in planning and executing movements and in motor learning. To remedy this dysfunction in motor learning, intervention within a meaningful context must occur to improve the ability of the central nervous system to process and integrate sensory inputs.[36]

In summary, sensory integration treatment encapsulates three areas: the theory, the evaluation, and the treatment. Each is vital in treating the child. A clinician can receive additional training in sensory integration theory and treatments.

SUMMARY

Therapists have a plethora of intervention techniques available to them. It is the responsibility of the therapist to use appropriate interventions that promote improved patient function and independence. Interventions should also be consistent with plan-of-care goals identified for each child.

CHAPTER DISCUSSION QUESTIONS

1. How can a child practice standing and weight shifting while in the family's kitchen/food preparation area?
2. Design two physical therapy–related treatment activities that focus on either dressing or feeding.
3. Describe the benefit of including typically developing peers within a treatment session.
4. Think of three community-based programs/resources that could be utilized by children/families to augment services.
5. What is the current recommendation for daily physical activity for children in the United States?
6. What are some methods utilized to promote strength and stability in children with CP?
7. What are the underlying foundational beliefs of conductive education?
8. What population benefits most from constraint-induced movement therapy?
9. What is aquatic therapy?
10. What are some of the benefits of hippotherapy?
11. What are the underlying foundational beliefs of NDT?
12. What are the underlying foundational beliefs of PNF?
13. How do strengthening and stability influence the ability of a child with CP to move independently?
14. How are TheraTogs and taping similar?

REFERENCES

1. World Health Organization. *International Classification of Functioning, Disability and Health (ICF) (website)*: Geneva; 2001. Accessed July 27, 2023. https://www.who.int/standards/classifications/international-classification-of-functioning-disability-and-health.
2. Van Sant AF. Movement system diagnosis. *J Neurol Phys Ther*. 2017;41(suppl 3):S10–S16.

3. Novak I, Morgan C, Fahey M. State of the evidence traffic lights 2019: systematic review of interventions for preventing and treating children with cerebral palsy. *Curr Neurol Neurosci Rep.* 2020;20(2):3.

4. Carbone PS, Smith P J, Lewis C, LeBlanc C. Promoting the participation of children and adolescents with disabilities in sports, recreation, and physical activity. *Pediatrics.* 2021;148(6):e2021054664.

5. Danzig JA, Katz EB. Musculoskeletal and skin considerations in children with medical complexity: common themes and approaches to management. *Curr Probl Pediatr Adolesc Health Care.* 2021;51(9):101074.

6. Aitchison B, Rushton AB, Martin P, Barr M, Soundy A, Heneghan NR. The experiences and perceived health benefits of individuals with a disability participating in sport: a systematic review and narrative synthesis. *Disabil Health J.* 2022;15(1):101164.

7. Ostendorf CG, Wolf SL. Effect of forced use of the upper extremity of a hemiplegic patient on changes in function. A single-case design. *Phys Ther.* 1981;61(7):1022–1028.

8. Chen YP, Pope S, Tyler D, Warren GL. Effectiveness of constraint-induced movement therapy on upper-extremity function in children with cerebral palsy: a systematic review and meta-analysis of randomized controlled trials. *Clin Rehabil.* 2014;28:939–953.

9. Gee BM, Leonard S, Lloyd KG. (2022). Exploring the intensity, frequency, and duration of pediatric constraint induced movement therapy published research: a content analysis. *Children.* 2022;9(5):700.

10. Gordon AM, Hung Y-C, Brandao M. Bimanual training and constraint-induced movement therapy in children with hemiplegic cerebral palsy: a randomized trial. *Neurorehabil Neural Repair.* 2011;25(8):692–702.

11. 2018 Physical Activity Guidelines Advisory Committee. *2018 Physical Activity Guidelines Advisory Committee Scientific Report, 2018.* US Department of Health and Human Services. Accessed July 27, 2023. https://health.gov/sites/default/files/2019-09/PAG_Advisory_Committee_Report.pdf.

12. Bjornson KF, Belza B, Kartin D, Logsdon R, McLaughlin JF. Ambulatory physical activity performance in youth with cerebral palsy and youth who are developing typically. *Phys Ther 2007.* 2007;87:248–257.

13. Caspersen CJ, Powell KE, Christenson GM. Physical activity, exercise, and physical fitness: definitions and distinctions for health-related research. *Public Health Rep.* 1985;100(2):126.

14. Kaur H, Singh T, Arya YK, Mittal S. Physical fitness and exercise during the COVID-19 pandemic: a qualitative enquiry. *Front Psychol.* 2020;11. Accessed July 27, 2023. https://www.frontiersin.org/articles/10.3389/fpsyg.2020.590172.

15. Verschuren O, Darrah J, Novak I, Ketelaar M, Wiart L. Health-enhancing physical activity in children with cerebral palsy: more of the same is not enough. *Phys Ther.* 2014;94:297–305.

16. American College of Sports Medicine. Liguori G, Feito Y, Fountaine C, Roy BA. *Acsm's Guidelines for Exercise Testing and Prescription.* 11th ed. Philadelphia: Wolters Kluwer; 2022.

17. Verschuren O, Peterson MD, Balemans ACJ, Hurvitz EA. Exercise and physical activity recommendations for people with cerebral palsy. *Dev Med Child Neurol.* 2016;58:798–808.

18. O'Shea R, Jones M, Lightfoot K. Examining conductive education: linking science, theory, and intervention. *Arch Rehabil Res Clin Transl.* 2020;2(4):100077.

19. Lai CJ, Liu WY, Yang TF, Chen CL, Wu CY, Chan RC. Pediatric aquatic therapy on motor function and enjoyment in children diagnosed with cerebral palsy of various motor severities. *J Child Neurol.* 2015;30:200–208.

20. Kelly M, Darrah J. Aquatic exercise for children with cerebral palsy. *Dev Med Child Neurol.* 2005;47:838–842.

21. Muñoz-Blanco E, Merino-Andrés J, Aguilar-Soto B. Influence of aquatic therapy in children and youth with cerebral palsy: a qualitative case study in a special education school. *Int J Environ Res Public Health.* 2020;17(10):3690.

22. Gorter JW, Currie SJ. Aquatic exercise programs for children and adolescents with cerebral palsy: what do we know and where do we go? *Int J Pediatr.* 2011;2011:1–7.

23. Abadi FH, Sankaravel M, Zainuddin FF, Elumalai G, Choo LA, Sattari H. A perspective on water properties and aquatic exercise for older adults. *International Journal of Aging Health and Movement.* 2020;2(2):1–10.

24. Martín-Valero R, Vega-Ballón J, Perez-Cabezas V. Benefits of hippotherapy in children with cerebral palsy: a narrative review. *Eur J Paediatr Neurol.* 2018;22(6):1150–1160.

25. Portaro S, Cacciola A, Naro A. Can individuals with Down syndrome benefit from hippotherapy? An exploratory study on gait and balance. *Dev Neurorehabil.* 2020;23(6):337–342.

26. Bierman JC, Franjoine MR, Hazzard CM, Howle J, Stamer M, eds. *Neuro-Developmental Treatment: A Guide to NDT Clinical Practice,* 1st ed. Thieme, New York; 2016.

27. Bly L, Whiteside A. *Facilitation Techniques Based on NDT Principles.* Laguna Beach, CA: NDTA Publishing; 1997.

28. Butler C, Darrah J, Adams R. Effects of neurodevelopmental treatment (NDT) for cerebral palsy: an AACPDM evidence report. *Dev Med Child Neurol.* 2001;43:778–790.

29. Voss D, Ionta M, Myers B. *Proprioceptive Neuromuscular Facilitation.* Philadelphia: Lippincott Williams & Wilkins; 1985.

30. Sharman MJ, Cresswell AG, Riek S. Proprioceptive neuromuscular facilitation stretching: mechanisms and clinical implications. *Sports Med.* 2006;36(11):929–939.

31. Smedes F, Heidmann M, Schäfer C, Fischer N, Stępień A. The proprioceptive neuromuscular facilitation-concept; the state of the evidence, a narrative review. *Phys Ther Rev.* 2016;21(1):17–31.

32. Kinesio Taping Association, Kase K, Hashimoto T, Okane T. *Kinesio Taping Perfect Manual: Amazing Taping Therapy to Eliminate Pain and Muscle Disorders.* Tokyo: Ken'i-Kai Information; 1996.

33. Kase K, Wallis J, Kase T. *Clinical Therapeutic Applications of the Kinesio Taping Method.* Albuquerque: Kinesio Taping Association; 2003.

34. MacDowall I, Sanzo P, Zerpa C. The effect of Kinesio taping on vertical jump height and muscle electromyographic activity of the gastrocnemius and soleus in varsity athletes. *Int J Sports Sci.* 2015;5(4):162–170.

35. Bundy AC, Lane SJ. *Sensory Integration: Theory and Practice.* 3rd ed. Philadelphia: FA Davis; 2019.

36. Long T, Battaile B, Toscano K. *Handbook of Pediatric Physical Therapy.* 3rd ed. Philadelphia: Wolters Kluwer; 2019.

37. Shumway-Cook A, Woollacott MH, Rachwani J, Santamaria V. *Motor Control: Translating Research into Clinical Practice.* 6th ed. Philadelphia: Lippincott Williams & Wilkins; 2022.

38. Merino-Andrés J, García de Mateos-López A, Damiano DL, Sánchez-Sierra A. Effect of muscle strength training in children and adolescents with spastic cerebral palsy: A systematic review and meta-analysis. *Clin Rehabil.* 2022 Jan;36(1):4–14. doi:10.1177/02692155211040199. Epub 2021 Aug 18. PMID: 34407619; PMCID: PMC9639012.

39. Taub E, Crago JE, Uswatte G. Constraint-induced movement therapy: A new approach to treatment in physical rehabilitation. *Rehabilitation Psychology.* 1998;43(2), 152–170. https://doi.org/10.1037/0090-5550.43.2.152.

40. Bourke-Taylor H, O'Shea R, Gaebler-Spira D. Conductive education: A functional skills program for children with cerebral palsy. *Phys Occup Ther Pediatr.* 2007;27(1), 45–62.

RESOURCES

American Hippotherapy Association, Inc.
2850 McClelland Drive #1600
Fort Collins, CO 80525
www.americanhippotherapyassociation.org

Animal Behavior Institute
Animal Behavior Institute, Inc.
4711 Hope Valley Road
Suite 4F-332
Durham, NC 27707
www.animaledu.com

American College of Sports Medicine
401 West Michigan Street
Indianapolis, IN 46202-3233
317-637-9200
www.ascm.org

Neurodevelopmental Treatment Association (NDTA)
1540 S. Coast Highway, Suite 203
Laguna Beach, CA 92651
800-869-9295
www.ndta.org

Conductive Education Information
www.conductive-ed.org.uk

InterAmerican Conductive Education Association (IACEA)
PO Box 3169
Toms River, NJ 08756-3169
800-824-2232
www.iacea.org

Certificate in the Principles of Conductive Education
Governors State University
PT Program
1 University Parkway
University Park, IL 60466
www.govst.edu/cecert

Kinesio Taping Association
3939 San Pedro Drive NE
Bldg C, Suite 6
Albuquerque, NM 87110
888-320-8273
www.kinesiotaping.com

Sensory Processing Disorder (SPD)
1901 W. Littleton Boulevard
Littleton, CO 80120
303-794-1182
www.spdnetwork.org

Sensory Integration International
PO Box 5339
Torrance, CA 90510-5339
310-787-8805
www.sensoryint.com

Pediatric Therapy Teams

Catherine Bookser-Feister, PT, DPT

"If you want to go fast, go alone. If you want to go far, go together."
African Proverb

LEARNING OBJECTIVES

At the end of the chapter, the reader will be able to do the following:

1. Understand why teams are important in pediatrics.
2. Understand the importance of the child's family or caregivers as part of the team.
3. Identify characteristics of effective teams and effective team members.
4. Identify the types of teams and models of intervention used in school, early intervention, and medical practice settings.

CHAPTER OUTLINE

KEY TERMS

Early Intervention (EI)
Educationally relevant
Free and appropriate public
  education
Individualized Education
  Program

Individualized Family Service
  Plan
Interdisciplinary
Least restrictive environment
Multidisciplinary
Related services

School-based physical therapy
Transdisciplinary
Unidisciplinary

All physical therapist assistants (PTAs) know how a physical therapist (PT) and PTA work together as a small unit or team. In pediatrics, however, PTs and PTAs usually work as part of a larger team that includes the child, the child's family or caregivers, and various professionals. In this chapter, we'll examine the types of teams that are common in pediatrics, and we'll explore some of the factors that make team members and their teams effective.

BACKGROUND

The center of any pediatric team is the child. Surrounding that child and the most essential part of the team is the child's family (or those who are caring for the child on a day-to-day basis). On a larger level, teams will include all the professionals who support the child and family, including but not limited to therapists and assistants, physicians, nurses, teachers, and social workers. In teams both large and small, each member brings a unique viewpoint and experience; each team member needs to be aware and respectful of the others' roles and contributions.

COORDINATED CARE AND EFFECTIVE TEAMS

In almost all pediatric practice settings, more than one adult will be involved with the child, and for the sake of that child, the adults need to cooperate with each other. The ability to "work with individuals of other professions to maintain a climate of mutual respect and shared values" is a basic competency for today's healthcare professionals.[1] Coordinated teamwork in pediatrics helps keep the focus on the child as a whole person and ensures that the many different needs of the child are addressed. The PTA, who engages in direct care and day-to-day interactions with other team members, can help ensure that care is coordinated and that teams are functional. Highly effective teams have well-defined roles and responsibilities, clear communication, and respectful interactions. Families and professionals from different disciplines have varying types and levels of expertise, and each team member understands and explains how they are best able to contribute. Professionals need to be open to new learning while having a clear understanding of their own skills and limits. Parents have a unique and central role on the pediatric team, as they are the adults who know the child best and are a constant presence in the child's life through many team changes.

Teams rely on clear communication, both oral and written, to prevent confusion and to help with team cohesion. When you are on a team, you should respond promptly to requests for information, as other team members may need your information before they can complete a task. Remember that communication is a two-way street, involving active listening as well as speaking. Allow pauses when you are talking, so others have a chance to process what you are saying and give their input. Strive for an open, professional tone in your interactions, so that everyone feels free to speak, and use simple, clear language that is easily understood by all. Be aware of and limit physical therapy jargon, which can make people outside of the profession feel excluded.[2]

If you do need to use terms that are specific to your discipline, be sure to define them for clarity. Be aware of cultural differences in communication and use an interpreter or translate written materials when there are language barriers.

> ### BOX 4.1   American Physical Therapy Association Core Values[4]
>
> Accountability
> Altruism
> Collaboration
> Compassion and Caring
> Duty
> Excellence
> Inclusion
> Integrity
> Social Responsibility

Reprinted from www.apta.org, with permission of the American Physical Therapy Association. © 2023 American Physical Therapy Association. All rights reserved.

The American Physical Therapy Association's (APTA's) core values for the PT and PTA can be a guide to professional behavior to help improve the team's functionality (Box 4.1). A PTA who demonstrates integrity, accountability, a willingness to collaborate, and a welcoming stance of inclusion, compassion and caring will be an asset to any team.[3]

MODELS FOR TEAMWORK

Models for teamwork vary across practice settings. Let's examine four models commonly used in pediatric therapy service delivery: unidisciplinary, multidisciplinary, interdisciplinary, and transdisciplinary (Box 4.2).

As the name suggests, in a unidisciplinary model, PTs and PTAs work with children and their families independently of other disciplines.[4] An example of this would be traditional outpatient sports-oriented therapy provided in a private practice physical therapy setting, where the PT evaluates the child and develops the plan of care, and the PTA and PT provide treatment. Although the PT and PTA may communicate with each other, the family, and the referring physician, there is no attempt to coordinate care with other types of professionals. Unidisciplinary care may be the only (and therefore the best) option in rural or underserved areas of the country, where healthcare professionals are scarce.

In multidisciplinary teams, many disciplines are involved with the child and the family, but each discipline works separately. The disciplines respect and value input from other disciplines, and there should be care coordination among the disciplines.[4] An example of multidisciplinary teamwork would be when a child is evaluated and treated separately by professionals from

BOX 4.2	Models of Pediatric Teams			
	Unidisciplinary	**Multidisciplinary**	**Interdisciplinary**	**Transdisciplinary**
Who is in it?	Child, family, and one discipline (i.e., PT)	Child, family, and several or many disciplines	Child, family, and several or many disciplines	Child, family, and several or many disciplines
Who makes the goals?	Goals limited to one discipline	Separate goals, set by each discipline	Shared goals, developed by team	Shared goals or outcomes developed by team
What happens with assessment and treatment?	All evaluations and treatments are in a setting with only one discipline.	Disciplines assess and treat independently but share information.	Disciplines may assess and treat jointly or independently but always plan and evaluate services together.	High level of collaboration among group members; some blurring of discipline roles, primary service provider.

physical, occupational, and speech language therapies, and later, the therapists exchange notes or communicate with each other to discuss the child's condition and progress. Remember to abide by the Health Insurance Portability and Accountability Act (HIPAA) or Family Educational Rights and Privacy Act (FERPA) when communicating with team members.

In an interdisciplinary model, the PT evaluation and treatment sessions may occur independently of the other disciplines, but team members work closely to plan and coordinate the examination, evaluation, and treatment of the child and evaluate the effectiveness of their services.[5] An example of this type of teamwork would be seen in a coordinated inpatient rehabilitation plan of care, where patients attend separate therapy sessions, but the medical team holds regular team meetings to discuss the patient's progress and plan discharge. This model may also be used in public school and early intervention settings.

In a transdisciplinary team, members are committed to working closely together and freely sharing all information. The child is usually evaluated in an arena assessment, a combined session by a group of professionals and the child's parents or caregivers. To ensure clear communication and to limit the stress to the child and family, one team member may act as the primary service provider, with other team members available for consultation when needed. In a transdisciplinary team, all therapists work toward all the goals of the team. For example, while helping the child learn to move and balance in standing, the PT may have the child practice pulling on clothing (traditionally an area

addressed by occupational therapy). This collaborative model involves some amount of role release, with overlapping of the professions' tasks. It can be effective, but team members may encounter challenges such as needing extra time for training and coordination.[4,8] PTs and PTAs using the transdisciplinary model need to be open, flexible and responsive, listening carefully and communicating clearly with the other disciplines. Although there is role-sharing, all professionals are responsible for making sure they are working safely and within the limitations of their state licensure laws. The transdisciplinary model is often used in state-sponsored early intervention and school teams.

With goodwill, coordination, and clear communication, most types of teams can be effective, but specific models may be preferred in particular PT practice environments.

PEDIATRIC PHYSICAL THERAPY PRACTICE SETTINGS

Pediatric medical rehabilitation teams are used in inpatient and outpatient hospital settings. Medical teams, which are usually multidisciplinary or interdisciplinary, are often led by a physician, with goals related to improving the child's health, wellness, or function. These teams can be large or small, depending on the complexity of the child's needs and the resources available in that facility. In addition to the parents, PT, PTA, and physician, team members may include occupational therapists, speech and language pathologists, audiologists, recreational therapists, child life specialists, nurse practitioners, physician assistants, bedside nurses, dieticians, nutritionists, chaplains, psychologists, and social workers. Assistive technology professionals, prosthetists, and orthotists may also consult with the team.

Outpatient therapy centers may opt for a very well-coordinated transdisciplinary model or a more medically oriented multi- or interdisciplinary team model, with team members such as speech or occupational therapists or, in the case of a sports clinic, athletic trainers. Some outpatient clinics provide only physical therapy and will use a unidisciplinary model. As in other settings, the outpatient therapist needs to communicate carefully with the parents or primary caregivers, whether by having the parents in the room during treatment or ensuring that there is collaboration with them before and after the session.

Pediatric physical therapy may also occur in the child's school. School-based physical therapy is fundamentally different from medical physical therapy because it is regulated by public education law and is financed primarily by the school district. To understand this crucial difference, it is helpful to know the history of education for children with special needs in the United States. Many years ago, children with serious cognitive or physical needs were denied the opportunity to get a publicly funded education. For example, a school district could refuse to serve a child who did not walk or was not toilet trained. In 1971, a group of Pennsylvania parents of children with intellectual disabilities felt that their children deserved more, and they brought and won a class-action lawsuit against their school district. Other parent-initiated lawsuits followed.[4]

Soon after this, a federal law (Public Law 94-142, the Education for All Handicapped Children Act of 1975) was passed that gave all children the right to a "free and appropriate public education." This law has been reauthorized several times, and its primary principles are still in effect. A more recent edition of the law is called the Individuals with Disabilities Education Act (IDEA). Part B of this law guarantees that children aged 3 to 21 years with exceptional educational needs can receive an appropriate evaluation and an Individualized Education Program (IEP), a yearly plan with team-based goals and objectives to guide the child's instruction. The educational team can be interdisciplinary or transdisciplinary, with the teacher as the team leader and with therapists, counselors, school nurses, instructional

assistants, and others also involved. Parents are part of the team and are legally entitled and encouraged to participate in developing the IEP.[4]

The law also mandates that children get their specially designed instruction in the least restrictive environment. (This means that children with disabilities must be included in classes with their same-aged, typically developing peers, unless they need to be in more restrictive or isolated classroom settings in order to learn.) It specifies that students receive related services (including physical therapy) if these services are needed to assist the student to benefit from special education. Because of the related services provision in the law, physical therapy may be provided by and in the school, but this therapy must be educationally relevant and must support the child's IEP goals. In other words, all children are eligible for a free and appropriate public education, but this does not mean that all children with physical therapy needs will be eligible for in-school therapy.[5–8]

What makes therapy educationally relevant? Let's consider an example of a third grader who can walk on level surfaces but is not yet independent in climbing stairs. If the elementary school is a one-story building, it might not be considered educationally relevant for the school therapists to work on stairclimbing, since the child doesn't have to walk on stairs to get to class. In that situation, the parent could take the child to outpatient therapy to work toward this skill, outside of school time. However, if the educational team writes an IEP goal that the child improve socialization with other students, the school therapist might justify working on steps so that the child could safely board the school bus and play with friends while climbing on the playground equipment.

Pediatric physical therapy can also be found in Early Intervention (EI) services, a state-based public program for infants and toddlers with developmental delays or risk of delays due to specific disabilities. EI services are mandated by federal education law (under Part C of the IDEA), and regulations specify where and how services are provided. Although EI services are federally authorized, each state develops its own program and eligibility criteria. These programs are designed so that children and their families receive comprehensive evaluations, support, and intervention early to take advantage of sensitive periods in development when tremendous improvement is possible. Physical therapy is just one of many services, across many disciplines, that can be

BOX 4.3 Early Intervention Services Included in IDEA

- Family training, counseling, home visits
- Special instruction
- Speech-language pathology
- Audiology, sign language, and cued language services
- Occupational therapy
- Physical therapy
- Psychologic services
- Service coordination
- Medical services (only for diagnostic or evaluation purposes)
- Early identification, screening, and assessment services
- Health services (if necessary to enable the infant or toddler to benefit from the EI process)
- Social work
- Vision services
- Assistive technology devices and services
- Transportation and related costs necessary to receive early intervention.

Source: Chiarello L, Catalino T. Infants, toddlers, and their families: early intervention services under IDEA. In: Palisano RJ, Orlin MN, Schreiber J, eds. *Campbell's Physical Therapy for Children.* 5th ed. Elsevier; 2017, pp. 703–722, Box 30.1.

provided in these family-centered programs (Box 4.3).[9] Teamwork models vary from state to state, but services must be coordinated. Family involvement is essential, and a transdisciplinary approach is often used. Educational relevance is not a requirement for early intervention, and physical therapy can be a primary service.

Some children are automatically eligible for EI services because they have conditions that are known to lead to developmental delays (such as very low birth weight, Down syndrome, or cerebral palsy). If a child is showing delays but does not have one of these specific conditions, they may still be eligible for EI services based on a percentage of developmental delay in the areas of physical, cognitive, communication, social-emotional, or adaptive development. Each state has its own definition of what is considered a significant delay, with some states offering services to children with 25% delay, and others limiting help to those with more than 50% delay.

After eligibility is established, the child's family and the evaluators meet to develop an Individualized Family Service Plan (IFSP). The IFSP states outcomes and strategies based on the family's priorities and concerns and specifies the type and amount of services to be provided.

An important concept in EI is that these services should be provided in the child's natural environment, so that children can be in settings where they are the most familiar and secure and where they demonstrate their usual behavior.[9] Most EI services are provided in the home; some are in a community setting (such as a daycare or playground) where typically developing children are also present.[10] A major benefit of providing therapy in the natural environment is that the PTA can ensure that therapeutic activities match the needs, priorities, and schedules of the child and family. However, the challenges of working in EI are also well documented in the literature.[11] When working in the home, PTAs may become uncomfortably aware of how a lack of resources (such as financial security, comfortable housing, safe neighborhoods) affect developmental progress. An effective PT or PTA recognizes how challenges impact each family and works with the family and other team members and community resources to help diminish the negative impacts on the child and family.

CASE STUDY: EARLY INTERVENTION TEAMWORK

Gabriela, a 2-year-old girl with Down syndrome, is referred to the local early intervention team. Gabriela lives with her parents, three older siblings, and aunt in a small, single-family home in a rural area. Spanish is the primary language spoken in the home.

Gabriela is automatically eligible for EI services because she has the qualifying health condition of Down syndrome. Her developmental skills are evaluated in an arena assessment in the home, with an interpreter, PT, occupational therapist, speech-language pathologist, developmental therapist, her mother, aunt, and siblings all participating. The atmosphere during the assessment is pleasant and collaborative.

The team observes that Gabriela is a happy child who eats well, says three single-syllable words, and enjoys playing with her toys. She is stable and safe when sitting up on a blanket, and she can move forward 6 feet by belly-down crawling. She is not yet standing without support, cruising, or walking. With the help of the rest of the team, Gabriela's mother fills out the Spanish version

Continued

CASE STUDY: EARLY INTERVENTION TEAMWORK—cont'd

of the Ages and Stages-3 Questionnaire to provide formal documentation of the need for services. The team uses additional standardized assessment tools, noting that scores are below the cut-off points in all the developmental areas, with lowest scores in gross motor skills.

Two weeks after the assessment, the team again meets in the home to develop the IFSP. The parents' primary concern is that Gabriela isn't standing and walking, so it's difficult for her to play with her siblings. They are also concerned that she can't ask for items when she wants them. Based on the family's priorities, the team writes an IFSP outcome that Gabriela will stand without support and take steps. An additional outcome is that she will speak or sign up to 20 words. The team decides that physical therapy will occur weekly for the next 6 months, with a joint session with the speech-language therapist once a month. Physical therapy services will be delivered by the PTA, with regular supervision by the PT as required by the state licensure regulations.

Prior to their first visit to the home, the PT and PTA meet to discuss the plan of care, using the International Classification of Functioning, Disability, and Health (ICF) model and the Movement Systems Analysis to help guide their clinical thinking. Using the ICF, they identify that Gabriela's health condition is Down syndrome, with hypotonia and weakness (a force production deficit) affecting her body structures and functions. She has activity limitations in standing, cruising, and walking, leading to decreased participation with her siblings during play. The PT and PTA agree that this child's cheerful disposition is a facilitating personal factor and the attentive and engaged family is a facilitating environmental factor. Because limited English proficiency is an environmental barrier that could complicate communication, the clinicians will use an in-person interpreter whenever possible, with a live video or phone interpreter as a back-up. Using the Movement Systems model, it is determined that Gabriela demonstrates force production deficits. Thus, a component of the plan of care will be strengthening Gabriela's lower extremities and trunk especially in antigravity and single leg stance positions.

On the first treatment visit, the PTA warmly and respectfully greets the family, then listens carefully while they describe their usual home routines. They discuss the most convenient times to work with Gabriela on standing balance activities and then plan to help her stand at the couch when the family is playing, in the playpen when the mom is cooking, and with hand-held assist while her older sister is helping her dress. During the session, the family members practice helping Gabriela stand. The PTA gives them tips on giving the right level of assistance and teaches them the sign language for "stand" and "walk."

The PTA documents the list of the family's routines in her visit note and then emails it to the rest of the team so that all can be informed and prepared for future visits.

DISCUSSION QUESTIONS

1. Why is the caregiver/family the primary member of the pediatric therapeutic team?
2. What are the key differences between interdisciplinary and transdisciplinary teams?
3. Which type of teams are most often used for medical rehabilitation? For schools? For early intervention programs?
4. Think about how you can communicate effectively with parents and professionals who are on your team. What are some ways that you can show that you are listening respectfully? What are ways that you can show respect when speaking?
5. What does it mean for physical therapy in schools to be a related service? How can physical therapy intervention help support a child's ability to move around the school environment? How could therapy help support a child within a classroom?

REFERENCES

1. Interprofessional Education Collaborative. *Core Competencies for Interprofessional Collaborative Practice: 2016 update.* Washington, DC: Interprofessional Education Collaborative; 2016.
2. Early Childhood Technical Assistance Center. *Teaming and Collaboration Practice Guide 2 of 3. Teaming Members Engaging in Quality Communication*; 2020. Accessed July 7, 2023. https://ectacenter.org/~pdfs/decrp/PGP_TC2_qualitycommunication_2018.pdf.
3. American Physical Therapy Association. *Core Values for the Physical Therapist and Physical Therapist Assistant*; 2021. September 28, 2022. https://www.apta.org/apta-and-you/leadership-and-governance/policies/core-values-for-the-physical-therapist-and-physical-therapist-assistant.
4. Effgen SK, Howman J. Serving the needs of children and their families. In: Effgen SK, Fiss ALF, eds. *Meeting the Physical Therapy Needs of Children*. 3rd ed. Philadelphia: FA Davis; 2021.

5. Effgen S, Kaminker MK. The educational environment. In: Palisano RJ, Orlin MN, Schreiber J, eds. *Campbell's Physical Therapy for Children*. 5th ed. St Louis: Elsevier; 2017.

6. Vialu C, Doyle M. Determining need for school-based physical therapy under IDEA: commonalities across practice guidelines. *Pediatr Phys Ther*. 2017;29(4):350–355.

7. Vialu C, Doyle M, Ruff A, et al. (2021) Fact sheet educationally relevant physical therapy—part II: determining a student's need for school-based PT under IDEA. Accessed September 28, 2022. https://pediatricapta.org/includes/fact-sheets/pdfs/Fact%20Sheet_EducationallyRelevantPhysicalThearpy-PartII_2021.pdf.

8. Chiarello L, Catalino T. Infants, toddlers, and their families: early intervention services under IDEA. In: Palisano RJ, Orlin MN, Schreiber J, eds. *Campbell's Therapy for Children*. 5th ed. Place: Elsevier; 2017.

9. Effgen SK, Fiss ALF. Early intervention. In: Effgen SK, Fiss ALF, eds. *Meeting the Physical Therapy Needs of Children*. 3rd ed. Philadelphia: FA Davis; 2021.

10. US Department of Education: *43rd Annual Report to Congress on the Implementation of the Individuals With Disabilities Education Act, 2021*. Accessed September 28, 2022. https://sites.ed.gov/idea/files/43rd-arc-for-idea.pdf.

11. Gmmash A, Effgen SK, Goldey K. Challenges faced by therapists providing services for infants with or at risk for cerebral palsy. *Pediatr Phys Ther*. 2021;32(2):88–96.

RESOURCES

Interprofessional Educational Collaborative (Core Competencies)
https://www.ipecollaborative.org/core-competencies

Early Childhood Technical Assistance Center
https://ectacenter.org/about.asp

US Department of Education's IDEA website
https://sites.ed.gov/idea/

Family Resources From the American Physical Therapy's Academy for Pediatric Physical Therapy
https://pediatricapta.org/consumers/

Best Practices for Communicating Through an Interpreter From the Refugee Health Technical Assistance Center
https://refugeehealthta.org/access-to-care/language-access/best-practices-communicating-through-an-interpreter/

The Movement System

Kristine (Tina) Chase, PT, DPT, PCS

LEARNING OBJECTIVES

At the end of the chapter, the reader will be able to do the following:

1. Define the movement system and its relevance to pediatric physical therapy practice.
2. Describe the five phases of movement and how each phase can be used to conduct movement analysis of tasks and activities frequently observed in pediatric clients.
3. Characterize movement system diagnoses for neuromuscular conditions by describing faulty movement patterns and common impairments.
4. Identify treatment principles to guide the selection of interventions when working with individuals with neuromuscular movement system dysfunction.

CHAPTER OUTLINE

KEY TERMS

Dysmetria
Execution
Force production deficit
Fractionated movement deficit
Hypokinesia
Initial conditions
Initiation

Modifier
Movement pattern coordination deficit
Movement system
Movement system diagnoses for neuromuscular conditions
Phases of movement

Postural vertical deficit
Preparation
Sensory detection deficit
Sensory selection and weighting deficit
Movement analysis
Termination

In 2013, the American Physical Therapy Association (APTA) established "transforming society by optimizing movement to improve the human experience" as the vision for the profession of physical therapy. The APTA simultaneously adopted eight guiding principles to support the achievement of the vision.[1,2] The first guiding principle asserts the physical therapy profession "will promote the movement system as the foundation for optimizing movement to improve the health of society" and "the physical therapist will be responsible for evaluating and managing an individual's movement system across the lifespan to promote optimal development, diagnose impairments, activity limitations and participation restrictions; and provide interventions targeted at preventing or ameliorating activity limitations and participation restrictions."[1] The physical therapist assistant has a role in supporting the physical therapist in providing services in accordance with movement system principles.

DEFINITION

The *movement system* is defined as the collection of systems—including cardiovascular, pulmonary, endocrine, integumentary, nervous, and musculoskeletal—that interact to move the body or its component parts.[1,2] Figure 5.1 is the APTA's graphic of the movement system.

The movement system includes movement at all levels of the human body including movement of the body from one position to another, segmental movement such as at a single joint, and movement at the molecular and cellular levels such as what occurs during tissue healing. A person's health is therefore determined by the collective health of the body's systems and each system's ability to contribute to movement at multiple levels of the human body. Physical therapy providers focusing on the movement system can address health conditions in ways that prioritize movement, physical function, overall wellbeing, and ultimately the ability to participate in and contribute to society.

PHYSICAL THERAPY PRACTICE AND MOVEMENT SYSTEM DIAGNOSES FOR NEUROMUSCULAR CONDITIONS

Physical therapy practice is grounded in several frameworks including the International Classification of Functioning, Disability and Health (ICF) model and The Guide's Patient-Client Management Model.[3,4] In 2015, the APTA House of Delegates endorsed the development of diagnostic labels and classification systems promoting the physical therapist's ability to manage disorders of the movement system.[1] The movement system diagnoses for neuromuscular conditions constitute a framework that can be used by physical therapy providers to understand, classify, and direct the care of children with neuromuscular dysfunction.[5] The diagnoses for neuromuscular conditions are a collection of eight descriptive diagnostic labels grounded in movement-related terms that characterize the condition of the movement system. The diagnostic framework is situated within the physical therapist's scope of practice aligning with and not replacing existing, well-established models of practice. Figure 5.2 is an example of representation for the relationship between APTA Patient/Client Management Model, ICF, and Movement-related Diagnosis.[6] Figure 5.3 is an example of a relationship between ICF and Movement-Related Diagnosis.[6]

USE IN PEDIATRICS

The movement system diagnoses for neuromuscular conditions allow pediatric physical therapists to examine, identify, and label movement-related dysfunction regardless of a child's health condition. Diagnosis of a movement system dysfunction is based on a physical therapy examination that includes tests for specific impairments as well as observation and analysis of movement during select tasks.[7] Movements often analyzed in pediatrics include rolling, crawling, moving

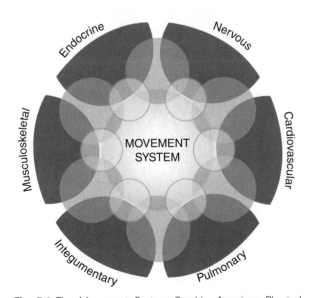

Fig. 5.1 The Movement System Graphic, American Physical Therapy Association, 2016. (Reprinted from www.apta.org, with permission of the American Physical Therapy Association. © 2023 American Physical Therapy Association. All rights reserved.)

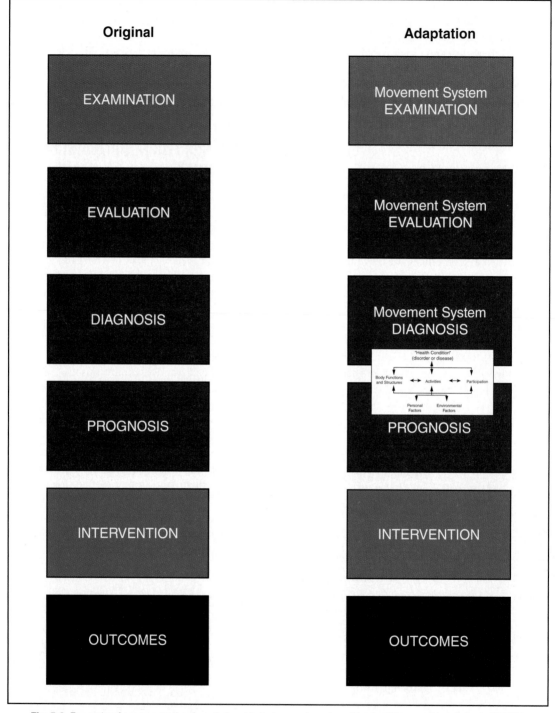

Fig. 5.2 Example of representation for relationship between American Physical Therapy Association's (APTA's) Patient/Client Management Model, the International Classification of Functioning, Disability and Health (ICF) model, and Movement-Related Diagnosis. (From Norton BJ. Diagnosis dialog: recap and relevance to recent APTA actions, *Int J Sports Phys.* 2017;12(6):870–883.)

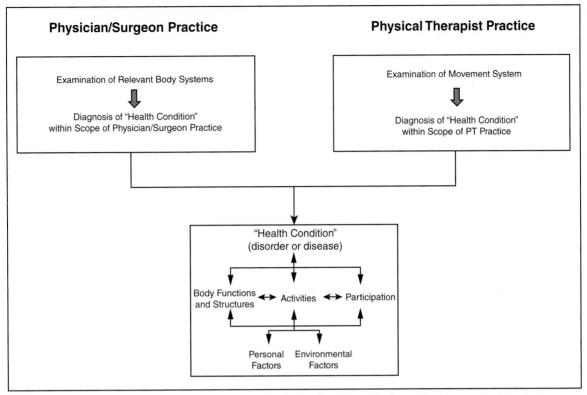

Fig. 5.3 Example of the relationship between the International Classification of Functioning, Disability and Health (ICF) model, and Movement-Related Diagnosis. (From Norton BJ. Diagnosis dialog: recap and relevance to recent APTA actions, *Int J Sports Phys.* 2017;12(6):870–883.)

from sit to stand, and standing. Additional movement tasks frequently analyzed in pediatrics are listed in Box 5.1.

MOVEMENT ANALYSIS AND PHASES OF MOVEMENT

Analysis of how an individual moves when performing a task or activity can be organized by considering phases of movement. Movement can be divided into five distinct phases beginning with a description of the conditions before movement starts and ending when movement stops.[8] The five phases including initial conditions, preparation, initiation, execution, and termination provide a framework to organize observations and describe movement when analyzing how a client moves when performing a task.[8] The components of each of the five phases of movement for movement analysis are outlined in Table 5.1.

MOVEMENT SYSTEM DIAGNOSES FOR NEUROMUSCULAR CONDITIONS

Eight movement system diagnoses serve as nomenclature to characterize movement of infants and children with neuromuscular conditions as well as movement of individuals across the lifespan.[5] When used in pediatrics, the descriptive nature of the diagnostic labels provides pertinent clinical information about the primary movement strategies used by infants and children regardless of their health conditions, allowing providers to understand the primary movement faults and select interventions that optimally address the identified movement system deficits. Although primary movement deficits and subsequent movement system diagnoses may change as a child matures, interventions can focus on optimizing movement to maximize participation and overall wellbeing based on the child's movement system needs at the given time.

BOX 5.1   Movement Tasks Analyzed in Pediatrics

For individuals with global or primary lower extremity involvement

Prone on elbows
Rolling
Pull to sit
Creeping/crawling
Floor to stand
Sit to stand
Standing
Standing feet together
Step up
Gait
Complex gait
Running
Jumping
Hopping

For individuals with primary upper extremity involvement

Reach
Grasp
In-hand manipulation

From Scheets PL, Bloom NJ, Crowner B, and others. *Movement System Diagnoses: Neuromuscular Conditions.* St Louis: Washington University; 2020.

Movement Pattern Coordination Deficit

Diagnosis description: The primary movement dysfunction in infants and children with movement pattern coordination deficit is poor timing and sequencing of either intersegmental movements or postural responses (anticipatory and reactive) relative to balance demands. In the lower extremity, the movement problem is primarily observed during tasks that require stability prior to and during limb or trunk movements. In the upper extremity, the movement problem is primarily observed during hand manipulation and grasp and release of different objects coupled with reach. Motor performance typically improves with practice and instruction.[5]

Subjective medical history: Movement pattern coordination deficit often accompanies diagnoses of developmental coordination disorder, developmental delay, autism spectrum disorder, idiopathic toe walking, and motor apraxia. Caregivers may describe children as delayed in achievement of independent walking, clumsy, frequently tripping and falling, being awkward, or delayed compared to peers, and performing poorly during sport activities.[5]

Tests and signs: When transitioning from sitting to standing, individuals may have an altered sequence of movement (such as insufficient dorsiflexion at execution) and demonstrate excessive posterior sway or

TABLE 5.1   Framework for Movement Analysis

Phase of Movement	Initial Conditions	Preparation	Initiation	Execution	Termination
Time period	State of the individual, task, and environment before the movement begins	When movement is organized within the central nervous system	When movement begins	When the body segments are moving	When movement stops
Body's response		Comprehension of instructions and understanding the requirements of the task	Overcoming inertia of the body at rest	Moving the center of mass into a new position	Deceleration of the center of mass Body stabilizes into a new position
Considerations for observation and analysis		May not be readily apparent but inferred based on response	Timing Direction Smoothness	Direction Amplitude Speed	Accuracy Timing Stability

Adapted from Hedman L, Rogers M, Hanke T. Neurologic professional education: linking the foundation science of motor control with physical therapy interventions for movement dysfunction. *Neurol Rep.* 1996;20:9–13; Quinn L, Riley N, Tyrell CM, and others. A framework for movement analysis of tasks: recommendations from the Academy of Neurologic Physical Therapy's Movement System Task Force. *Phys Ther.* 2021;101:1–8.

stepping strategy for balance at termination. Children will often demonstrate difficulty with single-limb balance, impacting their stability to negotiate stairs. They often demonstrate altered sequence, instability, or lack of fluidity when running, jumping, and skipping but are unlikely to require significant physical assistance.[5]

Treatment principles: Because children have relatively typical strength, segmental movement, and sensation, interventions focused on improving coordination, speed, amplitude, and efficiency of motor tasks are appropriate. Interventions should assist with successful completion of the missing but essential components of tasks and aim to increase consistency of performance with increased environmental demands. Performance should improve with practice and repetition.[5]

Expected outcome: Children can be expected to stand and walk independently without an assistive device, negotiate up and down stairs reciprocally, and achieve smooth coordinated upper extremity movement.[5]

Force Production Deficit

Diagnosis description: The primary movement fault of infants and children with force production deficit is weakness as illustrated in the performance of tasks and in testing of body structures and functions. The origin of the weakness may be muscle, neuromuscular junction, peripheral nerve, or central nervous system dysfunction. The presentation may be focal (one joint), segmental (generalized to an extremity or body region), or related to fatigue (of skeletal muscle rather than cardiopulmonary capacity).[5]

Subjective medical history: Force production deficit often accompanies diagnoses of prematurity, developmental delay, Down syndrome, fragile X syndrome, cerebral palsy (mild), myelomeningocele, muscular dystrophies, and hypotonia. Caregivers may describe children as needing caregiver assistance, experiencing excessive fatigue, being premature, and delayed in their acquisition of milestones.[5]

Tests and signs: Individuals will demonstrate one or more of the following: have less than 3+/5 to 4/5 muscle strength throughout a limb or limbs, have difficulty moving through full range of motion against gravity, focal weakness at one primary joint, or deterioration in range of motion/speed of movement with repetition. Infants may demonstrate a head lag with pull to sit and have difficulty maintaining head elevation to 90 degrees when prone on elbows beyond the appropriate age. Children may exhibit a positive Gower sign (using

upper extremities on thighs) when transitioning from floor to stand and may have difficulty or fail to initiate standing from sitting in a chair. An assistive device may be needed with gait, and deviations with walking are often significant. Individuals may have difficulty elevating their upper extremities overhead and maintaining adequate grip force on an object in the hand.[5] Limited improvement is noted with practice, and performance level may decrease with repetition.

Treatment principles: The prognosis for remediation of impairments is an important consideration when determining the appropriate intervention and is largely related to the child's health condition, time since onset, and interventions.[4] When potential for recovery of strength is good, resistance training performed at an intensity aligned with the literature based on the health condition is appropriate. When potential for recovery of strength is poor, interventions should be designed to teach adaptive and compensatory strategies and to assist with the acquisition of and training in the use of orthotics, assistive devices, and wheeled mobility consistent with the literature for individuals with the health condition.[5]

Expected outcome: Outcomes are variable and based on the extent of muscle weakness and prognosis for recovery. Some individuals may achieve independence with ambulation needing increased time, an ankle-foot orthosis (AFO), or assistive device; others may require a wheelchair and/or assistance to achieve mobility and functional upper extremity use. In severe forms, independent sitting and walking may not be achieved.[5]

Fractionated Movement Deficit

Diagnosis description: The primary movement system problem of infants and children with fractionated movement deficit is the inability to fractionate movement in the upper or lower extremities or both. The problem is associated with moderate or greater hyperexcitability and is always associated with central neurologic deficit.[5]

Subjective medical history: Fractionated movement deficit often accompanies diagnoses of intraventricular hemorrhage (IVH), periventricular leukomalacia (PVL), brain tumor, brain injury/hypoxia, and cerebral palsy/static encephalopathy. Caregivers may describe children having difficulty with mobility, stiffness of the limbs and/or pain, falls, slow walking, poor upper extremity use, or a complicated perinatal history.[5]

Tests and signs: Individuals will lack the ability to fractionate movement, generate force rapidly, and make rapid reversals in movement, which will be evident across multiple tasks and purposeful movements. Hypertonia will be present, and individuals may exhibit positive primitive reflexes (such as positive asymmetric tonic neck reflex [+ATNR] and positive symmetric tonic neck reflex [+STNR]) beyond age appropriate. Neck hyperextension with shoulder elevation may be present with pull to sit and prone on elbows. Children may use mobility patterns such as commando crawl and bunny hop rather than assuming quadruped and crawling, and excessive lower extremity extension may be present when transitioning to standing from the floor. Gait is often characterized by compensatory movement strategies such as hip hiking, vaulting, and circumduction to initiate swing, stiffness of hip and knee flexion during swing and scissoring, toe walking, and hip and knee flexion during stance. An assistive device may be required early in development or to maintain independent gait.[5]

Treatment principles: Because the acquisition of fractionated movement may not be possible, orthotic support to the foot, ankle, and knee to achieve proper alignment and safe weight-bearing and stepping may be necessary. Interventions may focus on compensatory or adaptive movement strategies and include repetition to improve speed, endurance, motor planning, and efficiency. Because some deficits may persist, education about the potential for secondary musculoskeletal pain and possible prevention strategies is important.[5]

Expected outcome: Outcomes are variable and based on the degree of involvement and ability to move against gravity. For forms with involvement of all four limbs and reduced antigravity movement, a wheelchair for locomotion may be necessary. When few limbs are involved and more antigravity movement is present, independent sitting and ambulation with or without an assistive device may be possible.[5]

Postural Vertical Deficit

Diagnosis description: The primary movement problem of infants and children with postural vertical deficit is inaccurate perception of vertical orientation resulting in postural control deficits and the tendency to resist correction of center of mass alignment, which may be medial/lateral or anterior/posterior.[5]

Subjective medical history: Postural vertical deficit often accompanies diagnoses of Rhett syndrome, brain injury, or stroke. Caregivers may report children tending

to fall backward or laterally, to have a fear of falling, or to have vision or visual perceptual deficits.[5]

Tests and signs: Infants and children will possess movement in at least 60% of the lower extremity muscle groups, although movement may not be fractionated. Individuals will have difficulty motor planning or organizing movement patterns into purposeful actions. Sensation to light touch and joint position sense may be impaired. Impulsivity, poor judgment, and fear avoidance behavior such as clutching or grabbing with upper extremities or shifting the base of support to avoid specific movements or alignments may be present.[5]

Treatment principles: Interventions focused on teaching controlled active movement and awareness of faulty movement patterns is appropriate. Principles related to maintaining the center of mass over the base of support during transitions and maintaining forward progression when walking can be emphasized.[5]

Expected outcome: Outcomes are related to the severity of the behavioral and cognitive deficits, motor function, and anticipated recovery of the perceptual deficits. Ambulation with a walker may be possible; however, in more severe forms, ambulation may not be possible and significant assistance with transfers may be required.[5]

Sensory Selection and Weighting Deficit

Diagnosis description: The primary movement problem of infants and children with sensory selection and weighting deficit is difficulty with postural stability, orientation, or both caused by decreased ability to screen for and attend to information from the sensory system. Sensory seeking or sensory avoidance behaviors may be present. Sensory processing issues are the primary movement system problem and may impact steady state, anticipatory and reactive postural control, and limb movement.[5]

Subjective medical history: Sensory selection and weighting deficit often accompany diagnoses of autism spectrum disorder, Asperger's syndrome, sensory processing disorder, and Rhett's syndrome. Caregivers may report children feeling unstable, losing their balance, or demonstrating instability when walking in crowds, in visually complex environments, or on compliant or moving surfaces. Children may demonstrate repetitive, nonpurposeful movements, impaired social behaviors, aversion to a variety of sensory stimuli, or delayed acquisition of motor milestones appropriate for their age.[5]

Tests and signs: Infants and children may demonstrate increased instability or postural sway during motion that includes head movement or changes in sensory conditions such as closing their eyes. They may deviate their line of progression, lose their balance, or become dizzy when turning, turning around, or moving fast. Signs of gaze aversion and self-stimulation behaviors such as rocking, spinning, and banging may be observed.[5]

Treatment principles: The overarching goal is optimal, purposeful movement and postural stability in both simple and complex sensory environments.[5] Appropriate interventions may include exposure to and practice of movement in progressively challenging sensory environments and adaptation of sensory stimuli and environments to promote optimal motor performance.[5]

Expected outcome: Ambulation in a straight line without loss of balance in all regular sensory environments can be achieved, although prolonged exposure in highly visually stimulating environments may be limited. Mild symptoms including instability may occur with tasks involving rotation of the head or body.

Sensory Detection Deficit

Diagnosis description: The primary movement problem of infants and children with sensory detection deficit is the inability to execute intersegmental movement due to a lack of joint position sense or multisensory failure affecting joint position sense, vision, and/or the vestibular system. A loss of joint position sense involving one or more upper or lower extremities is the primary movement system problem.[5]

Subjective medical history: Sensory detection deficit can accompany diagnoses of peripheral polyneuropathy or multisystem failure and can occur with exposure to childhood cancer treatments such as vincristine. Caregivers may report children having difficulty standing still, walking loudly due to foot slap, frequently tripping and falling, and being unable to run.[5]

Tests and signs: Individuals may demonstrate impaired joint position sense and impaired sensation to touch in one or more of the extremities, contributing to poor timing and coordination of limb movement during tasks. Transitioning from sit to stand is characterized by hyperextension of the knees before the hips during execution and instability of the ankles and use of stepping strategy to maintain the base of support upon termination. Gait is characterized by variable foot placement, knee hyperextension during stance, and foot slap due to a loss of eccentric control at the ankle. Balance and quality of movement may improve with visual guidance.[5]

Treatment principles: Interventions should be specific to the degree and type of sensory loss and can focus on providing compensatory and adaptive strategies to facilitate alignment and motor performance despite limited sensory input. Examples include reducing speed of movement and using orthotics, vision, and an assistive device or hands for guidance during ambulation.[5]

Expected outcome: Standing stability for functional tasks may be limited, especially on uneven surfaces and when lighting is poor. Ambulation with an assistive device and hand function is possible with visual guidance.[5]

Dysmetria

Diagnosis description: The primary movement system problem of infants and children with dysmetria is the inability to grade forces appropriately for the distance and speed required for a task. Rapid movements are generally too large, and slow movements are generally too small for their intended purpose, and performance deteriorates with faster speeds. Dysmetria may involve upper extremities, lower extremities, or both and is associated with cerebellar dysfunction.[5]

Subjective medical history: Dysmetria can accompany diagnoses of cerebral palsy, agenesis of the corpus callosum, fragile X syndrome, and ataxia. Caregivers may report children being clumsy, falling and being injured frequently, and being messy during fine motor tasks such as eating.[5]

Tests and signs: Individuals frequently demonstrate difficulty directing movement toward a target resulting in undershooting or overshooting, which makes tasks such as reaching to targets challenging. Abnormal rhythm and incoordination during rapidly alternating movements is common, and coordinating movement to grasp small or light objects can be difficult. During transitions, excessive sway, a wide base of support, and use of the upper extremities to achieve stability may be observed. Individuals may demonstrate variable foot placement and require assistance when walking. Practice does not change performance.[5]

Treatment principles: Interventions appropriate for children with cerebellar disorders are likely appropriate for this children with dysmetria. Examples may include promoting stability during movement such as by reducing the degrees of freedom using fixed ankle orthoses, decreasing the speed and amplitude of movement, or providing an assistive device during gait.[5]

Expected outcome: Independent sitting and household ambulation with a device and bracing can be expected. A wheelchair may be necessary in the community. Independence with activities of daily living is limited.[5]

Hypokinesia

Diagnosis description: The primary movement system problem for infants and children with hypokinesia is related to slowness in initiating and executing movement and may be associated with stopping of ongoing movement.[5]

Subjective medical history: Hypokinesia can accompany diagnoses of intraventricular hemorrhage, seizure disorder, and stroke. Caregivers may report slow movement, difficulty with initiation, or an inability to sustain ongoing movement.[5]

Tests and signs: Antigravity movement is possible; however, arrests in ongoing movement during functional tasks occur. Postural adjustments are delayed or absent, and posterior loss of balance is common.[5]

Treatment principles: Interventions may focus on both development of skills and compensation for movement challenges. Interventions designed to increase speed and amplitude of movement and improve coordination and balance relative to the demands of the task are likely appropriate.[5]

Expected outcome: Ambulation with or without an assistive device may be possible; however, supervision may be needed to reduce fall risk associated with loss of balance. Individuals may learn adaptive strategies to improve both independence and safety.[5]

Modifiers

Modifiers can be used to indicate an impairment that is not included in the description of a movement system diagnosis. Individuals can be assigned one or more modifiers in addition to a movement system diagnosis to highlight personal factors that help characterize and clarify their health condition. Examples of modifiers can be found in Box 5.2.

SUMMARY

The movement system diagnoses for neuromuscular conditions provide a framework for describing the clinical presentation and movement strategies used by infants and children with neuromuscular conditions.

BOX 5.2   Modifiers That May Accompany a Movement System Diagnosis for a Neuromuscular Condition
Biomechanical deficit Cognitive deficit Disregard/neglect Agitation Confusion Decreased attention span Memory loss Pain Decreased ability to dual/multi-task Structural joint deformity Other….

From Scheets PL, Bloom NJ, Crowner B, and others. *Movement System Diagnoses: Neuromuscular Conditions.* St Louis: Washington University; 2020.

The movement system diagnoses are grounded in the description of movement and can be used to inform decisions surrounding interventions and outcome expectations.

CHAPTER DISCUSSION QUESTIONS

1. Define the movement system.
2. Describe the benefits of applying movement system diagnoses for neuromuscular conditions to infants and children with neurologic dysfunction in physical therapy practice.
3. Describe the five phases of movement.
4. What are the primary characteristics of movement pattern coordination deficit?
5. What are the primary characteristics of force production deficit?
6. How does a neuromuscular movement system diagnosis of sensory selection and weighting deficit differ from sensory detection deficit?
7. How are modifiers used in conjunction with the neuromuscular movement system diagnoses?

REFERENCES

1. American Physical Therapy, 2015. Association: Vision, mission, and strategic plan. Accessed June 16, 2021. https://www.apta.org/apta-and-you/leadership-and-governance/vision-mission-and-strategic-plan.

2. American Physical Therapy Association. Physical Therapist Practice and the Human Movement System: 1–4 [White paper]. Alexandria, VA: American Physical Therapy Association; 2015.

3. World Health Organization. *International Classification of Function, Disability and Health*. Geneva, Switzerland: World Health Organization; 2001.

4. American Physical Therapy Association. *Guide to Physical Therapy Practice*. Alexandria, VA: American Physical Therapy Association; 2014.

5. Scheets PL, Bloom NJ, Crowner B, et al. *Movement System Diagnoses: Neuromuscular Conditions*. St Louis: Washington University; 2020.

6. Norton BJ. Diagnosis dialog: recap and relevance to recent APTA actions. *Int J Sports Phys.* 2017;12(6):870–883.

7. Scheets PL, Sahrmann S, Norton B. Use of movement system diagnoses in the management of patients with neuromuscular conditions: a multiple patient case report. *Phys Ther.* 2007;87:654–669.

8. Hedman L, Rogers M, Hanke T. Neurologic professional education: linking the foundation science of motor control with physical therapy interventions for movement dysfunction. *Neurol Rep.* 1996;20:9–13.

RESOURCES

Scheets PL, Bloom NJ, Crowner B, and others. *Movement System Diagnoses: Neuromuscular Conditions. Description of Categories*. St Louis: Washington University; 2014. https://download.lww.com/wolterskluwer_vitalstream_com/PermaLink/JNPT/A/JNPT_39_2_2015_01_28_LATHAN_JNPT-D-12-00002R4_SDC3.pdf.

American Physical Therapy Association. Physical therapist practice and the human movement system [White paper]. 2015

Scheets PL, Sahrmann S, Norton B. Use of movement system diagnoses in the management of patients with neuromuscular conditions: a multiple patient case report. *Phys Ther.* 2007;87:654–669.

6

Cerebral Palsy

Shruti V. Joshi, PT, DPT, PCS

LEARNING OBJECTIVES

At the end of the chapter, the reader should be able to do the following:

1. Understand the pathophysiology and causes of cerebral palsy.
2. Identify the various types of cerebral palsy and their characteristics.
3. Understand the various sensory, medical, motor, and cognitive impairments associated with cerebral palsy.
4. Understand the role of evaluation and ongoing assessment in the treatment of a child with cerebral palsy.
5. Identify appropriate treatment strategies for the entire age span of a child with cerebral palsy.
6. Understand the roles of other healthcare professionals in the management of a child with cerebral palsy.
7. Be familiar with the various assistive technologies that may be used for intervention.

CHAPTER OUTLINE

KEY TERMS

Cerebral palsy

Diplegia

Gross Motor Functional
   Classification System

Hemiparesis

Hypertonia

Hypotonia

Spasticity

Spastic quadriplegia

Tetraparesis

Triplegia

DEFINITION

Cerebral palsy (CP) is a permanent, nonprogressive neurologic disorder of motor function. In other words, *cerebral palsy* is a broad term used to describe a group of chronic conditions impairing control of posture and movement. Motor disturbances appear in the first few years of life and generally do not worsen until later in life. Cerebral palsy is a result of faulty development, injury, or damage to motor areas in the brain, disrupting the brain's ability to control movement and posture. Early signs of CP usually appear before 3 years of age. Some characteristic signs are spasticity, muscle weakness, ataxia, rigidity, and atypical movement patterns. Infants with CP are frequently slow to reach developmental motor milestones.

Cerebral palsy affects joint motion, muscle strength, balance, and coordination (Fig. 6.1). These problems are first noted in early childhood and continue into adult life. The muscles of speech, swallowing, and breathing may be involved. Intellectual disabilities and seizures can also occur.

The prevalence of CP is about 3 per 1000 children between the ages of ages 3 and 17 years.[1] Cerebral palsy is 16 times more common in children who had low birthweight (<2500 g) and 48 times more common in children who had very low birth weight (<1500 g) than in children with normal birthweight (>2500 g).[2] The Centers for Disease Control and Prevention estimates the cost of care for individuals with CP born in the year 2000 to be $11.5 billion.[3]

PATHOPHYSIOLOGY

Cerebral palsy is a medical condition caused by a permanent brain insult during pregnancy (prenatal period), delivery (perinatal period), or shortly after birth (postnatal period). Premature birth is associated with an increased risk of CP. Brain damage may be traced to several factors, depending on the type of CP, its onset, and the health history of mother and child. Cerebral palsy is either congenital (present at birth) or acquired after birth within the first few years of life. In many cases, the actual cause may be unknown.

Congenital CP results from brain damage during pregnancy or around the time of birth. Infants with very low birthweight and premature infants are at increased risk for CP. Improved neonatal intensive care

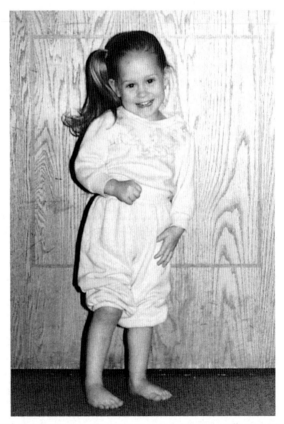

Fig. 6.1 Children with cerebral palsy often have affected joint motion, muscle strength, balance, and coordination. (From Zitelli BJ, Davis HW. *Atlas of Pediatric Physical Diagnosis.* 5th ed. Philadelphia: Mosby; 2007.)

has resulted in increased survival rates for these at-risk infants. Children born of multiple gestations (twins, triplets, or more) are also at increased risk for congenital CP.[4] Congenital CP can be caused by a variety of conditions including the following:

- Infection during pregnancy: A number of infections can affect both mother and child; for example, rubella, cytomegalovirus, Epstein-Barr virus, and bacterial urinary tract infections can cause damage to the nervous system of the developing fetus.
- Jaundice: Severe, untreated jaundice (known as *neonatal hyperbilirubinemia*) can result in brain damage and athetoid CP.
- Neonatal encephalopathy: Neonatal encephalopathy is a syndrome of altered neurologic function in an infant born at or later than 35 weeks' gestation; it includes features such as seizures, difficulty breathing, reduced tone, and depressed reflexes. It may be associated with acute events during labor and delivery or shortly after birth that reduce blood/oxygen supply to the brain, a condition called *hypoxic-ischemia encephalopathy* (HIE).[5] Placental abruption, uterine rupture, and umbilical cord prolapse are some of conditions associated with HIE.[5]
- Stroke: Women who have coagulation disorders may be at increased risk for stroke in the fetus. Premature infants have immature brain tissue that is susceptible to cerebrovascular injury as well.
- Other conditions associated with CP are inborn errors of metabolism, placental pathology, multiple pregnancies, intrauterine growth restriction, tight nuchal cord at delivery, and congenital anomalies such as schizencephaly.
- Bleeding: Prolonged bleeding in an infant's brain shortly after birth can cause brain damage.

Acquired CP results from brain damage in the first few months or years of life and can be caused by conditions such as brain infections (e.g., encephalitis or meningitis) or head trauma or injury (e.g., falls, automobile accidents, or child abuse). While the causes of CP are multifactorial and often linked to maternal or child health history or accidents that result in brain damage, not all children who have CP have experienced an interruption in oxygen supply to the brain.[6] Undocumented antenatal events may cause brain damage or increase an infant's vulnerability to future events. The prevalence of CP has remained relatively constant, and recent evidence indicates that there may be genetic factors that predispose some infants to developing CP.[4]

CLINICAL SIGNS

Children with CP sustain damage in the areas of the brain that control movement and muscle tone. While the brain lesion does not change over time, the clinical manifestations may change as the child grows. Many of these children have normal intelligence, even though they have difficulty with motor control and movement. In some children, muscle tone is generally increased (spasticity or hypertonia), whereas in others, muscle tone is decreased (hypotonia). Speech may be affected as well. Typically, children with hypertonia in the extremities may have hypotonia in the trunk and neck region. Hypertonia can lead to joint contractures and postural malalignment. The primary clue that a child might have CP is a delay in achieving developmental motor milestones such as learning to roll over, sit, crawl, smile, or walk. Some specific warning signs are given in Table 6.1.

CLINICAL SIGNS OF CP
• Difficulty with motor control and movement
• Difficulty maintaining normal posture
• Altered muscle tone
• Impaired speech

Other signs of CP typically include involuntary movements, difficulty with fine motor tasks (e.g., writing or using scissors), and difficulty with gross motor skills such as maintaining balance, sitting, crawling, or walking. The symptoms differ from person to person and may change over time. Because there are many different types of CP and the severity of the disability can vary tremendously, there is a wide range of signs and symptoms to consider when making the diagnosis. The clinical presentation of CP is highly variable, and it can affect each child differently.

CLINICAL FEATURES AND PRESENTATION

Cerebral palsy has been classified in several ways, according to the quality of muscle tone or movement, pattern of motor impairment, and severity. *Muscle tone* is the amount of resistance to movement in a muscle. Muscle tone keeps the body in a certain posture or position (e.g., sitting upright) to maintain balance (e.g., standing with feet together) and to move against gravity (e.g., standing up from the floor). The tone in different muscle groups

TABLE 6.1   Modified Ashworth Scale

Grade	Description
0	No increase in muscle tone
1	Slight increase in muscle tone, manifested by a catch and release or by minimal resistance at the end of the ROM when the affected part(s) is moved in flexion or extension
1+	Slight increase in muscle tone, manifested by a catch, followed by minimal resistance throughout the remainder (less than half) of the ROM
2	More marked increase in muscle tone through most of the ROM, but affected parts move easily
3	Considerable increase in muscle tone; passive movement difficult
4	Affected part(s) rigid in flexion or extension

body are stiff and tight and do not allow normal movement. There is increased resistance to passive stretch, which may be velocity dependent (spasticity), and in many cases, there is also the presence of abnormal neurologic reflexes, such as clonus, hypersensitivity to sensory stimuli, and hyperactive deep tendon reflexes. Hypertonia can be so severe that joint movement is difficult or impossible; this leads to abnormal posturing and joint deformities. Frequently, a child with spastic quadriplegia, for example, may have increased tone and spasticity in the arms and legs but decreased underlying tone of the trunk and head and neck.

When children exhibit decreased tone throughout their bodies, they may be classified as having *hypotonic CP*. Typically, they will present with poorly defined muscles, decreased responses to deep tendon reflexes, and hypermobile joints. They also typically have decreased ability to generate enough force for a sustained muscle contraction. This diagnosis may be made in infancy or when the child is a toddler. As children grow, abnormal movement patterns that would place them in a different classification, such as athetoid CP, may develop.

A child with *athetoid CP* typically shows signs of fluctuating tone, muscles that stiffen on their own to cause abnormal postures of the arms or legs, and/or writhing movements. Children with *ataxic CP* have poor balance

must be balanced to allow for smooth movement. Cerebral palsy has been classified into types of muscle tone or movement: spastic (hypertonic), hypotonic, ataxic, and athetoid (dyskinetic). The Modified Ashworth Scale (Table 6.2) provides a standard method of describing tone.

Spastic CP is the most common form under this classification. In most cases, the involved muscles of the

TABLE 6.2   Gross Motor Functional Classification System

	Infancy	Childhood	Adolescence
Level 1	Independent head control, moves in and out of sitting independently	Independent ambulation, rises from floor independently, manages steps independently	Independent ambulation, runs and jumps, reduced speed, balance, and agility
Level 2	Uses upper extremity (UE) support to maintain sitting	Continues to use UE for support in sitting, independently rises from floor, reciprocal crawling, ambulates with assistive technology	
Level 3	Maintains floor sitting when low back is supported, can roll and creep forward on stomach	"W" sits, may require adult assistance to assume sitting, creeps on stomach or crawls on hands and knees, may pull to stand on a stable surface and cruise short distances, walks short distances indoors using an assistive mobility device, sits independently	Community ambulation with an assistive device, climbs steps using a railing, uses wheeled mobility for longer distances
Level 4		Ambulates short distances, wheeled mobility in community	Uses wheeled mobility
Level 5	Limited voluntary control		Extensive use of adaptive equipment

and coordination, and the gait pattern typically requires a wide base of support.

The second type of classification of CP indicates the pattern of motor involvement. Some children have weakness and poor motor control of one arm and one leg on the same side of the body. This is called hemiparesis. Many have problems in all four extremities, or tetraparesis. Another category, diplegia, describes involvement primarily in the legs, with little or no involvement in the arms. Less frequently, there may be a diagnosis of triplegia, in which one arm and hand are virtually uninvolved, whereas all other limbs are. These two classification schemes can be combined for a more descriptive diagnosis such as spastic quadriplegia.

The third type of classification is a Gross Motor Functional Classification system (Table 6.3), which classifies children by degree of severity of CP or functional capability. This system provides a qualitative, objective measure of prognosis for gross motor skills. A child can be classified at one of five levels, depending on the child's skill level, not age.[7] About 60% of children with CP in 2010 were walking independently, 7.8% were walking with a handheld mobility device and 33% had limited or no walking ability.[1]

Level I

An infant in this category can move in and out of sitting, floor sit independently, and manipulate objects with their hands before 18 months. This same child is able to independently ambulate before 2 years of age without an assistive device. By 4 years of age, the child can get up from the floor into standing without assistance. By 6 years of age, the child can climb stairs. By age 12 years, a child performing at this level is able to ambulate without assistance on all surfaces and can successfully complete tasks that require more advanced gross motor skills. The Level I child can run and jump with reduced speed, balance, and coordination.

Level II

An infant who is classified as functioning at Level II is able to maintain floor sitting but needs to use their hands to maintain balance. This child is "commando" or belly crawling, pulling to stand by using furniture, and beginning to cruise before the age of 2 years. By age 4 years, the child continues to require one or two hands to balance in floor sitting, so the hands are not free to manipulate objects bilaterally in space. Transitions in and out of sitting are accomplished independently; the child can pull to stand on a stable surface (Fig. 6.2). Crawling is accomplished with a reciprocal pattern, and ambulation can be accomplished with an assistive device. At 6 years, the child can sit on the floor independently with both hands free, can get up from the floor using a stable surface, and can ambulate short distances without an assistive device. These children usually require an assistive device when walking outdoors and in the community until about age 12 years. They can climb stairs using the railing but cannot run or jump. By age 12 years, uneven surfaces, inclines, and crowds are still difficult for these children to negotiate. Under most conditions, they are able to ambulate without an assistive device.

Level III

Infants are able to maintain floor sitting when their lower back is supported. These children are able to roll and creep forward on their stomachs. Between the ages of 2 and 4 years, these children often "W" sit (sitting between flexed and internally rotated hips and knees)

TABLE 6.3 **Common Warning Signs of Cerebral Palsy**	
Age of Infant	**Signs**
Over 2 months	Head lags with pull to sit
	Muscle or joint movement feels stiff
	Generally feels floppy, hypotonic, or joints are hypermobile
	Extensor tendencies: the child seems to overextend the back and neck, constantly acts as if he or she is pushing away from you when held in a cradled position
	Legs may get stiff and they cross or "scissor" when the child is picked up
Over 6 months	Continues to have the asymmetric tonic neck reflex
	Reaches out with only one hand while keeping the other fisted
Over 10 months	Crawls in a lopsided manner, pushing off with one hand and leg while dragging the opposite hand and leg
	Scoots around on buttocks or hops on knees but does not crawl on all fours

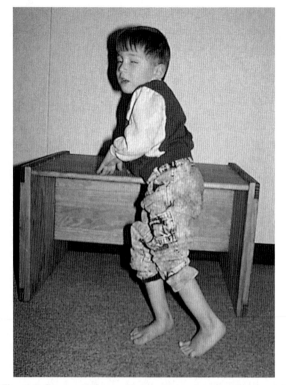

Fig. 6.2 Some children with cerebral palsy are able to pull themselves into a standing position by using a stable surface, such as a piece of furniture, as leverage. (From Zitelli BJ, Davis HW. *Atlas of Pediatric Physical Diagnosis.* 5th ed. Philadelphia: Mosby; 2007.)

and may require adult assistance to assume an optimal sitting position. These children creep on their stomachs or crawl on hands and knees (often without reciprocal leg movements). They may pull to stand on a stable surface and cruise short distances. They may walk short distances indoors using an assistive mobility device but need assistance for steering and turning. By age 6, these children sit independently in a chair, transfer using a stable object, walk with an assistive device, and climb stairs with assistance. By age 12, they can independently ambulate in the community with the help of an assistive device, climb steps using a railing, and use a wheelchair for longer distances.

Level IV

Infants and toddlers in this category have head control, but truncal support is needed for sitting. These children can usually roll independently by age 2 years. By age 4, they can sit when placed, but they need both hands on the floor to maintain balance. These children need adaptive devices to accomplish sitting and standing. They are able to roll and creep but do not use reciprocal leg movements. By their 6th birthday, these children can sit independently in a chair but require truncal stabilization to maximize hand function. Transfers require minimal adult assistance. Ambulation is accomplished using assistive devices for short distances, but adult supervision is required, and difficulty persists in negotiating turns and uneven surfaces. These children use wheeled mobility systems in the community and may achieve independence using a powered mobility system. By age 12, these children may accomplish higher levels of function but may still rely on wheeled mobility systems.

Level V

Before their 2nd birthdays, children functioning at this level have limited voluntary control of movement. They are unable to hold up their head or trunk against gravity and require adult assistance to roll. By age 12, these children cannot sit, stand, or walk. Adaptive equipment and assistive technology are used extensively to attempt to compensate for a child's motor deficits. Some children are able to use power mobility systems.

DIAGNOSIS OF CEREBRAL PALSY

A diagnosis of CP is typically assigned when an infant or child appears to have difficulty learning typical movements over time and is delayed in achieving milestones such as sitting, rolling, and walking. Parents may report concerns such as delayed head control, stiffness of the legs and arms, or difficulty using one or both hands in reaching for and playing with objects.

Many infants born prematurely—especially those with a history of HIE, intraventricular hemorrhage (IVH), or risk factors associated with CP such as perinatal stroke—are followed up in special clinics where their growth and overall health and development are monitored. Recent research has revealed that it is possible to identify infants at high risk for CP using clinical observations and measurement tools that assess postural control and patterns of movement. Professionals who have specialized training can use the General Movements Assessment (GMA) to look for "fidgety movements," which are spontaneous, small movements present at rest and may be observed in the trunk, neck, and extremities from 7 to 8 weeks through almost 6 months of age.[8]

The absence of these movements in infants at around 3 months' corrected age is highly indicative of an injury to the brain, and these infants have been found to have a higher likelihood of having moderate or severe CP.[9]

A consultation from a developmental pediatrician or pediatric neurologist is also recommended to assist in the diagnosis. Magnetic resonance imaging (MRI) of the brain is usually performed to determine whether an abnormality exists. Reduced myelination of the posterior limb of the internal capsule, which indicates abnormalities in the corticospinal tract,[9] is detectable via MRI and so are abnormalities in basal ganglia, cystic periventricular leukomalacia, IVH grade IV, and stroke involving the motor cortex—all of which may predispose a child to developing CP.[10] An MRI can detect these changes as early as the 2nd day after birth, and the optimal time for visualizing perinatal cerebral injury is between 7 and 21 days after birth in an infant with HIE.[5] In a recent study during which infants with HIE were followed up, a small number of children who did not have any concerning findings on MRI and GMA went on to develop mild CP. They were all functioning at the highest level (Gross Motor Function Classification System [GMFCS] level I), indicating that milder forms of CP may take longer to diagnose because the signs are harder to detect early on.[9]

Another tool that has a high value in the diagnostic process is the Harris Infant Neurological Examination (HINE).[11] At 3 months' corrected age, 96% of infants later diagnosed with CP had absent fidgety movements on the GMA, and the HINE scores at this age were also lower, with the lowest scores belonging to the children with the most severe forms of CP.[10] When the findings from the GMA, HINE, and neuroimaging were combined, 98.74% of infants that later went on to develop CP were correctly identified at 3 months of age. Physical therapists trained in administering, scoring, and interpreting these clinical measures have an important role in the diagnostic process as their expertise in observing and analyzing movement can assist physicians in identifying infants at risk of CP, and making referrals for appropriate services.

In many cases, infants and children with CP do not receive a diagnosis until the age of 2 years, even though early detection of movement characteristics and brain abnormalities that predict a future diagnosis of CP using a combination of the previously described tools is now the gold standard.[9,12] Not all children are followed up in a highly specialized clinic with providers trained in these evidence-based instruments, and some children with no perinatal risk factors who go on to develop CP may be missed because they do not have this frequency and quality of surveillance. Alternative models have proposed that trajectories of motor development that indicate worsening motor delays between 6 and 12 months of age[12] are suggestive of a diagnosis of CP between 24 and 36 months of age. For infants and children being followed up by their primary care provider or pediatrician, specific findings such as early handedness (<12 months), irritability, poor feeding, persistent head lag beyond 4 months of age, delayed sitting (>9 months), rolling (>4–6 months), and walking (>15–18 months), tone abnormalities such as hypertonia or hypotonia, persistent primitive reflexes, clonus, fisting of hands and stiffness of extremities, are all indicative of the need for further investigation and referral for specialist follow-up to rule out CP.[13,14] The Test of Infant Motor Performance (TIMP) is another tool that can assist therapists and medical teams in identifying abnormal movements and delays in postural and head control before 17 weeks' postconceptional age so that infants can be referred for services to address these delays.[15]

The advantage of early detection and identification of delayed motor skills and postural control is that while a final diagnosis is pending, the child can be assigned a diagnosis of *developmental delay* and referred to the state's Early Intervention (Part C) program, and therapy services (physical, occupational, speech, nutrition, vision) can be initiated as soon as possible.

SECONDARY CONDITIONS

The disabilities associated with CP can vary greatly in severity. For example, one child with mild CP may have no obvious impairment other than a slight lack of coordination, which may impact the child's ability to perform higher-level motor skills such as running, jumping, and going up and down stairs (GMFCS level I), while another child with a severe form may be unable to walk (GMFCS levels IV and V), talk, see, or eat by mouth. Some children with CP are also affected by other medical disorders, including seizures or intellectual disability (ID). This section will outline some common problems associated with CP.

INTELLECTUAL DISABILITY

Intellectual disability ID, also known as cognitive delay or cognitive disability, is usually diagnosed when a child achieves a score less than 70 on a standardized measure of intellectual functioning (memory, thinking, problem-solving).[16] There is wide variation in estimates of children with CP who have problems with intellectual functioning; this can be partially explained by the reliance on measures of intelligence that comprise items requiring motor coordination, speed, and verbal or fine motor skills that may be difficult for children with CP to execute. However, a few recent studies utilizing population-based samples across the world indicate higher rates of ID in children with greater severity of physical involvement (GMFCS levels III–V),[17] and in teenagers with poor manual and gross motor function.[18] Higher rates of ID have been reported in children with CP who have epilepsy,[18] congenital brain malformations,[17] and other impairments such as blindness, deafness, and reduced verbal abilities.[17] Studies in Sweden that have started to include older adults with CP indicate that the rate of ID increased as individuals with CP aged; one of the possible reasons is that ID may not have been detected in childhood or adolescence.[19] The presentation of ID can range from mild to profound. Individuals with mild ID have some ability to read and can perform most daily functions on their own, but at the other end of the spectrum, individuals with profound ID require maximal support for all everyday life activities.

Seizures

One of every three individuals with CP has or will develop seizures. Approximately 40% of children with CP have seizures.[1] Some children start having seizures years after the brain is damaged. Many different types of seizures may occur. In most cases, these seizures are controlled with anticonvulsant medications; however, a small number of children and adolescents may have a condition called *intractable epilepsy* in which seizures occur frequently despite medication.

Vision Impairments

The coordination of the eye muscles is often affected by the brain damage causing CP. More than three out of four children with CP have *strabismus*, a problem with one eye turning in or out, with or without nearsightedness, and children at lower levels of the GMFCS have more severe strabismus.[20] If this problem is severe and not corrected early, the vision in the affected eye will get worse. It is extremely important to encourage families to have their child's eyes checked by 1 year of age and then annually if impairments are present. Cortical visual impairment is present in children who have a history of HIE and seizures, and other vision disorder such as nystagmus, anomalies, or atrophy of the optic nerve may also be present.[21]

Orthopedic Issues

In most cases, a decrease in a child's joint range of motion (ROM) is detected first; the decrease may be functional or fixed. This decrease in ROM at the joint is most often caused by asymmetric tone, spasticity, or muscle tension. A functional shortening is generally caused by increased tone and passive resistance to stretch or irritability of the child (which can be an active resistance to the stretch), or it may be position dependent. A fixed-muscle shortening is referred to as a *contracture*. An orthopedic surgeon should be consulted if a contracture is noticed. If untreated, contractures may lead to other orthopedic deformities, such as hip subluxation or dislocation, scoliosis, foot equinus, equinovarus, and moderate to severe functional limitations of the upper and lower extremities.

Many infants and children with CP do not get the variety of movement that their typically developing peers do; therefore, they may not experience the bony modeling that happens in childhood, for example, deepening of the acetabulum from crawling on hands and knees and loss of varus angulation of the tibiae with standing and walking experience. Among children with hemiparesis, many will develop a shortening of the involved leg and arm. The difference between the legs is rarely more than 2 inches, but an orthopedic surgeon should be consulted if shortening is noticed. Depending on the degree of difference between the legs, a heel or sole lift may be prescribed to fit into the shoe on the shorter side to facilitate more even distribution of body weight, improve posture and gait, and prevent a tilt of the pelvis. Also orthotics, splinting, casting, or medication may be used to improve joint mobility and stability.

In children with typical development, at 12 months of age, the radiologic angle between the femoral head and shaft is about 168 degrees, and it decreases to 158 degrees by 8 years of age.[22] As a result of lack of weight-bearing through the legs, children in GMFCS levels IV and V spend long periods in seating devices and do not walk or stand supported or independently. In children with CP, the head-shaft angle does not decrease at the same rate with age due to muscle imbalances,[23] especially with the overpowering impact of the adductor and ilio-psoas muscles, and is associated with hip subluxation or dislocation.[22] Dislocations of the hip (unilateral and bilateral) have a strong linear association with GMFCS level; are associated with reduced hip abduction range, pelvic obliquity, and scoliosis[24]: and can happen as early as 2 years of age. Worsening of hip displacement can also occur after puberty and in adulthood and can cause pain,[25] reduced function, and reduced ambulation as some individuals with CP become less physically active over time[26]; this can impact quality of life.

Worldwide evidence indicates that hip surveillance programs are effective and decrease the frequency of hip dislocation in children with CP.[23,25,27] These programs collect data on the type of CP and the GMFCS level, and based on these data, obtain radiographs at specific frequencies to monitor the migration of the hip joint. When the migration percentage reaches 30% of more, children are referred for orthopedic treatment and management, which may include surgical procedures to prevent worsening dislocation.

Like children with hip deformities, children with CP at lower functional levels of the GMFCS (III–V) have a higher incidence of more severe scoliotic curves. These curves are often C shaped and may progressively worsen with growth and puberty.[25]

Other common orthopedic issues affect the knee and include *crouch gait* characterized by bilateral knee flexion during standing and walking, patella alta, and genu varum or valgum. Many children with quadriplegic and diplegic CP have shortening of the gastrocnemius-soleus muscle complex from chronic spasticity, and children with diplegia may walk on their toes. Unilateral toe walking is seen in children with hemiplegic CP because of spastic overactivation of the gastrocnemius-soleus muscle complex is on the involved lower extremity.

Dental Problems

It is difficult for some individuals with CP to brush their own teeth and move food around in their mouth and chew effectively; therefore, they may tend to retain food particles in the oral cavity and saliva. This places them at risk for poor oral health. In addition, they also have enamel defects more frequently than healthy children, making their teeth more susceptible to decay, and dental erosion may be increased by the presence of gastroesophageal reflux disease (GERD).[28] Dental caries, tooth

wear, and bruxism are other common dental problems among individuals with CP.[29]

Hearing Loss

Some children with CP have a complete or partial hearing loss; it is often bilateral, and the degree of hearing loss varies by severity of motor disability, with more severe disability associated with worse hearing.[30] If an infant does not blink in response to loud noises by 1 month, turn the head or otherwise respond to sound by 3–4 months, or say words by 12 months, referral for a hearing screen or assessment is recommended.

Oral Motor Dysfunction

Children with spastic diplegia, quadriplegia, athetosis, or ataxia may have difficulty with tongue movements, swallowing, eating, creating sounds, babbling, and talking. Poor nutrition, dehydration, and lack of weight gain are often related to feeding and swallowing problems.[31] However, the extent of a child's oral motor dysfunction may not be predicted by their physical disability. A child may be severely impaired physically with spastic quadriplegia yet still be able to talk, eat, and communicate effectively.

Problems With Spatial Awareness

Over half the children with hemiparesis cannot sense the position of their arm or hand on the affected side. For example, when the involved hand is relaxed, the child cannot tell whether the fingers are pointing up or down without looking at them. When this problem is present, the child will rarely attempt to use the involved hand, even if the motor disability is minimal.

Gastroesophageal Reflux Disease

Gastroesophageal reflux (GER) is the passage of stomach contents into the esophagus with or without vomiting. Although considered physiologic in infancy, its frequency is steadily reduced once typically developing infants start sitting independently because of increased abdominal strength, maturation of the lower esophageal sphincter (LES), and consumption of more solid foods. However, GER is described as pathologic when it causes troublesome symptoms and/or complications such as esophagitis and anemia and is labeled as GERD.[32] It can be associated with projectile vomiting, poor weight gain, feeding difficulties, irritability, frequent regurgitation, choking episodes, and apneic spells.[32] Children with CP may have persistent GERD; some contributing factors are poor postural control, altered rib cage alignment, and altered muscle tone that affects LES function.

Normally, GERD in children is diagnosed based on clinical findings and subjective reports by an infant's family or symptoms of heartburn and pain reported by children. However, investigative methods such as pH and intraluminal impedance monitoring (which involves measuring the pH of the esophagus through a probe) are available. In children with CP, GERD may be difficult to recognize because it may exacerbate or cause spasmodic or dystonic movements of the head and neck (a condition called *Sandifer syndrome*)[32] and be mistaken for epilepsy.[33] Children with speech delays or those who are nonverbal may not report symptoms of heartburn, chest pain, or epigastric pain clearly. In school-age children and adolescents with quadriplegic CP with severe involvement, GERD has been found to be one of several contributing factors to frequent respiratory illnesses and hospitalizations[34] because it increases the risk of aspiration. Feeding difficulties and poor weight gain may be concurrently present; therefore, children with CP may need referral to a pediatric gastroenterologist for ongoing management.

MANAGEMENT OF CEREBRAL PALSY

There is no standard therapy that works for all patients. Medications can be used to control seizures and muscle spasms. Custom orthotics can compensate for muscle imbalances. Surgery may be warranted to correct musculoskeletal deformities. Assistive technology devices can help a child overcome impairments. Physical, occupational, speech, and behavioral therapy and counseling for emotional and psychologic needs are necessary to help many individuals with CP achieve optimal functioning in daily life.

Medical Management

Because of the vast array of potential associated disorders, a multidisciplinary approach is necessary in the management of CP. In addition to having a pediatrician for primary care, a child with CP may be seen by specialty physicians such as a developmental pediatrician, a neurologist, an orthopedic surgeon, or a physiatrist. Other providers of the child's care may include an optometrist or developmental optometrist, physical therapist, occupational therapist, speech and language pathologist, developmental therapist, audiologist, or dietician to address individual needs.

Pharmaceutical Intervention

Pharmaceuticals are used for a number of conditions, such as spasticity, management of seizures, and GERD. Treatment to reduce hypertonia or spasticity may include intervention with medications such as baclofen and diazepam.[35] These medicines can be taken by mouth, but baclofen may also be delivered directly into the cerebrospinal canal through an intrathecal pump.[36] Intrathecal administration is the preferred route because it does not produce the systemic adverse effects (drowsiness, dizziness, weakness, confusion, upset stomach) that occur with oral administration of baclofen.[37] Also, because oral baclofen does not cross the blood-brain barrier effectively, maintaining optimum levels of the drug requires larger doses, whereas much smaller intrathecal doses can produce the desired therapeutic effect. The intrathecal baclofen pump is surgically implanted under the subcutaneous fat of the abdomen and administers a constant flow of medication into the cerebrospinal fluid to reduce spasticity. Baclofen should never be suddenly stopped because this can cause acute withdrawal in the form of more severe spasticity and hallucinations and can be life-threatening.[37]

Injections of botulinum toxin are a treatment for chronic hypertonia in CP, spasticity, and other disorders.[35] Often, pediatric physiatrists perform Botox injections with or without the use of an electromyogram (EMG), depending on the location and size of the muscle to be injected. If ROM is significantly diminished, a child may be sent to a physical therapy team to receive serial casting 2 to 3 weeks after the injections to maximize the functional benefits of Botox administration. Alternatively, some physicians may inject phenol into the nerve innervating the spastic muscle. The phenol strips the myelin from the nerve sheath and thus reduces the input to the muscle, reducing the muscle tone. Postinjection rehabilitative treatment may involve ROM, active stretching, functional training, and strengthening programs.

Seizure disorders are also treated with pharmaceutical interventions.[38] The seizure medications work via various mechanisms: influencing the release of neurotransmitters such as gamma-amino-butyric acid (GABA); changing the exchange of ions such as sodium across the cell membranes; or altering the excitability and activation of neurons in the brain. Valproic acid, which has several mechanisms of action, and clobazam, which belongs to a class of drugs called *benzodiazepines*, are often a first line of treatment for children with seizure disorders. Lamotrigine, a new medication, is combined with valproic acid and rufinamide and used as an adjunct treatment for children with severe, intractable seizures. Other medications that act by changing neurotransmitter release are levetiracetam and perampanel. While many children have their seizures managed with a single medication (monotherapy), some require more than one medication (polytherapy) for effective control.

When infants and children with CP are experiencing GERD, lifestyle modifications are the first line of treatment. For infants, these include increasing the thickness of feeds, elimination of cow's milk, increasing frequency/reducing volume of feeds, and eliminating exposure to cigarette smoke. Prone positioning when awake is effective at reducing frequency of reflux episodes for infants.[32,39] Additionally, for older children, eliminating spicy foods, elevating the head of the bed, and use of the side-lying position for sleep have been known to reduce GERD symptoms. For children with CP who are not ambulatory and have scoliosis, ensuring optimal seating and trunk posture may be key to reducing the impact of GERD. When GERD persists in school-aged children and adolescents, a 4- to 8-week course of proton pump inhibitors, which have emerged as a medication of choice in recent years, may be prescribed[40] by their primary care provider or a pediatric gastroenterologist.

Surgical Intervention

Surgical intervention may be used to manage various associated medical complications that individuals with CP might experience. The most common use of surgical intervention is to correct or prevent orthopedic deformities, such as hip dislocation, hip subluxation, and scoliosis. After several years of using an assistive device such as a wheelchair or walkers, some children may require surgical releases to address contractures of the hamstrings, hip adductors, or gastrocnemius and soleus muscles; tendon lengthening; or tendon transfers to improve functional capabilities.[41] Other children may have surgery for neurologic intervention; for example, shunt placement and revisions if hydrocephalus is present in infancy or selective dorsal rhizotomy surgery[42] for spasticity management. Some children with CP have oral motor dysfunction, which impairs safe and effective chewing or swallowing. These children may benefit from a gastrostomy tube (G-tube)[43] to augment or replace their oral nutritional intake. For children with

neurologic impairments and GERD symptoms that persist despite medication and lifestyle changes, surgical procedures such as gastric fundoplication and esophagogastric disconnection may be considered on an individual basis,[32] and these may reduce hospitalizations and positively impact feeding, growth, and quality of life.[44]

Physical Therapy Management

The five elements of client management are examination, evaluation, diagnosis, prognosis, and intervention. The physical therapist is responsible for the completion of the first four elements prior to intervention by a physical therapist assistant. The *examination* should include the following components: a history, a systems review, and selection and administration of specific appropriate tests and measures with focus on understanding the body structure and function impairments and activity limitations the child may be experiencing. The history should include any significant occurrences during prenatal and labor/delivery care, current health status, developmental milestones achieved, social history, and identification of patient/family expectations and desired outcomes. This history assists in guiding the physical therapist through a relevant systems review, which should include the physiologic status of the musculoskeletal, neuromuscular, cardiopulmonary, and integumentary systems and the child's overall affect and general cognition ability to communicate, and ability to follow directions.

The history and systems review are analyzed to develop hypotheses about the child's impairments and functional limitations so the appropriate tests and measures can be selected. There are a number of different styles of assessments that may be performed. A multidisciplinary assessment is a form of developmental assessment in which several professionals with different kinds of training and experience work with a child and family, directly or indirectly. Multidisciplinary assessments are common in Early Intervention (Part C) programs where a team of therapists (physical, occupational, speech, developmental) may simultaneously assess a young child with CP. This type of assessment can be helpful because professionals with different kinds of training are skilled in observing and interpreting different aspects of a child's development and behavior.

Standardized assessment tools appropriate to examination of a child with CP during various stages of development are available. The TIMP, HINE, GMA, and the Alberta Infant Motor Scale (AIMS)[45] are all used to assess movement in infants, especially those with a complex medical history and conditions such as extreme prematurity, respiratory depression, IVH, and HIE. These infants are often considered at high risk for CP, and there is robust research evidence to support the use of the TIMP in identifying abnormal movement patterns.[15] It is used to identify infants younger than 17 weeks' postconceptional age who have delays in head and trunk control and to examine key antigravity movements such as lower extremity kicking. The Gross Motor Function Measure (GMFM), and Pediatric Evaluation of Disability Inventory (PEDI)[46] may be used with children aged 2 years and older. The GMFM is a criterion-referenced measure used to assess ROM, reflexes, tone, strength, balance, and any atypical movement patterns.[47]

The next element of patient management is the *evaluation*, a dynamic process in which the physical therapist makes clinical judgments based on the information gathered during the examination. The results of the tests and measures are used to confirm the potential impairments, functional limitations, and disabilities of the child with a developmental delay. These potential impairments may be decreased or increased tone, decreased strength, diminished or poor balance, diminished bilateral coordination, reduced movement against gravity, decreased arousal and attention, and clumsiness during play. Delayed motor skills, delayed oral motor development, impaired locomotion, and poor sensory integration are also potential functional limitations. Cutoff values and percentile ranks on norm-referenced tests such as the TIMP, AIMS, and PEDI establish the extent of delay in movement skills for an infant or child compared with peers and can serve as justification that a child requires services such as physical therapy.

Another framework that may be used to describe impairments in movement quality and their impact on a child's functional limitations is the movement system diagnosis. The type and severity of CP will also influence the selection of the movement system analysis and help to establish the physical therapy *diagnosis.*

Once the impairments and functional limitations are identified, the *prognosis* is determined. The prognosis will include the predicted optimal level of functional improvement, recommendation for amount of service, and establishment of a plan of care. The prognosis will depend on the severity of the CP, impairments, and activity and participation limitations. The recommended amount of therapy and the establishment of a plan of care are the critical elements to establish before the start of intervention by a physical therapist or a physical therapist assistant.

INTERVENTION

Intervention is defined as the purposeful and skilled interaction with the patient/client, including coordination, communication, documentation, patient/client-related instruction, and procedural interventions. The physical therapy intervention will address the identified impairments or functional limitations of the child. Physical therapy may focus on reducing tone, increasing ROM, increasing strength, improving functional motor skills and mobility, and caregiver education regarding interventions, including positioning and handling issues. It is vital to the success of therapy that both the child, if appropriate, and the caregiver be fully educated in the interventions occurring in physical therapy. If the family does not understand how to perform the interventions, carryover outside of therapy sessions will be diminished. Furthermore, great effort should be made to embed therapy into the family's naturally occurring routines. For example, range-of-motion and stretching activities could occur in conjunction with diaper changing or dressing activities. If a child is working on transitional movements (sit-to-stand, standing, and squatting), the child's home environment should be set up to encourage these activities. Toys can be moved up onto a low table top or cabinet instead of left on the floor. The child can stand at the sink and help with rinsing the dishes or preparing food. Additionally, therapy might also focus on limiting or minimizing the child's disability within the community. This would involve identifying barriers in the home or community and recommending modifications that will make the environment more accessible.

CEREBRAL PALSY INTERVENTIONS

- Address impairments and functional limitations
- Reduce tone
- Increase ROM
- Increase strength
- Improve functional motor skills and mobility
- Educate caregivers
- Identify barriers and recommend modifications to make environment more accessible

PROGNOSIS

Even when a firm diagnosis is made during the early years, it is often difficult to predict how severe the disability will be in the future. Gross motor growth curves that were determined based on population samples of children with CP in Canada may help healthcare teams and families understand how the movement abilities of children with CP in each GMFCS level change with age and predict the level of independence children are likely to achieve.[48] For example, children at GMFCS level V may reach a plateau in terms of maximal motor function by the time they are 4 years old, whereas children at GMFCS level I may continue to acquire new movement skills until the age of 8 or 9 years.[49]

At this time, CP cannot be cured, but many individuals with CP can enjoy high levels of active participation in home, school, and community settings if their primary and secondary impairments are managed through access to a multidisciplinary team of expert health providers, assistive equipment, caregiver education, and programs for community integration. When children with CP are young, the emphasis of therapy services may be the acquisition of motor skills such as sitting, walking, eating on their own, and achieving maximal functional independence in activities such as toileting and dressing. However, as they grow, the focus may have to shift,[50] especially for children at lower levels of the GMFCS, toward managing assistive devices and supports such as walkers, wheelchairs, orthotics, and modifications of activities of daily living (ADLs) so that the impact of pain and impairments such as spasticity, contractures, and scoliosis on posture and alignment and on mobility that the child has already acquired can be minimized. Reduced mobility and lack of opportunities for exercise and physical recreation can put them at risk for atherosclerotic changes and cardiovascular disease.[51] Participation in family routines, social and educational environments, and life as an adult including housing and employment should be the focal points through the child's journey to adulthood.

CASE OF A CHILD WITH CEREBRAL PALSY

Examination

History

Amy was born prematurely at 28 weeks' gestation. She was hospitalized for a total of 3 months. After her first month of life, a computerized tomography (CT) scan of her brain was performed. Enlarged ventricles were reported, and hydrocephalus was diagnosed. She received a ventriculoperitoneal (VP) shunt for treatment of the hydrocephalus and recovered well. Amy underwent additional tests and procedures for diagnosis and treatment. She was prescribed anticonvulsant medication after an electroencephalogram (EEG) detected abnormal/seizure activity. She was discharged home at the end of the 3-month hospital stay and referred to the local early intervention program.

Amy's diagnoses were spastic quadriplegic CP, cortical blindness, and a seizure disorder. When she was 1 year old, she had bilateral tympanostomy tubes placed in her ears to relieve the symptoms of chronic ear infections. When she was 4 years old, she was evaluated for VP shunt malfunction. A CT scan at the time indicated that her ventricles had shrunk or collapsed. Her neurosurgeon stated that the shunt was overcompensating, but the shunt was not removed.

Based on her initial outpatient evaluation, Amy received physical therapy, speech, and occupational early- intervention services until she was 3 years old. She received the following equipment while at the clinic: stroller base with adaptive seating, supine stander, adapted table and chair, and bilateral solid ankle foot orthotics (AFOs).

She was transitioned out of Early Intervention (Part C) and began receiving services at an outpatient clinic when she was 3 years old. At that time, Amy's family had grown from one child to four. Amy's father was in law school when she was born and initially attended all her therapy sessions. After he took the bar exam and began to work, he was unable to attend the sessions but visited occasionally. Amy's mother worked full-time, but she attended therapy sessions whenever she had days off. Amy's extended family was extremely helpful in providing assistance whenever needed. One aunt eventually became Amy's primary caregiver.

Tests and Measures

Amy was reassessed at 3 years of age to develop fresh goals and a treatment plan. Assessment consisted of ROM, tone and strength assessment, tolerance of and response to handling and various developmental positions; assessment findings were determined using clinical observations and professional judgment. The outcome measure used to document functional performance was the WeeFIM System, and the evaluator was certified to administer the test. Amy was dependent for all items in the mobility, self-care, and communication domains, with the exception of exhibiting maximal assistance in

Continued

CASE OF A CHILD WITH CEREBRAL PALSY—cont'd

comprehension and social interaction. She assisted with rolling supine to side-lying or prone by bringing her non-weight bearing arm around to the front of her body, but she could not independently perform any transitions or mobility skills. Joint passive ROM (PROM) was within normal limits, except for moderately decreased PROM of bilateral hamstrings and decreased PROM of bilateral adductors. Amy displayed poor head and trunk control. She kept her head turned to the right 75% of the time. She also had decreased left neck rotation and lateral flexion ROM. Amy did not actively bear weight in her upper or lower extremities and had spasticity of bilateral upper and lower extremities and underlying hypotonia, particularly in the trunk. She tolerated handling well and enjoyed being talked to by the therapist. According to the GMFCS scale, Amy's functioning is categorized as level V—severely limited in self-mobility, even when using assistive technology.

Evaluation

Weekly physical therapy was recommended. Amy also began to receive weekly occupational and speech therapy in the same outpatient clinic. She seemed frail and lethargic at times. Her seizure medications were adjusted; she was weaned off phenytoin and phenobarbital and prescribed Topamax. Within 3 to 4 weeks, she appeared much more alert and interactive during therapy sessions. Her parents and caregivers were concerned with how thin she was, despite the amount of food she consumed. Amy underwent G-tube placement to help increase the number of calories she ingested and improve her nutritional status. She began receiving a continuous drip of PediaSure while she slept. Increased care was required with feedings at night, as well as the care and cleaning of the surgical site, which was not healing. This placed an additional strain on the family dynamics. Amy spent at least 50% of her time with her maternal aunt and uncle.

Prognosis

Given the extent and severity of Amy's impairments and functional limitations, she will likely require extensive assistance to meet her daily needs. Ongoing weekly physical, occupational, and speech therapies were recommended. Assistive technology will be crucial for Amy to maintain musculoskeletal alignment.

Direct Intervention

Coordination/Communication

At this time, the family had been battling with the school system to provide appropriate care and education for Amy. Two school therapists and a teacher insisted that she was

functioning at a "brainstem" level and refused to provide the services the parents thought were appropriate. Amy reportedly spent the majority of her time in school sitting/lying in a beanbag chair because she had outgrown the adapted chair. Amy's parents refused to sign the individualized education program (IEP) at the end of the 2000–2001 school year and requested independent evaluations to assess her cognitive, visual, and communicative capabilities.

Amy was referred to a pediatric physiatrist and a pediatric orthopedic surgeon for spasticity management and contractures. She also needed prescriptions for adaptive equipment. Various options to manage spasticity were discussed, but ultimately, orthopedic surgery was recommended to lengthen the hamstrings and hip adductors to address her lower extremity contractures. Amy's parents decided they wanted a second opinion and asked her therapist and other parents for recommendations. The same recommendations came from several parents and other physical therapists at the center: consultation with a well-regarded local orthopedic surgeon. The parents were concerned that Amy had also begun to develop a scoliosis, so the physical therapist agreed to attend the consultation with the family for support. After the initial consultation and findings from and MRI were obtained, several surgical interventions were recommended. They included bilateral hamstring, adductor, and hip flexor tenotomies; right varus derotation osteotomy; and pelvic osteotomy. These interventions would address the contractures, femoral anteversion, acetabular dysplasia, and hip subluxation with migration of 70% on the right. The orthopedic surgeon concluded that with the migration index of her left hip at 40%, the contractures of her left lower extremity, the abnormal forces of spasticity, and her abnormal movement patterns, Amy most likely would eventually need the varus derotation osteotomy. He recommended she have both hips done at the same time.

The decision to consent to the surgery was difficult for the family. They really did not want to subject Amy to such an extensive procedure. However, the surgeon felt strongly that since he was going to perform the surgery, he might as well do it all at the same time. Based on his extensive research and experience, the osteotomies were inevitable. Finally, the family agreed and scheduled the surgery. The day before the surgery, Amy's parents got a call from the surgeon's office. Because of irregularities in her preoperative blood tests, Amy's surgery was postponed until her blood coagulation levels could be normalized. After months of blood work and testing, they found out that the initial report was a lab error, and the surgery could go forward. In the interim (during the

CASE OF A CHILD WITH CEREBRAL PALSY—cont'd

summer), Amy's aunt began hippotherapy and aquatics for Amy while she continued all other therapies.

Therapeutic Exercise

Amy's PROM was good, with the exception of her hamstrings, until she turned 4. She began to grow and "bulk up" after insertion of the G-tube. She outgrew her stander and chair at home and had maxed out the adjustability of the stroller. Increased tightness and deformities began to develop. Significant tightness was noted in her neck and bilateral upper and lower extremities. Specifically, the popliteal angle was 40 to 50 degrees bilaterally. She began to develop a "windswept" posture of her pelvis and lower extremities and would not actively bear weight on her lower extremities, nor would she take steps in her gait trainer.

Assistive Devices

Physical and occupational therapy sessions were increased to twice weekly. Amy began responding very well to a light box that was introduced in therapy, and she was beginning to functionally use her vision. The team also began to work on appropriate positioning and use of her left upper extremity for communication devices and switch activation. Amy's aunt became very involved in this whole process, purchasing any necessary tools or equipments not approved by insurance (e.g., gait trainer, light box, switches) and working with her on an almost daily basis. Amy began to identify pictures, letters, and concepts (big/small) with accuracy varying from 30% to 70%. With physical fatigue, Amy became less accurate.

Presurgical Goals

Short-term goals for Amy prior to surgery were:
1. Amy will long sit on the floor while maintaining head in midline for 20 seconds; maximal support at her trunk and knees in no more than 30 degrees of flexion.
2. Amy will activate quads in supported standing for 2 out of 5 trials.
3. Amy will sit on a bench for 60 seconds with upper extremities supported on a table and support only at her pelvis.
4. Amy will roll from supine to prone with moderate assist through her pelvis for 2 out of 5 trials, initiating the movement by lifting her right or left arm.

New Episode: Plan of Care

Amy underwent extensive bilateral orthopedic surgery just prior to her 5th birthday. She was immobilized with a hip spica cast for 6 weeks. This was a very difficult time for Amy's parents. The hospital was about 90 minutes

away from their home, and Amy experienced some minor postoperative complications. The parents alternated who stayed overnight at the hospital with her. She was hospitalized for a week. Amy's parents did not own a van and were unsure of how they were going to transport her from the hospital to home, so before surgery the physician's office assisted with the preparation for postoperative transport and care. Her parents opted to keep Amy home from school for the 6 weeks she was in a cast. They attempted to rent a handicap-accessible van without success and became concerned that Amy would have to be transported lying on the back seat of the car secured by pillows and seat belts. Fortunately, Amy's aunt sold her car and bought a van that could be used to transport the child to and from the hospital and therapy. Amy's parents were able to rent a reclining wheelchair for her.

Reevaluation

Two days after surgery, in physical therapy, Amy began weight-bearing exercises as tolerated while in the hip spica cast. The therapists instructed her parents on care and hygiene related to the cast. One week after discharge, Amy resumed outpatient physical and occupational therapy twice a week for trunk strengthening and improving hand/arm use and head control. She also received speech therapy once a week. When the spica cast was removed, the orthopedic surgeon ordered physical therapy five times per week for 4 weeks, with a decrease to four times per week for 4 weeks, then three times per week for 4 weeks. Amy's goals also changed after the surgery.

Once the intensive postoperative rehabilitation was completed, therapy continued twice weekly. Amy's aunt reported that Amy had begun to wake up several times during the night crying and had muscle spasms. Massage helped alleviate the spasms and calmed Amy. She began to see a massage therapist weekly and receive increased water/fluids through her G-tube, but after 6 weeks, she was still having muscle spasms every night. Amy started taking a multivitamin and within 2 days, the spasms had stopped completely and Amy now, more than a year later, takes a multivitamin daily and sleeps well through the night without muscle spasms. The most dramatic postoperative improvement was Amy's ability to sit with her legs extended.

Direct Intervention
Orthotics

While wearing a thoracolumbosacral orthosis (TLSO) brace, which had been modified into a sitting brace, Amy was able to sit with her arms on a support surface while activating a switch and keep her head up in midline for

Continued

CASE OF A CHILD WITH CEREBRAL PALSY—cont'd

short periods. She began to accept weight on her lower extremities, with active pushing approximately 30% of the time. With prepping and use of her TLSO, Amy has actually demonstrated full weight-bearing with hands held for up to 5 seconds.

Goals

After surgery, Amy was reassessed, and her goals were revised as follows:

1. Once placed, Amy will long sit utilizing a TLSO with supervision for 20 seconds while activating a switch toy with her left upper extremity.
2. Amy will stand with bilateral knee immobilizers, AFOs, and a TLSO with upper extremities on a support surface and minimal cues to maintain midline for 10 seconds.
3. Amy will ambulate in her Pony gait trainer for 20 feet with assist to turn or avoid obstacles.
4. Amy will roll to left and right side-lying independently.
5. Amy will perform sit-to-stand from a bench with maximal assistance at her trunk for 4 out of 5 trials.

Outcomes

Amy responded very well to her orthopedic surgery. In an attempt to determine whether the surgical intervention and therapy had research-based evidence, an article published by O'Donnell and Roxborough[52] gave descriptions of the best sources of research evidence. According to these authors, the best sources of evidence are systems in which the latest professional evidence is integrated from an electronic health record with the client's current circumstances. In Amy's case, a website, www.evidence.org, was searched without success in locating any information on children with CP. The second best source reported was review articles. According to a review article by Gormley,[53] the evidence supports the use of orthotics to minimize the potential abnormal positioning of the foot and contractures. The authors also discussed the use of orthopedic surgery for correction of contractures and torsional deformities of the long bones (i.e., femur). Logan[54] discussed that diet and biomechanics are essential parts of the treatment for children with CP. G-tube surgery, orthotic use, and orthopedic intervention were all a part of Amy's care.

Logan[15] also discussed the need for therapists to have training in a variety of treatment options available and to approach treatment of the child as a whole. In Amy's therapy sessions, the clinic staff had attempted various treatment approaches. Many specific treatment approaches are lacking in true research-based evidence. There are no stringent research articles regarding the effects of myofascial release, cranial sacral therapy, Feldenkrais, or sensory integration on the functional improvements of a child with CP. There have been a few research studies regarding the positive outcomes of children with spastic quadriplegic CP with neurodevelopmental treatment (NDT)[16,17] and horseback riding,[18] but they lack quality research design, adequate sample size, and control groups.

On the other hand, outcomes of the specific surgical interventions (e.g., varus derotation osteotomy and pelvic osteotomy) for children with CP have been reported in several journals.[19-22] Surgical intervention for contractures, subluxed hips, and torsional deformities for a child with CP is well accepted in the medical community.[19-23] Amy did demonstrate a positive outcome overall, and the only surgical intervention that may be necessary in the next 2 decades is surgical fusion if her scoliosis continues to progress despite bracing.

Analysis of Case Using the ICF Model (After Surgery)

Body functions: Lower extremity deformities requiring surgery bilaterally, hip spica cast, pain, decreased trunk strength, decreased head and neck control, decreased volitional hand/arm use, decreased communication skills, decreased ROM.

Activity limitations: Decreased lower extremity weight-bearing, decreased ability to play and interact with peers, limited independence, decreased sitting tolerance, difficulty with mobility.

Participation restrictions: Could not attend school, difficulty participating in family routines, difficulty in accessing environmental stimuli and playing with toys.

Environmental factors: Difficulty in finding transportation, limited resources, changes in nutritional needs, modifications required for toys.

Movement System Analysis

Amy exhibits severe deficits in force production in all limbs and trunk.

CHAPTER DISCUSSION QUESTIONS

1. What are the hallmark signs of CP? List the measurement tools that can be used in identifying children at risk for CP.

2. Which specialty referrals and diagnostic methods are most appropriate for infants at risk for motor delays to confirm a diagnosis of CP?

3. Describe the medical conditions that may co-occur with CP.

REFERENCES

1. Centers for Disease Control and Prevention. Data and statistics for cerebral palsy. Updated May 2, 2022. Accessed October 23, 2022. https://www.cdc.gov/ncbddd/cp/data.html.

2. McGuire DO, Tian LH, Yeargin-Allsopp M, Dowling NF, Christensen DL. Prevalence of cerebral palsy, intellectual disability, hearing loss, and blindness, National Health Interview Survey, 2009–2016. *Disabil Health J.* 2019;12(3):443–451.

3. Honeycutt A, Dunlap L, Chen H, al Homsi G. Economic costs associated with mental retardation, cerebral palsy, hearing loss, and vision impairment—United States, 2003. *MMWR.* 2004;53(03):57–59. Accessed October 23, 2022. https://www.cdc.gov/mmwr/preview/mmwrhtml/mm5303a4.htm.

4. MacLennan AH, Thompson SC, Gecz J. Cerebral palsy: causes, pathways, and the role of genetic variants. *Am J Obstet Gynecol.* 2015;213(6):779–788.

5. American College of Obstetricians and Gynecologists' Task Force on Neonatal Encephalopathy. *Neonatal Encephalopathy and Neurologic Outcome.* 2nd ed. Washington, DC: American College of Obstetricians and Gynecologists; 2014.

6. Nelson KB. Causative factors in cerebral palsy. *Clin Obstet Gynecol.* 2008;51(4):749–762.

7. Palisano R, Rosenbaum P, Walter S, et al. Gross motor function classification system for cerebral palsy. *Dev Med Child Neurol.* 1997;9:214.

8. Einspieler C, Bos AF, Krieber-Tomantschger M, et al. Cerebral palsy: early markers of clinical phenotype and functional outcome. *J Clin Med.* 2019;8(10):1616.

9. Glass HC, Li Y, Gardner M, et al. Early identification of cerebral palsy using neonatal MRI and General Movements Assessment in a cohort of high-risk term neonates. *Pediatr Neurol.* 2021;118:20–25.

10. Morgan C, Romeo DM, Chorna O, et al. The pooled diagnostic accuracy of neuroimaging, general movements, and neurological examination for diagnosing cerebral palsy early in high-risk infants: a case control study. *J Clin Med.* 2019;8(11):1879.

11. Hay K, Nelin M, Carey H, Chorna O, Moore-Clingenpeel M, Maitre N. Hammersmith Infant Neurological Examination asymmetry score detects hemiplegic cerebral palsy from typical development. *Pediatr Neurol.* 2018;87:70–74.

12. Byrne R, Noritz G, Maitre NL. Implementation of early diagnosis and intervention guidelines for cerebral palsy in a high-risk infant follow-up clinic. *Pediatr Neurol.* 2017;76:66–71.

13. Boychuck Z, Andersen J, Bussières A, et al. International expert recommendations of clinical features to prompt referral for diagnostic assessment of cerebral palsy. *Dev Med Child Neurol.* 2020;62(1):89–96.

14. Garfinkle J, Li P, Boychuck Z, Bussières A, Majnemer A. Early clinical features of cerebral palsy in children without perinatal risk factors: a scoping review. *Pediatr Neurol.* 2020;102:56–61.

15. Peyton C, Schreiber MD, Msall ME. The Test of Infant Motor Performance at 3 months predicts language, cognitive, and motor outcomes in infants born preterm at 2 years of age. *Dev Med Child Neurol.* 2018;60(12):1239–1243.

16. Committee to Evaluate the Supplemental Security Income Disability Program for Children with Mental Disorders; Board on the Health of Select Populations; Board on Children, Youth, and Families; Institute of Medicine; Division of Behavioral and Social Sciences and Education; The National Academies of Sciences, Engineering, and Medicine. In: Boat TF, Wu JT, eds. *Mental Disorders and Disabilities Among Low-Income Children.* Washington, DC: National Academies Press; 2015.

17. Reid SM, Meehan EM, Arnup SJ, Reddihough DS. Intellectual disability in cerebral palsy: a population-based retrospective study. *Dev Med Child Neurol.* 2018;60(7):687–694.

18. Bertoncelli CM, Altamura P, Vieira ER, Bertoncelli D, Thummler S, Solla F. Identifying factors associated with severe intellectual disabilities in teenagers with cerebral palsy using a predictive learning model. *J Child Neurol.* 2019;34(4):221–229.

19. Jonsson U, Eek MN, Sunnerhagen KS, Himmelmann K. Changes in walking ability, intellectual disability, and epilepsy in adults with cerebral palsy over 50 years: a population-based follow-up study. *Dev Med Child Neurol.* 2021;63(7):839–845.

20. Jeon H, Jung JH, Yoon JA, Choi H. Strabismus is correlated with gross motor function in children with spastic cerebral palsy. *Curr Eye Res.* 2019;44(11):1258–1263.

21. West MR, Borchert MS, Chang MY. Ophthalmologic characteristics and outcomes of children with cortical visual impairment and cerebral palsy. *J Am Assoc Pediatr Ophthalmol Strabismus.* 2021;25(4):223.e1–223.e6.

22. van der List JP, Witbreuk MM, Buizer AI, van der Sluijs JA. The head–shaft angle of the hip in early childhood: a comparison of reference values for children with cerebral palsy and normally developing hips. *Bone Joint J.* 2015;97-B(9):1291–1295.

23. Chougule S, Dabis J, Petrie A, Daly K, Gelfer Y. Is head–shaft angle a valuable continuous risk factor for hip migration in cerebral palsy? *J Child Ortho.* 2016;10(6):651–656.

24. Hägglund G. Association between pelvic obliquity and scoliosis, hip displacement and asymmetric hip abduction in children with cerebral palsy: a cross-sectional registry study. *BMC Musculoskelet Disord.* 2020;21(1):464.

25. Hägglund G, Alriksson-Schmidt A, Lauge-Pedersen H, Rodby-Bousquet E, Wagner P, Westbom L. Prevention of dislocation of the hip in children with cerebral palsy. *Bone Joint J.* 2014;96(11):7.

26. Otjen JP, Sousa TC, Bauer JM, Thapa M. Cerebral palsy—beyond hip deformities. *Pediatr Radiol.* 2019;49(12):1587–1594.

27. Wynter M, Gibson N, Willoughby KL, et al. Australian hip surveillance guidelines for children with cerebral palsy: 5-year review. *Dev Med Child Neurol.* 2015;57(9):808–820.

28. Guaré RO, Ferreira MCD, Leite MF, Rodrigues JA, Lussi A, Santos MTBR. Dental erosion and salivary flow rate in cerebral palsy individuals with gastroesophageal reflux: GERD, dental erosion, and salivary flow rate in cerebral palsy. *J Oral Pathol Med.* 2012;41(5):367–371.

29. Lansdown K, Irving M, Mathieu Coulton K, Smithers-Sheedy H. A scoping review of oral health outcomes for people with cerebral palsy. *Spec Care Dentist.* 2022;42(3):232–243.

30. Weir FW, Hatch JL, McRackan TR, Wallace SA, Meyer TA. Hearing loss in pediatric patients with cerebral palsy. *Otol Neurotol.* 2018;39(1):59–64.

31. Speyer R, Cordier R, Kim J, Cocks N, Michou E, Wilkes-Gillan S. Prevalence of drooling, swallowing, and feeding problems in cerebral palsy across the lifespan: a systematic review and meta-analyses. *Dev Med Child Neurol.* 2019;61(11):1249–1258.

32. Rosen R, Vandenplas Y, Singendonk M, et al. Pediatric gastroesophageal reflux clinical practice guidelines: joint recommendations of the North American Society for Pediatric Gastroenterology, Hepatology, and Nutrition and the European Society for Pediatric Gastroenterology, Hepatology, and Nutrition. *J Pediatr Gastroenterol Nutr.* 2018;66(3):516–554.

33. Bayram AK, Canpolat M, Karacabey N, et al. Misdiagnosis of gastroesophageal reflux disease as epileptic seizures in children. *Brain Dev.* 2016;38(3):274–279.

34. Vianello A, Carraro E, Pipitone E, et al. Clinical and pulmonary function markers of respiratory exacerbation risk in subjects with quadriplegic cerebral palsy. *Respir Care.* 2015;60(10):1431–1437.

35. Reilly M, Liuzzo K, Blackmer AB. Pharmacological management of spasticity in children with cerebral palsy. *J Pediatr Health Care.* 2020;34(5):495–509.

36. Hasnat MJ, Rice JE. Intrathecal baclofen for treating spasticity in children with cerebral palsy. *Cochrane Database Syst Rev.* 2015;2015(11):CD004552.

37. Delhaas EM, Huygen FJPM. Complications associated with intrathecal drug delivery systems. *BJA Educ.* 2020;20(2):51–57.

38. Moon JU, Cho KO. Current pharmacologic strategies for treatment of intractable epilepsy in children. *Int Neurourol J.* 2021;25(suppl 1):S8–S18.

39. Lightdale JR, Gremse DASection on Gastroenterology, Hepatology, and Nutrition, et al. Gastroesophageal reflux: management guidance for the pediatrician. *Pediatrics.* 2013;131(5):e1684–e1695.

40. Berg EA, Khlevner J. Treatment of gastroesophageal reflux disease in children. *Pediatr Rev.* 2021;42(1):51–53.

41. Church C, Biermann I, Lennon N, et al. Walking activity after multilevel orthopedic surgery in children with cerebral palsy. *Dev Med Child Neurol.* 2022;64(10):1289–1296.

42. Tedroff K, Hägglund G, Miller F. Long-term effects of selective dorsal rhizotomy in children with cerebral palsy: a systematic review. *Dev Med Child Neurol.* 2020;62(5):554–562.

43. Sullivan PB, Juszczak E, Bachlet AM, et al. Impact of gastrostomy tube feeding on the quality of life of carers of children with cerebral palsy. *Dev Med Child Neurol.* 2004;46(12):796–800.

44. O'Loughlin EV, Somerville H, Shun A, et al. Antireflux surgery in children with neurological impairment: caregiver perceptions and complications. *J Pediatr Gastroenterol Nutr.* 2013;56(1):46–50.

45. Fuentefria R do N, Silveira RC, Procianoy RS. Motor development of preterm infants assessed by the Alberta Infant Motor Scale: systematic review article. *J Pediatr Versao En Port.* 2017;93(4):328–342.

46. Shore BJ, Allar BG, Miller PE, Matheney TH, Snyder BD, Fragala-Pinkham M. Measuring the reliability and construct validity of the Pediatric Evaluation of Disability Inventory–Computer Adaptive Test (PEDI-CAT) in children with cerebral palsy. *Arch Phys Med Rehabil.* 2019;100(1):45–51.

47. Russell D, Rosenbaum PL, Wright M, Avery LM. *Gross Motor Function Measure (GMFM-66 & GMFM-88) User's Manual.* 2nd ed. Philadelphia: Wiley; 2013.

48. Rosenbaum PL, Walter SD, Hanna SE, et al. Prognosis for gross motor function in cerebral palsy: creation of motor development curves. *Obstet Gynecol Surv.* 2003;58(3):166–168.

49. Hanna SE, Bartlett DJ, Rivard LM, Russell DJ. Reference curves for the Gross Motor Function Measure: percentiles for clinical description and tracking over time among children with cerebral palsy. *Phys Ther.* 2008;88(5):596–607.

50. CanChild. Motor growth curves. Accessed October 23, 2022. https://www.canchild.ca/en/resources/237-motor-growth-curves.

51. Hammam N, Becher H, Andersen J, Manns PJ, Whittaker JL, Pritchard L. Early indicators of cardiovascular disease are evident in children and

adolescents with cerebral palsy. *Disabil Health J.* 2021;14(4):101–112.

52. O'Donnell ME, Roxborough L. Evidence-based practice in pediatric rehabilitation. *Phys Med Rehabil Clin N Am.* 2002;13(4):991–1005.

53. Gormley ME Jr. Treatment of neuromuscular andmusculoskeletal problems in cerebral palsy. *Pediatr Rehabil.* 2001;4(1):5.

54. Logan LR. Facts and myths about therapeutic interventionsin cerebral palsy: integrated goal development. *Phys Med Rehabil Clin N Am.* 2002;13(4):979.

RESOURCES

National Institute of Neurological Disorder and Stroke
www.ninds.nih.gov

American Academy of Cerebral Palsy and Developmental Medicine
www.aacpdm.org

National Disability Sports Alliance
25 W. Independence Way
Kingston, RI 02881
401-792-7130
www.ndsaonline.org

United Cerebral Palsy
1600 L Street NW #700
Washington, DC 20036
800-872-5827
www.ucp.org

Easter Seals
230 W. Monroe Street #1800
Chicago, IL 60606-4802
800-221-6827
www.easter-seals.org

March of Dimes Birth Defects Foundation
1275 Mamaroneck Avenue
White Plains, NY 10605
888-663-4637
www.marchofdimes.com

Children's Hemiplegic and Stroke Association
4101 West Green Oaks Boulevard
PMB #146
Arlington, TX 76016
817-492-4325
www.hemikids.org

Pediatric Traumatic Brain Injury

Maryleen K. Jones, PT, DHSc, NCS, CSRS, CLT

LEARNING OBJECTIVES

At the end of the chapter, the reader should be able to do the following:

1. Identify causes of traumatic brain injury.
2. Identify types of traumatic brain injury.
3. Differentiate between traumatic brain injury and acquired brain injury.
4. Characterize traumatic brain injury by severity.
5. Describe the importance of the Glasgow Coma Scale and the Rancho Los Amigos Levels of Cognitive Functioning.
6. Describe characteristics of movement systems diagnosis related to traumatic brain injury.
7. Identify components of a treatment plan for a patient with a traumatic brain injury.

CHAPTER OUTLINE

KEY TERMS

Acceleration-dependent injury

Contrecoup injury

Coup injury

Diffuse axonal injury

Glasgow Coma Scale

Heterotopic ossification

Movement systems approach

Pediatric Glasgow Coma Scale

Rancho Los Amigos Levels of
  Cognitive Functioning

Rotational injury

Translational injury

Traumatic brain injury

Traumatic brain injury (TBI) in infants and children (Fig. 7.1) is a fairly common occurrence, although the mechanisms of injury, presentation, and resultant impairments may be quite varied. In this chapter, mechanisms, incidence, demographics, and management and treatment of brain injuries are outlined and discussed. The effects of a TBI can be quite devastating, not only to the infant or child but also to the family, including siblings, parents, and/or caregivers. Depending on the severity of the TBI, the lifelong implications for a particular infant or child can be mild, moderate, or severe; in some cases, full-time nursing care will be required. Understanding all the potential mechanisms and outcomes is vital to meeting the rehabilitation needs of these infants and children and to the education of their families and/or care providers.

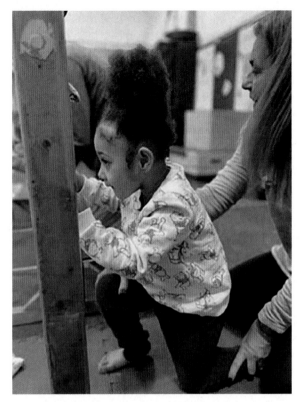

Fig. 7.1 Although traumatic brain injury is a fairly common occurrence in children, resultant injuries and impairments can be varied.

DEFINITION

TBI is classified as a traumatically induced physiologic alteration of brain functioning, resulting in partial or total impairment of one or more areas of functioning caused by an external force.[1] The areas of functioning potentially affected include, but are not limited to, the following: cognition, memory, attention, reasoning, abstract thinking, judgment, problem-solving, information processing, speech and language, psychosocial behavior, sensory processing and integration, perceptual and motor abilities, and physical functioning. Acquired brain injury (ABI) is a brain injury that results from an internal factor, such as a hypoxic event (e.g., cardiac arrest, near drowning), exposure to a toxic substance, compression from a tumor, or an infectious disease process that causes encephalopathy.[2]

INCIDENCE AND PREVALENCE

According to the Centers for Disease Control and Prevention, TBI is the leading cause of disability for children and adolescents in the United States. Infants and children from birth to age 4 years and between the ages of 15 and19 years are at the greatest risk for injury.[3] Of the estimated 830,000 children who experience a brain injury, more than 62,000 require hospitalization, with approximately 3% succumbing to their injuries. Mechanisms responsible for pediatric brain injuries include motor vehicle accidents (MVAs), falls, sports injuries, and physical abuse.[3]

EPIDEMIOLOGY AND PATHOLOGY

For children between the ages of 1 and 18 years, TBIs are classified as mild, moderate, or severe using the Pediatric Glasgow Coma Scale (PGCS) and the Glasgow Coma Scale (GCS), which will be discussed in further detail later in this chapter. An estimated 75% to 80% of children who are seen in emergency departments because of suspected head injury return home with mild injury (GCS score of 13–15). Approximately 15% of all children who present to an emergency department are hospitalized with a moderate (13%) or severe (2%) brain injury, with GCS scores of 9 to 12 and less than 8, respectively.[4,5] Sadly, it is reported that 3.4% of children brought to the emergency department with brain injuries each year succumb to their injuries.[5] Every year in the United States, 61% of children with moderate to severe brain injuries experience permanent disability,[6] and 14% of children classified as having mild brain injury experience persistent disability.[6] Across all pediatric age groups and types of brain injuries, boys are more likely than girls to present with a TBI.[6]

The potential mechanisms of injury that result in TBI include MVAs, either with the infant or child restrained or unrestrained in a vehicle or an MVA when the child is a pedestrian; anoxia; seizure disorders or epilepsy; shaken baby syndrome (SBS) and assault/abusive head trauma (ABT); cerebrovascular accidents (CVAs); tumors/neoplasms; infections; penetrating injuries; near-drowning injuries; neurotoxic events; and hydrocephalus. The classification of TBI does not include brain dysfunctions that result from congenital or degenerative disorders or birth trauma. Falls followed by abuse-related brain injuries are the most common mechanisms of injuries among children from birth to 4 years of age, comprising 72% of all TBI-related injuries for that age range.[6]

SBS and ABT as mechanisms of injury have increased in prevalence in the past few years in the United States, and SBS is a leading cause of morbidity and mortality among infants.[6] SBS and ABT result in diffuse brain damage due to the shaking of the infant and also result in cerebral tissue bruising as the cerebral tissue repeatedly makes contact with the rough inner surface of the skull. Violent shaking can also produce rotational "shearing" forces that result in diffuse axonal injury (DAI). DAI often results in retinal hemorrhage, bilateral cortical involvement, and significant neurologic injury without signs of external trauma.[7] Blood vessels that supply the brain can also be torn, causing additional intracranial bleeding. Infants younger than 6 months are susceptible to injury for several reasons, including but not limited to the following: head to body size proportion, weak neck musculature, underdeveloped brains, and strength differences between the child and the perpetrator.[7]

Falls and injuries associated with MVAs are quite common among school-aged children. Often, children in this age group are not properly restrained while riding in a vehicle, or they are not closely supervised while playing outdoors and are struck when they run out into the street to retrieve a ball or toy. In the school-aged population (5–14 years), MVAs and MVAs involving pedestrians, falls, sports-related injuries, and recreational injuries such as bicycle-related accidents are the most common causes of morbidity and mortality.[6] Sports-related and recreation-based activities are also implicated in the most common injuries to children in the early adolescent and adolescent age groups and contribute to the high number of mild brain injuries reported each year in the United States.[8]

CLINICAL SIGNS

The short- and long-term effects of these injuries to the brain are highly dependent on their location within the brain, the age of the infant or child, and the length of time elapsed since the injury. The pathophysiology of TBI is related to the deformation of the brain's parenchyma and the vasculature related to the anatomical site of attachment. Because of the diverse mechanisms of TBI previously mentioned, many patients present with a combination of comorbidities. For example, a patient may sustain a skull fracture in addition to injury to the cerebral cortex. The pediatric population, especially children younger than 3 years, may also experience leptomeningeal cysts (growing skull fractures) as a complication of the initial injury, resulting in encephalomalacia (Fig. 7.2).[9] TBIs involve both primary (site of impact or penetrating injury) and secondary injuries (blood vessel and/or cellular changes in brain tissue that evolve after the primary injury).

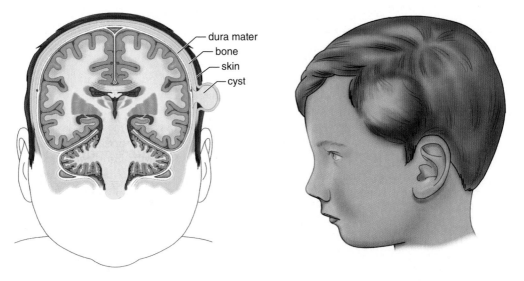

— dura mater
— bone
— skin
— cyst

Fig. 7.2 Leptomeningeal cysts (growing skull fractures) may be a complication of the initial injury, resulting in encephalomalacia.

Primary injuries are a result of the injury's initial impact related to the external forces applied to the head.[7] An acceleration-dependent injury is related to the effects that occur when a force is applied to a movable head. It may be either translational or rotational in nature.[6] A translational injury causes lateral movement of both the skull and the brain in response to a force applied to the side of the skull. As the skull is impacted, it rapidly decelerates, but the brain inside does not. Rather, it continues to move until it is stopped by the skull on the side opposite the impact. A coup injury occurs at the point of impact, and when the brain strikes the skull opposite the area of direct impact (secondary to the initial force/injury), a contrecoup injury occurs.[6] Both coup and contrecoup injuries can cause significant brain damage. A rotational injury occurs when the brain remains stationary in a moving, rotating skull. As a result, the forces on the brain are rotational in nature. Rotational injuries are related to shearing trauma, which has also been associated with diffuse axonal injuries.[6]

Secondary injuries occur because of processes induced in response to the initial trauma. These secondary injuries account for a significant amount of the overall damage that occurs with a TBI. Examples of secondary lacerations include scalp lacerations, skull fractures, cerebral edema, epidural hematomas, acute subdural hematomas, subarachnoid hemorrhages, increased intracranial pressure, and organ damage.[2] Medical management of secondary injuries attempts to minimize the damage resulting from the primary injury, mostly with surgical intervention, pharmacologic management, and mechanical ventilation. The main goal of all of these interventions is to sustain life and medically stabilize the patient to prevent further injury.

TBIs are classified as mild, moderate, or severe (Box 7.1), typically based on a standardized classification system used by emergency medical personnel at the time of the injury. The GCS and PGCS are observational scales used in emergency departments and intensive care units following TBI to rate brain injury in a newly injured infant or child.[3] If the child is younger than 2 years, the PGCS may be used because it utilizes age-appropriate responses to rate the severity of the child's injury. These scales are used to determine a prognosis for the child's possible outcome. The items rated include eye opening, motor response, and verbal response (Table 7.1). Based on a total from all three categories, scores of 3 to 8 are defined as a severe injury, 8 or 9 to 12 as a moderate injury, and 13 to 15 as a mild injury.

BOX 7.1 TBI Classifications

Mild TBI

Early-appearing signs and symptoms: headaches, nausea and vomiting, blurred vision, tinnitus, dizziness, stiff neck, fatigue, and light and noise sensitivity

Late-appearing signs and symptoms: slowed or impaired information processing, disorganization, reduced frustration tolerance, rapid mood changes and increased irritability, difficulties retrieving previous information, increased sensitivity to noise, and reports of being overloaded or overwhelmed

Moderate TBI

Loss of consciousness and/or posttraumatic amnesia of more than 30 minutes but less than 24 hours and/or the presence of a skull fracture

Severe TBI

Loss of consciousness or posttraumatic amnesia lasting more than 24 hours, a GCS score of less than 8, extensive physical impairments with possible respiratory compromise, and a slowed overall recovery

---

Mild TBI is the most common type of brain injury and describes the initial insult relative to its neurologic severity. Concussions and whiplash injuries are often consistent with a diagnosis of a mild brain injury, but often, in the sports medicine literature, they are not described as such. Mild brain injuries are currently increasing in number for both boys and girls because of increased participation in recreational and contact sports in the United States.[6] Certain activities and sports place children, especially preteens and teens, at risk. Forty-five percent of emergency department visits related to TBIs are attributed to football, bicycling, basketball, soccer, ice hockey, lacrosse, and playground activities.[8] The use of helmets in many recreational and sporting activities has increased in recent years and is thought to have aided in decreasing the severity of brain injuries.[8] In addition to the increased use of helmets in sports activities, successful prevention initiatives such as increased awareness, improved on-the-field screening, and rule changes in contact sports and care-seeking behavior may have led to a decline in incidence among adolescent boys in recent years.[8]

Mild TBI is defined by any period of a loss of consciousness, any loss of memory for events immediately before or after the accident, any alteration in mental status at the time of the accident, any focal neurologic deficit that

TABLE 7.1	Comparison of Glasgow Coma Scale and Pediatric Glasgow Coma Scale		
Sign	**Glasgow Coma Scale**	**Pediatric Glasgow Coma Scale**	**Score**
Eye Opening	Spontaneous	Spontaneous	4
	To command	To sound	3
	To pain	To pain	2
	None	None	1
Verbal Response	Oriented	Age-appropriate vocalization, smile, or orientation to sound; interacts (coos, babbles); follows objects	5
	Confused, disoriented	Cries, irritable	4
	Inappropriate words	Cries to pain	3
	Incomprehensible sounds	Moans to pain	2
	None	None	1
Motor Response	Obeys commands	Spontaneous movements (obeys verbal command)	6
	Localizes pain	Withdraws to touch (localizes pain)	5
	Withdraws	Withdraws to pain	4
	Abnormal flexion to pain	Abnormal flexion to pain (decorticate posture)	3
	Abnormal extension to pain	Abnormal extension to pan (decerebrate posture)	2
	None	None	1
Best Total Score			15

The Glasgow Coma Scale (GCS) is scored between 3 and 15, with 3 being the worst and 15, being the best. It is composed of 3 parameters: best eye response (E), best verbal response (V), and best motor response (M). The components of the GCS should be recorded individually; for example, E2V3M4 results in a GCS score of 9. A score of 13 or higher correlates with mild brain injury, a score of 9 to 12 correlates with moderate injury, and a score of 8 or less represents severe brain injury. The Pediatric Glasgow Coma Scale (PGCS) was validated in children 2 years of age or younger.
Data from:
1. Teasdale G, Jennett B. Assessment of coma and impaired consciousness. A practical scale, *Lancet* 2:81, 1974.
2. Holmes JF, Palchak MJ, MacFarlane T, Kuppermann N. Performance of the pediatric Glasgow Coma Scale in children with blunt head trauma, *Acad Emerg Med* 12:814, 2005.

may or may not be transient in nature but does not exceed a loss of consciousness of approximately 30 minutes, an initial GCS score of 13 to 15 after 30 minutes, and/or post-traumatic amnesia of no more than 24 hours.[10] Common symptoms of mild TBI are divided into "early" and "late" symptoms.

Common early symptoms, described as those symptoms present at the time of the injury, are headaches, nausea and vomiting, blurred vision, tinnitus (ringing in the ears), dizziness, stiff neck, fatigue, and light and noise sensitivity. These symptoms can have an adverse impact on a child's academic performance and interpersonal skills. Because children with mild brain injuries do not typically have associated physical injuries, their behavior in school or at home may be misconstrued as attention problems, increased negative behaviors, poor motivation, or a negative attitude.

Late symptoms are those that may develop over the next 72 hours and may include cognitive, emotional, and sleep disturbances in addition to the early physical symptoms. Cognitive symptoms may involve difficulty thinking, decreased concentration, poor recall of new information, perseveration, and delayed processing. Symptoms that are emotional in nature include irritability, sadness, increased sensitivity, nervousness, and unexplained anxiety. Sleep patterns may also be altered by an increase or decrease in the typical amount of sleep or difficulty falling asleep. These symptoms within the cognitive domain may manifest when the child is in a more challenging, cognitively demanding environment such as school and psychosocial environments.[11]

Moderate brain injury is characterized by a loss of consciousness and/or posttraumatic amnesia lasting more than 30 minutes but less than 24 hours and/or the presence of a skull fracture. As stated earlier, it is typically differentiated by a GCS score of 8 or 9 to 12. A severe brain injury is characterized by a loss of consciousness or posttraumatic amnesia lasting more than 24 hours, a GCS score of less than 8, extensive physical impairments with possible respiratory compromise, and a slowed overall recovery.[2] The extensive physical impairments are often the result of brainstem or more diffuse cortical damage.[11]

In both moderate and severe brain injuries, common impairments are noted in the physical, cognitive, sensory, speech and language, personality, and behavioral domains. Neurologic, musculoskeletal, and sensory impairments vary depending on the location of the injury, the severity of the injury, and the age of the child. Disturbances typically involve limitations in independence with mobility, impaired strength, limited range of motion, impaired motor planning and coordination, vision deficits (including visual field deficits), decreased perceptual abilities, hearing impairment or loss, impaired sensation (including decreased kinesthetic awareness and proprioception), impaired balance (both static and dynamic), decreased safety awareness, and increased impulsivity. There is also the possibility of seizure activity.

Timely intervention and management of children with TBI may prevent negative sequelae and resultant secondary complications such as deep vein thrombosis, pressure injuries, the onset of pneumonia, muscular and cardiovascular deconditioning, genitourinary issues, urinary and bowel incontinence, peripheral nerve injury or entrapment, contractures, and development of chronic pain or complex regional pain syndrome.[6,12–15] The development of heterotopic ossification (HO) is a common risk for children who experience brain injury. In HO there is pathologic bone formation around a joint in the pericapsular space.[11] This often causes pain, decreased range of motion, and swelling of the joint. The etiology of HO is unclear, but it appears to be caused by increased muscle tone around a joint.[1] Approximately 3% to 20% of children who sustain a brain injury will develop HO.[5,16] If suspected or diagnosed, HO should be treated aggressively by physical therapists (PTs); the use of splinting can be included, if required.

Speech and language problems often result from brain injury, and these include difficulty with articulation and fluency of speech; echolalia; aphasia (both expressive and receptive); and difficulties with organizational and executive functioning, listening and reading comprehension, and word finding. Feeding and swallowing issues also commonly occur and require comprehensive assessment by a speech-language pathologist.[17]

Cognitive impairments for children with moderate and severe brain injuries are typically long-lasting and, in some cases, very devastating. As with physical impairments, cognitive impairments vary but often include arousal problems, poor/diminished concentration and attention, long- and short-term memory deficits, limited insight into one's own deficits, organizational deficits, executive functioning deficits, problem-solving deficits, and impaired ability for new learning.[17] Early in the rehabilitative process, sustaining arousal is of primary focus. Arousal is controlled by the reticular activating system, and with moderate to severe brain injury, this system is often impaired, resulting in difficulty with sensory modulation of both internal and external environmental stimulants.

An overlooked aspect of recovery from TBI is related to the social/emotional and behavioral changes, which are prevalent. Social/emotional and behavioral changes observed after TBI include increased anxiety, emotional lability, low self-esteem, increased restlessness, increased agitation, increased mood swings, excessive emotional shifts, depression, lack of motivation, lowered frustration tolerance, lack of inhibition and increased impulsivity, difficulty with peer relationships, and poor or diminished social skills.[18] Areas of the brain—such as the prefrontal cortex, anterior cingulate cortex, temporal-parietal junctions, posterior temporal sulcus, insula, and amygdala—are responsible for the primary regulation of social behavior and functioning in daily life. When social and emotional regulation are impacted, the children as well as their parents experience a sense of grief and loss (Table 7.2).

TABLE 7.2   Resultant Impairments of Traumatic Brain Injury

Partial or total impairments of one or more of the following areas of functioning:
- Cognition and reasoning
- Memory and attention
- Abstract thinking
- Judgment
- Problem-solving
- Information processing
- Receptive and expressive language
- Psychosocial behavior
- Sensory and perceptual abilities
- Motor function
- Physical functioning including balance and coordination

MEDICAL INTERVENTION

Once an infant or child is medically stable in the acute care setting, deciding what will be the most appropriate next step for that child's recovery and rehabilitation is paramount. As part of an interdisciplinary approach, physical therapy, as well as occupational and speech therapy, are often ordered in the acute care setting. Interdisciplinary team members may include physicians, often a physiatrist and neurologist; a surgeon, if surgical intervention is necessary; rehabilitation nurse; case manager/team coordinator; social worker; neuropsychologist; respiratory therapist; and recreational therapist.

One option for furthering the child's recovery is transitioning the child to an inpatient rehabilitation program. This option offers the child the benefits of intensive and comprehensive therapies. Depending on the nature and extent of the child's injuries, the length of stay for this course of treatment is variable.

For children who do not require the intensive nature of an inpatient rehabilitation program, other options include day rehabilitation programs, outpatient therapies, and early intervention therapy for those younger than 3 years. Day rehabilitation programs offer intensive daily therapies in a clinic environment but allow children to be at home at night with their caregivers and family. For many children, less often for infants with brain injury, day rehabilitation programs may be a natural progression from more intensive inpatient rehabilitation programs, with the goal of transitioning back to school or outpatient services. Outpatient therapies are often appropriate for an infant or child with deficits in only one or two areas and allow for specifically focused services for those deficits (e.g., outpatient occupational and physical therapy for right hemiplegia without cognitive deficits). Early intervention services, either home- or center-based, can be implemented for infants from birth to 3 years of age. However, early intervention services focus primarily on the achievement of developmental milestones, rather than rehabilitation from a traumatic injury. Several day rehabilitation programs are now accepting infants younger than 3 years for a modified day rehabilitation program, such as two to three times per week for 1 to 2 hours a day. More traditional day rehabilitation programming often involves daily therapy for 4 to 6 hours a day.

Figure 7.3 shows the variety of pathways a child's rehabilitation journey may follow after sustaining a TBI.

Physical Therapy Assessment

The physical therapy examination is a comprehensive assessment and testing process that leads to a diagnostic classification, and in some cases, referral to another medical/healthcare professional. Components of the physical therapy examination include a thorough patient history; systems review; and in-depth assessment of the child's cognition, including orientation, Rancho Los Amigos Levels of Cognitive Functioning, attention, alertness, memory, agitation level, and safety awareness; range of motion; neuromuscular assessment, including muscle tone, reflexes, neurologic signs, and posturing; muscle strength assessment; endurance; balance; posture; pain assessment; skin and skull integrity; coordination; sensory functioning, including tactile, auditory, olfactory, vestibular, visual, proprioceptive, and stereognostic; and motor control of functional movements including the initiation, sequencing, execution, quality of movement, planning, grading, termination, compensatory patterns, and asymmetries. The movement continuum illustrated in Fig. 7.4 contains a set of core functional movement tasks, which may need to be modified to recognize an infant or child's appropriate motor development levels, such as assessing a 4-month-old's ability to initiate and complete the task of rolling over and maintaining head control while being propped in the prone position. Anthropometric characteristics, circulation, cranial and peripheral nerve integrity, gait and locomotion, neuromotor development, and sensory integration are examined and assessed as part of the PT's evaluation. The interdisciplinary team may meet to make recommendations and to determine the need for assistive technology, adaptive devices, orthotics, or prosthetic devices and discuss any potential environmental, home, school, and play barriers. On completion of the physical therapy evaluation, a physical therapy diagnosis is established. Under the movement systems framework, movement systems diagnoses that are relevant to the medical diagnosis of TBI are movement pattern coordination deficit, force production deficit, fractionated movement deficit, postural vertical deficit, sensory selection and weighting deficit, sensory detection deficit, and cognitive deficit (Table 7.3). The movement systems diagnosis is discussed in further detail in Chapter 5.

The Rancho Los Amigos Levels of Cognitive Functioning (Table 7.4) is a multi-level scale of cognitive

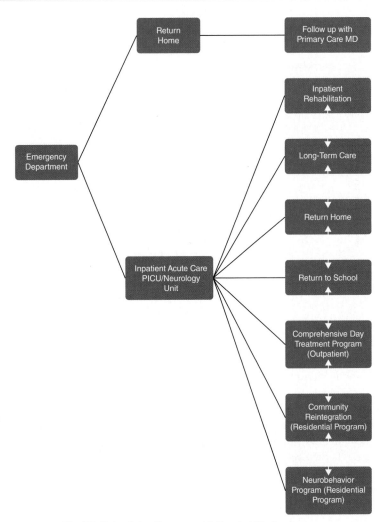

Fig. 7.3 Potential pathways a child's rehabilitation journey.

recovery developed by the professional staff of the Rancho Los Amigos Hospital in Downey, California.[3] This scale is used for assessment of recovery, communication between medical professionals and facilities, and measurement of change and progress during the rehabilitation course.

Additionally, outcome measures that may be appropriate for the pediatric patient with a TBI include measures that monitor hemodynamic responses to physical activity (blood pressure, heart rate, and respiratory rate), balance (pediatric Berg balance), postural stability (segmental assessment of trunk control), coordination (finger to target, heel to shin), gait (Timed Up and Go), and transitional movements (Timed Floor to Stand).

Physical Therapy Intervention

Based on this thorough examination, the PT completes the evaluation, synthesizing the data and making clinical judgments. A physical therapy diagnosis is then determined, in which the primary dysfunctions are identified and become the focus of direct interventions. Then the plan of care is created, through which the functional and measurable goals and expected outcomes are established in addition to any necessary referrals to other disciplines. It is of great importance to include in this process the goals of the family/caregivers and even the child, if appropriate, to promote their full participation in the recovery process.

A variety of treatment approaches exists for infants and children with brain injuries. Each patient should

Movement Continuum

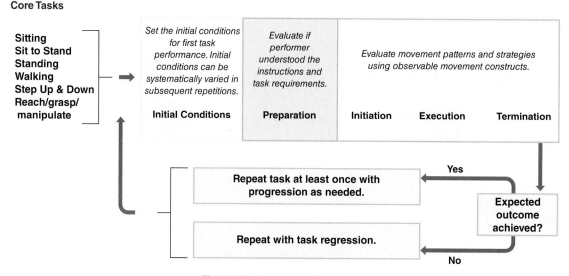

Fig. 7.4 The Movement Continuum.

have an individualized program created to address specific needs, inclusive of any cultural needs to make the most of the potential for recovery. Treatment planning should include addressing the identified primary and secondary impairments, with the ultimate goal of maximizing independence in mobility, self-care, and reintegration of the patient into their family, school, and community. Allowances must also be made for preinjury functional abilities, age, interests, and activities, especially in the case of school-aged children.

Primary impairments are atypical components of any individual system that contribute to abnormal or lack of movement (neuromuscular), neurobehavioral, or cognitive functioning and/or secondary impairments. These include insufficient force generation (i.e., strength), spasticity (velocity-dependent increased resistance to passive movement), abnormal extensibility/range of motion, dysautonomia (i.e., elevated sympathetic nervous system activity, increased heart rate, blood pressure, respiratory rate), and exaggerated or hyperactive reflexes. *Secondary impairments* are postures or movements observed during the performance of a task; these are compensatory due to the lack of the normal or adequate component. They include malalignment issues such as increased hip flexion, adduction and internal rotation with knee flexion, and ankle dorsiflexion during "crouch" gait patterns.[14] Additional complications and secondary impairments

include pressure injuries, decreased endurance/deconditioning, pneumonia, and contractures.

Once the primary and secondary impairments are identified, this knowledge can allow the PT to create and the physical therapist assistant [PTA] to execute effective interventions for treatment. Based on the Rancho Los Amigos Levels of Cognitive Functioning score, if appropriate, coma stimulation interventions can be initiated to promote increased arousal with modulation, increased attention and following of simple one-step commands, increased eye contact on request, and activation of trunk and extremity musculature with purpose and intention of movement. These therapeutic interventions can be progressed in difficulty and demand on the infant or child, depending on the patient's responses and ability to maintain an alert, modulated state while receiving auditory, visual, tactile, olfactory, and/or gustatory input. Providing a variety of sensory input, albeit one type of input at a time initially to avoid overstimulation, will assist in activating various centers within the brain, increasing arousal, and promoting the maximization of the neural plasticity potential of the damaged areas. Environmental modifications can also be made to ensure an infant or child does not experience overstimulation, especially during the early stages of coma recovery (Rancho Los Amigos Levels I–V). Limiting outside noises (television, radio, music), decreasing direct lighting, modulating

TABLE 7.3 Movement Systems Diagnosis

Movement Systems Diagnosis Descriptors Related to TBI

Movement System Diagnosis	Patient Subjective Reports	Key Signs
Movement Pattern Coordination Deficit	• Feels unsteady; possible fall • Fear of falling, clumsiness • Occasional falls • Delay in fine motor tasks • Overly messy when eating and dressing • Delay in walking • Awkward compared with peers • Poor performance in sports activities	Sit to stand • Altered sequence of movement components during execution (usually insufficient DF of leg over foot) • Posterior sway at ankle and may step at termination • Unlikely to require significant physical assistance Transitional movements and advanced motor skills • Altered sequence, instability, and lack of fluidity when executing transitional movements appropriate to age (or adjusted age) Gait • Variable foot placement or line of progression or may be guarded with slow, small steps • Assistance for balance • Ataxia with reciprocal movements
Force Production Deficits	• Increased need for caregiver assistance • Fatigue • History of prematurity Delay in acquisition of motor milestones appropriate for age	• Less than 3+/5–4/5 muscle strength throughout a limb or limbs or • Difficulty moving through full range against gravity or • Focal weakness at one primary joint or • Deterioration in range of motion/speed of movement with repetition Prone on elbows • Unable to maintain head at 90 degrees when age appropriate Floor to stand • Exhibits a + Gower sign or requires use of UEs via half kneel after age appropriate Sit to stand transition • Failure during initiation phase typically requiring assistance or accommodation • Extension of knees before hips during first half of execution Gait • May need manual assistance or a device to bear weight and maintain upright • Deviations are often significant • In severe forms will be unable to attempt ambulation

Continued

TABLE 7.3   Movement Systems Diagnosis—cont'd

Movement Systems Diagnosis Descriptors Related to TBI

Movement System Diagnosis	Patient Subjective Reports	Key Signs
Fractionated Movement Deficit	• Stiffness of the limbs and/or pain • History of hypoxia/ischemic event • Complicated perinatal history, (i.e., documented PVL, IVH)	Movement • Unable to fractionate movement • Slow; unable to make rapid reversals in movement • Unable to generate force rapidly Muscle Tone • Moderate or greater hyperexcitability • Grade 3 or 4 on the modified Ashworth Scale Reflexes • May exhibit previously integrated reflexes such as ATNR or STNR Pull to Sit • Neck hyperextension with shoulder elevation • May exhibit LE extension, adduction, and hip medial rotation (LE extensor pattern) Floor to Stand • Pulls up with UEs with LEs extended; unable to fractionate or dissociate LE movements Sit to stand • Slower movements • Stiff limbs • Lack of segmental joint mobility Creeping • May exhibit bunny hopping or commando crawling rather than assuming a 4-point position Gait • Compensatory movement strategy of hip hiking, vaulting, or circumduction to initiate swing of involved extremities • Stiffness of hip/knee flexion during swing • Scissoring • "Toe walking" or "equinus gait" • Hip and knee often flexed during stance of involved extremities • Likely to require AFO to control foot position for weight bearing • Likely to require assistive device at least early in course

TABLE 7.3 Movement Systems Diagnosis—cont'd

Movement Systems Diagnosis Descriptors Related to TBI

Movement System Diagnosis	Patient Subjective Reports	Key Signs
Postural Vertical Deficit	• Backward falls • Fear of falling • Visual or visual perceptual deficits	**Postural control** • Shifts center of mass beyond limits of stability to side or backward without weight acceptance • Resists correction or becomes fearful/agitated when center of mass alignment is corrected **Perception** • Sensation of "falling" when shifted toward correct vertical alignment • May have disregard or neglect of involved extremities **Behavior** • Impulsive • Poor judgment • Fear avoidance behavior such as clutching or grabbing with UE and shifting base of support **Motor Planning** • May have difficulty planning or organizing movement patterns into purposeful actions
Sensory Selection and Weighting Deficit	• Symptoms when riding in a car, when walking along patterned walkways, or in visually stimulating environments • Repetitive nonpurposeful movements • Impaired social behaviors • Aversion to a variety of sensory stimuli • Delayed acquisition of motor milestones appropriate for age	**Gait** • Deviation in line of progression to one or both sides • Instability with head turning **Turning** • Loss of balance or increased ankle or hip sway at termination • Worse with faster movement • Dizzy **Postural Control** • Able to stand unsupported but may require practice • Increased sway or instability with eyes closed or other change in sensory conditions • May demonstrate hip strategy during static standing tasks • Postural responses may be delayed or exaggerated; exaggerated responses lead to postural instability
Cognitive Deficit	• Lack of arousal • Lack of response to stimuli • Absent attention to examiner and situation • Absent ability to apply meaning to situation	**Movement:** • May demonstrate loss of spontaneous or voluntary movement • May be able to move against gravity but not in relationship to situational demands

Information excerpted from Scheets PL, Bloom NJ, Crowner B, et al. *Movement System Diagnoses: Neuromuscular Conditions. Description of Categories.* St Louis: Washington University; 2014. (permission needed from author –)

AFO, ankle-foot orthosis; *ATNR*, asymmetric tonic neck reflex; *DF*, dorsiflexion; *IVH*, intraventricular hemorrhage; *LE*, lower extremity; *PVL*, periventricular leukomalacia: *STNR*, symmetric tonic neck reflex; *UE*, upper extremity.

TABLE 7.4	**The Rancho Los Amigos Levels of Cognitive Functioning**
Levels of Recovery	**Description**
Level I	No Response—to pain, touch, sound, or sight
Level II	Generalized Response—to pain
Level III	Localized Response—Blinks to strong light, turns toward/away from sound, responds to physical discomfort, inconsistent response to commands
Level IV	Confused-Agitated—Alert, very active, aggressive or bizarre behaviors, performs motor activities but behavior is non-purposeful, extremely short attention span
Level V	Confused-Non-Agitated—Gross attention to environment, highly distractible, requires continual redirection, difficulty learning new tasks, agitated by too much stimulation. May engage in social conversations but with inappropriate verbalizations
Level VI	Confused-Appropriate—Inconsistent orientation to time and place, retention span/recent memory is impaired, begins to recall past, consistently follows simple directions, and goal-directed behavior with assistance
Level VII	Automatic-Appropriate—Performs daily routine in highly familiar environment in a non-confused but automatic, robotlike manner; skills noticeably deteriorate in unfamiliar environments. Lacks realistic planning for own future
Level VIII	Purposeful-Appropriate

Data from Rancho Los Amigos National Rehabilitation Center, Downey, California.

auditory input from staff and family members, and providing therapy in a small, quiet, stimulation-controlled environment are all helpful approaches.

Treatment sessions should be mindfully planned to consider the patient's learning capabilities, with practice structured accordingly. During the acute phase, a distributed practice schedule with frequent rest periods will allow for cognitive as well as physical rest. Physical and mental fatigue may lead to increased irritability and decreased engagement in the therapy session. Restoration of trunk and extremity strength, static and dynamic sitting and standing balance, and reeducation of developmental motor skills appropriate for the infant or child's age are vital treatment strategies for infants and children with brain injury. The restoration of motor functioning should include eliciting improved motor control, planning and sequencing skills, and addressing any sensory impairments such as decreased kinesthetic awareness and decreased proprioception. In an effort to promote the restoration of function, principles of neuroplasticity should be incorporated into each therapy session.[19,20] Sensory integration treatment can be implemented, if appropriate, including the use of swinging, swaddling, various textures for sensitization or desensitization, and garments (e.g., Benik vests, TheraTogs) or weighting of the trunk or extremities to increase kinesthetic awareness. Along with the use of compression garments to increase kinesthetic awareness, Kinesio taping and the use of wraps such as Fabrifoam are other available adjunctive treatment measures.

Treatment interventions should also address any truncal or extremity asymmetries caused by the brain injury or by limitations in strength, power, or endurance. In the case of an infant or child with hemiplegia, the resultant musculoskeletal deformities that can develop if appropriate treatment is not provided can be long-lasting and lead to more aggressive treatment requirements in the future (e.g., orthopedic surgery). As the child's functional and cognitive skills improve, providing more challenging cognitive tasks while performing more challenging motor tasks will test the child's ability to multitask using a variety of sensory inputs. The child will learn to process various, possibly conflicting, information while improving motor planning and sequencing and executive functioning skills.

When range-of-motion or flexibility concerns are present, a variety of treatment interventions can be implemented. Orthotics, splinting, knee immobilizers, and serial casting are available treatment interventions for range-of-motion impairments and can be used to prevent contractures.[6] Aquatic therapy interventions can also be very effective for the treatment of children with brain injury. However, if any hemodynamic or temperature abnormalities are present, aquatic therapy is contraindicated. For infants and children with more severe impairments, increasing tolerance to handling and sensory input, upright antigravity movement activities, and maintaining and improving range of motion for basic hygiene and functional tasks are appropriate interventions.

A task-oriented approach to interventions augments the neuroplasticity principles of salience, repetition, intensity, and specificity to promote motor control and learning in efforts to promote recovery of function. Body weight–supported gait training (both over ground and with a treadmill) as well as constraint-induced movement therapy (CIMT) have shown restorative potential.[21,22] Locomotor training with body weight support involves using a harness to off weight the client while the therapist provides assistance at the client's trunk and pelvis or lower extremities to promote advancement/stepping (Fig. 7.5).[22] Constraint-induced movement therapy has shown promising results for pediatric patients. Improvements have been shown to be maintained for more than 12 months after the conclusion of treatment. Constraint-induced movement therapy involves the patient wearing a mitten or removable arm cast on the uninvolved or less involved hand while completing functional tasks with the involved upper extremity for 3 to 4 weeks for multiple hours each day (Fig. 7.6).[23]

Depending on the appropriateness for each child, adaptive equipment can be utilized to augment functional mobility; it may be a temporary measure or provide modified independence for the future. Adaptive equipment includes walkers, crutches, canes, adaptive strollers, wheelchairs (both manual and powered mobility), standers, and gait trainers. The decision to utilize adaptive equipment should be based on the individual child's needs and potential abilities for recovery, with the goal of restoring the greatest level of independence, given functional mobility. In some instances, a wheelchair may be used temporarily to transport a child to and from the therapy gym until the child can ambulate the requisite distance with or without assistance and possesses the required endurance.

In addition to physical and sensory issues, physical therapy treatment may also have to incorporate strategies for modifying inappropriate behavior and emotional responses. Adaptations for cognitive delays and memory loss may also be an integral part of physical therapy.[18] Special education programs are well equipped to assist the child with community reintegration and cognitive therapy. In order to minimize objectionable behaviors and assist with

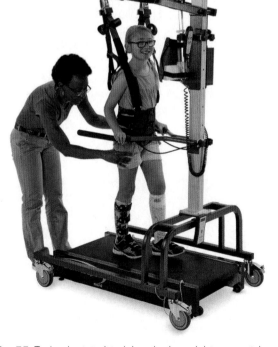

Fig. 7.5 Task-orientated training: body weight support locomotor training.

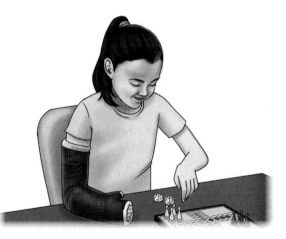

Fig. 7.6 Task-oriented training: CIMT.

regaining memory, therapy schedules, routines, and expectations and strategies should be consistent across disciplines. Rewards and consequences must be carefully and repeatedly explained and reinforced with the child. Clear, simple expectations explained in a cognitively appropriate manner will benefit children who have sustained a TBI. Schedules, personal identification, and family members' names should be written out for the child who can read. Older children and adolescents may benefit from a "helper book" or technology applications in a smartphone that can record all daily routines; important phone numbers; and lists of family, friends, and therapeutic/medical staff.[18] Some children may require picture charts and color organization to assist them in remembering important facts and routines. Regular periods of unrestricted physical activity will help the child release excessive energy and impulsivity. All adults should be behavioral role models so that the child's learned skills can be reinforced; positive reinforcement of acceptable behaviors is essential. Referral to a behavioral specialist may be required if behavioral disruptions persist.[6,18]

Involving family and caregivers in the recovery process is vital to the infant or child with a brain injury. Their ability to participate in the therapy sessions and to carry over the treatment interventions to the home environment, or during nontherapy times if a child is hospitalized, will exponentially influence and benefit the child's therapy process. It is the therapist's responsibility to include the family/caregivers and empower them to again feel as though they are effective caregivers for their infant or child with a brain injury (Box 7.2).

BOX 7.2   Traumatic Brain Injury Interventions

- Provide a variety of sensory input to assist in activating various centers within the brain
- Modify the environment to ensure the infant or child does not experience overstimulation
- Use orthotics, splints, knee immobilizers, and/or serial casting for range-of-motion limitations
- Augment functional mobility with adaptive devices and/or assistive technologies
- Incorporate strategies for modifying inappropriate behavior and emotional responses
- Involve family and caregivers in the recovery process

SUMMARY

Traumatic brain injuries in infants and children are very common and occur through a variety of mechanisms. The potential outcomes following brain injury are highly dependent on the severity and location of the actual injury. According to Hsia and colleagues,[24] at discharge, approximately 19% of those with mild brain injury exhibited neurologic sequelae, 94% of those with moderate brain injury exhibited neurologic sequelae, and 100% of those with severe brain injury exhibited neurologic sequelae. With effective early treatment, the functional abilities of these children can be highly improved. Treatment for TBI should focus on minimizing primary and secondary impairments, reintegrating the infant or child into the family unit as soon as possible, and providing the family/caregivers with effective methods for interacting with the child. All members of the interdisciplinary team should work together with the family/caregivers to facilitate the child's ability to return school and other preinjury activities.

CASE STUDY OF A CHILD WITH TRAUMATIC BRAIN INJURY

Examination

History

R.J. is a 6-year-old boy who fell from a playground jungle gym, striking his head on the ground, losing consciousness, and sustaining a TBI. On initial examination in the emergency department, R.J. was given a GCS score of 5. He was diagnosed with a left temporal subdural hematoma, a skull fracture, and a fractured left femur.

He was in the pediatric intensive care unit (PICU) for 2½ weeks following his injuries, during which time he was intubated for 3 days and then extubated without complication. R.J. underwent open reduction and internal fixation surgery for his left femur fracture, a procedure completed by the orthopedic surgeon. He had his intracranial pressure (ICP) monitored while in the PICU, and he underwent placement of a nasogastric tube for nutrition because of concerns about his ability to swallow effectively and safely. Physical therapy services were initiated in the PICU following the removal of the intracranial pressure bolt 8 days after his TBI. After 2½ weeks in the PICU, R.J. was transferred from the acute care pediatric hospital to a

CASE STUDY OF A CHILD WITH TRAUMATIC BRAIN INJURY—cont'd

small rehabilitation program within a specialized pediatric hospital.

He did not have a cast in place, but he was not to bear weight on the left lower extremity according to the recommendation of the orthopedic surgeon. This non-weight-bearing status was in place for 3 weeks, at which time he was seen for reevaluation by orthopedics, and his weight-bearing status was changed to weight-bearing as tolerated. R.J. had excellent callus formation of the left femur fracture during these 3 weeks.

R.J. lived at home with his mother and 4-year-old and 1-year-old sisters in a public housing project on the south side of a large metropolitan area. According to his mother, R.J. was developing typically until this accident and was not yet attending kindergarten, although she was planning on enrolling him in the fall. At the time of the initial evaluation, R.J.'s mother was able to identify several of his current limitations and stated three goals for his treatment:

1. R.J. will eat by mouth with assistance.
2. R.J. will walk with or without assistance.
3. R.J. will tell me what he needs by talking.

Review of Systems

On initial examination of R.J., the following items were noted:

1. R.J. responded to pain by grimacing.
2. R.J. was able to open his eyes on request in three of five attempts, but he was unable to make eye contact with the therapist. When R.J.'s eyes were open, he maintained his visual gaze to the left.
3. R.J. demonstrated an increased heart rate and respiratory rate when the therapist provided verbal or tactile input. He also began to yawn and make munching movements with his mouth.
4. R.J. was able to move his left upper extremity independently, but in a random, inconsistently purposeful fashion.
5. R.J. was able to move his left foot and ankle independently and tolerated gentle range of motion of his left knee and hip (as was approved by orthopedics).
6. R.J. was unable to move his right upper and lower extremity, except for inconsistent movement of his right hand, which was noted only twice.
7. R.J. was unable to independently perform any functional gross motor skills.
8. R.J. was unable to control his secretions.
9. R.J. was unable to vocalize.

At the time of admission to the inpatient rehabilitation program, referrals for occupational and speech therapy were written. It was recommended that R.J. receive these therapies to address feeding/swallowing, cognition, developmental skills, and activities of daily living.

Tests and Measures
Impairments

R.J. was noted to have a flaccid right upper and lower extremity, and his left upper extremity exhibited spontaneous movement, although not with consistent purpose. His left lower extremity exhibited movement at his foot and ankle, and he tolerated gentle range of motion of the left hip and knee joints. His muscle tone throughout his trunk was decreased significantly, as was tone in the right upper and lower extremities. Tone was decreased slightly in the left upper and lower extremities. He was unable to demonstrate upright head control and maintained his head in a position of left cervical spine lateral flexion and slight right cervical spine rotation. Hemodynamically, he displayed increases in his heart and respiratory rates when verbal and tactile input was provided, but his oxygen saturation remained stable throughout the examination. R.J. responded with a grimace to pain and was able to open his eyes on request in three of five attempts, but he was unable to make eye contact with the therapist. When his eyes were open, he maintained a strong left visual gaze.

Functional Limitations and Disability

R.J. was examined with the Rancho Los Amigos Levels of Cognitive Functioning to determine his current level of coma recovery during the initial evaluation. He was found to be at a Rancho Los Amigos level III, which is "localized response," indicating he turns away from/responds to sound, responds to physical discomfort, and exhibits inconsistent response to commands.

Diagnosis

On synthesis of the examination information, the following movement systems diagnoses were established: cognitive deficit and force production deficit. Additional physical therapy diagnoses determined for R.J. included impaired arousal, attention, and cognition; impaired motor functioning; impaired sensory integration; and impaired functional mobility.

Prognosis

Because of the severity of R.J.'s initial GCS score of 5 (indicating a severe brain injury) and his extensive left femur fracture, his overall prognosis for recovery of function was guarded. Because his injury occurred only 2½ weeks before his transfer to an inpatient rehabilitation program, it was thought he would have the possibility of some motor recovery but would likely have long-term cognitive impairments.

Continued

CASE STUDY OF A CHILD WITH TRAUMATIC BRAIN INJURY—cont'd

Plan of Care

R.J.'s length of stay in the intensive rehabilitation program was estimated at the time of the examination to be approximately 8 to 12 weeks to best maximize his potential for motor and cognitive recovery. The following goals and outcomes for physical therapy were determined:

Goals

1. R.J. will tolerate various types of stimulation for a period of 25 minutes without exhibiting signs of overstimulation or significant hemodynamic changes in order to begin integration into a simulated school setting.
2. R.J. will maintain independent sitting at the edge of the bed or bench for 5 minutes in order to participate in self-care activities.
3. R.J. will maintain lower extremity weight-bearing with assistance and least restrictive assistive device once cleared by orthopedics to perform weight bearing as tolerated (WBAT) in order to return to standing activities and initiate locomotion.
4. R.J. will use all extremities in play in order to participate in play with siblings and peers.
5. R.J. will complete an activity following a two-step direction in order to initiate return to age-appropriate interactions.

Outcomes

1. R.J. will participate in his daily care with modifications and assistance.
2. R.J.'s mother and other family members will increase their understanding of TBI and its effects, the anticipated goals, and the expected outcomes.
3. R.J. will participate in age-appropriate social interactions with modifications, as required.
4. R.J. will stand with assistance and ambulate short distances with or without an assistive device.

Intervention

R.J. received extensive physical therapy services in an inpatient rehabilitation program for 12 weeks, with physical therapy services delivered twice daily Monday through Friday, daily on Saturdays, and no therapies on Sundays. Intervention included weekly staffing/care conferences and multidisciplinary rounds, reintegration of R.J. into child life activities one to two times daily, and extensive family training.

The focus of treatment was on increasing modulated arousal, attention and focus, trunk and extremity muscle strengthening, postural stability, improving motor control of his extremities with functional play activities, and reestablishing mobility options. Because of his weight-bearing restrictions initially, no standing activities were done until the order was changed by the orthopedic surgeon to WBAT. Often, physical therapy sessions were in co-treatment with both occupational and speech therapy. R.J. responded well to the focus on increasing modulated arousal and attention and began to vocalize and communicate with single words, especially during movement activities. R.J. was evaluated for a customized pediatric manual wheelchair with tilt-in-space features and was also evaluated for specialized bath equipment, both of which were submitted to the insurance company for approval. He was also evaluated for and received bilateral ankle-foot orthoses (AFOs), which assisted in providing both knee and ankle/foot control during standing and ambulation activities and helped maintain his range of motion.

Outcomes

R.J. was discharged from the inpatient rehabilitation program after a 12-week stay. He was discharged home to his mother and then began attending a day rehabilitation program 5 days a week for 4 hours a day to continue his rehabilitation progress.

At the time of discharge, R.J. was able to independently roll from prone to supine, independently sit at the edge of a mat table or bench with upper extremity propping, transfer from sit to stand with moderate assistance, complete a stand-pivot transfer with minimal to moderate assistance, and ambulate 5 feet with moderate assistance and a posterior rolling walker. He exhibited antigravity movement of his right upper and lower extremity, although strength limitations persisted. He was able to tolerate increased environmental stimulation without exhibiting signs of overstimulation, although with increased environmental stimulation, R.J.'s attention to task would decrease significantly. Verbal cueing and redirection were required in those situations to assist R.J. to stay on task. He continued to exhibit increased impulsivity and decreased safety awareness, requiring direct supervision at all times when in his wheelchair. He was able to self-propel his wheelchair 150 to 200 feet with use of bilateral upper extremities for propulsion and was able to communicate his basic wants and needs. His mother and other family members stated they were very pleased with the progress he made while in the intensive in-patient rehabilitation program and were looking forward to future progress with the continuation of therapy services in the day rehabilitation setting.

CASE STUDY OF A CHILD WITH TRAUMATIC BRAIN INJURY—cont'd

Analysis of Case Using the ICF Model (At Discharge)
Body functions
Recovering from TBI, decreased strength in all extremities and trunk, decreased attention span, decreased cognitive processing

Activity limitations
Requires constant supervision and monitoring, limited ambulation and wheeled mobility skills, limited endurance

Participation restrictions
Decreased independence, limited ability to participate in age-appropriate community athletic activities, requires

wheeled mobility to participate in community events and family outings

Environmental factors
Required special-education learning environment, special recreation programming, calm and quiet environment for optimal interactions

Movement Systems Diagnosis at Discharge
R.J. continues to present with cognitive deficit with the need for a structured environment for optimal participation; his limited function in antigravity positions also led to an additional diagnosis of force production deficit.

CHAPTER DISCUSSION QUESTIONS

1. List three possible causes of TBI.
2. How are TBIs classified?
3. What are the possible effects on a child's long-term health and quality of life?
4. On the PGCS, as the scores increase in the motor response category, what does this indicate about the child's level of function?
5. If a person has a score of a 3 on the verbal skill portion of the GCS, what would you expect to see?
6. On your home health caseload, you receive a referral for a 12-year-old boy who has been at home for 3 days. He was an inpatient for 32 days, which included 15 days in the rehabilitation unit. He currently demonstrates the following abilities:
   - Propels a manual wheelchair with his feet
   - Responds inconsistently to yes and no questions
   - Cannot complete a two-step self-care–related task
   - Can walk 50 steps but cannot climb stairs to access his bedroom
   a. What is the classification on the Rancho Los Amigos Levels of Cognitive Functioning?
   b. What might be four challenges associated with direct care delivery? Give one strategy to overcome each challenge.

REFERENCES

1. Greenes DS, Madsen JR. Neurotrauma. In: Fleisher GR, Ludwig S, eds. *Textbook of Pediatric Emergency Medicine*. 4th ed. Philadelphia: Lippincott Williams & Wilkins; 2000.
2. Brain Injury Association of America. Incidence of brain injury in children. Accessed December 18, 2022. https://www.biausa.org/brain-injury/about-brain-injury/children-what-to-expect/incidence-of-brain-injury-in-children.
3. Centers for Disease Control and Prevention: TBI data. Updated April 24, 2023. Accessed December 15, 2023. https://www.cdc.gov/traumaticbraininjury/data/.
4. Araki T, Yokota H, Morita A. Pediatric traumatic brain injury: characteristic features, diagnosis, and management. *Neurol Med Chir (Tokyo)*. 2017;57(2):82–93.
5. Centers for Disease Control and Prevention. Report to Congress on the management of TBI in children. Updated January 22, 2016. https://www.cdc.gov/traumaticbraininjury/pubs/congress-childrentbi.html.
6. Schuchat A, Houry D, Baldwin G. Report to Congress. The management of traumatic brain injury in children: opportunities for action. Accessed December 22, 2022. https://www.cdc.gov/traumaticbraininjury/pdf/reportstocongress/managementoftbiinchildren/TBI-ReporttoCongress-508.pdf.
7. Haydel MJ, Weisbrod LJ, Saeed W. Pediatric head trauma. Updated November 12, 2022. In: Abai A, et al., eds. *StatPearls*. Treasure Island, FL: StatPearls Publishing; 2022.
8. Sarmiento K, Thomas KE, Daugherty J, et al. Emergency department visits for sports- and recreation-related traumatic brain injuries among children – United States, 2010-2016. *MMWR Morb Mortal Wkly Rep*. 2019;68(10):237–242.
9. Guler I, Buyukterzi M, Oner O, Tolu I. Post-traumatic leptomeningeal cyst in a child: computed tomography and magnetic resonance imaging findings. *J Emerg Med*. 2015;48(5): e121–e122.
10. McLaughlin M, Lisenby S, Sharma S. Pediatric rehabilitation: mild to moderate pediatric traumatic brain injury. Updated April 5, 2017. Accessed December 15, 2023. https://now.aapmr.org/mild-to-moderate-pediatric-traumatic-brain-injury/.

11. Bijur PE, Haslum M, Golding J. Cognitive and behavioral sequelae of mild head injury in children. *Pediatrics*. 1990;86(3):337.

12. Goya K, Hazarika A, Khandelwal A, et al. Non-neurological complications after traumatic brain injury: a prospective observational study. *Indian J Crit Care Med*. 2018;22(9):632–638.

13. Ostahowski PJ, Kannan N, Wainwright MS, et al. PEGASUS (Pediatric Guideline Adherence and Outcomes) Study: variation in seizure prophylaxis in severe pediatric traumatic brain injury. *J Neurosurg Pediatr*. 2016;18(4):499–506.

14. Safaz I, Alaca R, Yasar E, Tok F, Yilmaz B. Medical complications, physical function and communication skills in patients with traumatic brain injury: a single centre 5-year experience. *Brain Inj*. 2008;22(10):733–739.

15. Hurvitz EA, Mandac BR, Davidoff G, et al. Risk factors for heterotopic ossification in children and adolescents with severe traumatic brain injury. *Arch Phys Med Rehabil*. 1992;73:459.

16. Simonsen L, Sonne-Holm S, Krasheninnikoff M, Engberg AW. Symptomatic heterotopic ossification after very severe traumatic brain injury in 114 patients: incidence and risk factors. *Injury*. 2007;38(10):1146–1150.

17. Allison KM, Turkstra LS. Navigating medical speech-language pathology reports for children with TBI. *Perspectives on School-Based Issues*. 2012;13(3):63–69.

18. Greene RK, Rich-Wimmer N, Williams CN, Hall TA. Social functioning and autistic behaviors in youth following acquired brain injury. *Children*. 2022;9(11):1648.

19. Quinn L, Riley N, Tyrell CM, et al. A framework for movement analysis of tasks: recommendations from the Academy of Neurologic Physical Therapy's Movement System Task Force. *Phy Ther*. 2021;101(9):101–108.

20. Kleim JA, Jones TA. Principles of experience-dependent neural plasticity: implications for rehabilitation after brain damage. *J Speech Lang Hear Res*. 2008;51(1):S225–S239.

21. Burnfield JM, Cesa GM, Buster TW. Feasibility of motor-assisted elliptical to improve walking, fitness and balance following pediatric acquired brain injury: a case series. J Pediatr Rehabil Med. 2021;14(3):539–551.

22. Peri E, Panzeri D, Beretta E, Reni G, Strazzer S, Biffi E. Motor improvement in adolescents affected by ataxia secondary to acquired brain injury: a pilot study. *BioMed Research Int*. 2019;2019:8967138.

23. Malone LA, Felling RA. Pediatric stroke: unique implications of the immature brain on injury and recovery. *Pediatr Neurol*. 2020;102:3–9.

24. Hsia RY, Mannix RC, Guo J, et al. Revisits, readmissions, and outcomes for pediatric traumatic brain injury in California, 2005–2014. *PLoS One*. 2020;15(1):e0227981.

RESOURCES

Brain Injury Association of America
(Support groups can be found on the BIA website)
www.biausa.org

Centre for Neuro Skills Website
(Go to the "TBI Bookstore" on neuroskills.com for all the latest texts for professionals)
www.neuroskills.com

National Resource Center for Traumatic Brain Injury
www.neuro.pmv.vcu.edu

Traumatic Brain Injury National Data Center (TBINDC)
www.tbindc.org

Shaken Baby Syndrome
Coping With Mild Traumatic Brain Injury, by Diane Stole
Brainlash, 2nd ed., by Gail Denton
Over My Head by Claudia Osborn
I'll Carry the Fork! by Kara Swanson
Where Is the Mango Princess? by Cathy Crimmins
A Winner in Every Way by Jewel Claude Allen
Neurological Rehabilitation, 5th ed., by Darcy Umphred
Dizziness and Balance Disorders, edited by I. Kaufman Arenberg
Traumatic Brain Injury Rehabilitation, 2nd ed., edited by Mark J. Ashley and David K. Krych

Rheumatic Disorders

Yasser Salem, PT, PhD, MS, NCS, PCS
Howe Liu, PT, PhD, MD, FGSA

LEARNING OBJECTIVES

At the end of the chapter, the reader will be able to do the following:

1. Identify the different types of juvenile arthritis.
2. Identify intervention techniques for juvenile arthritis.
3. Identify appropriate long- and short-term treatment objectives.

CHAPTER OUTLINE

KEY TERMS

Autoimmune disease
Iridocyclitis
Joint inflammation
Micrognathia

Pauciarticular juvenile
  rheumatoid arthritis
Polyarticular juvenile rheumatoid
  arthritis

Scleroderma
Systemic juvenile rheumatoid
  arthritis

DEFINITION

Juvenile rheumatoid arthritis (JRA) is the most common rheumatic disease in childhood. The annual incidence rate of JRA in the United States is 7.4 cases per 100,000 children. It is a disorder causing joint inflammation and stiffness for more than 6 weeks in children younger than 16 years (Fig. 8.1). It is estimated that between 30,000 and 50,000 children in the United States have JRA, making it the most common rheumatic disorder among this age group.[1] Incidence of JRA has two distinct peaks: early onset with the symptoms developing between the ages of 1 and 3 years and early adolescence with the symptoms developing in the early teenage years.

PATHOLOGY

Like adult rheumatoid arthritis, JRA is an autoimmune disease in that the body mistakenly identifies some of its own cells and tissues as foreign.[2] The immune system, which normally helps to fight off harmful invaders such as bacteria or viruses, begins to attack healthy tissues. The

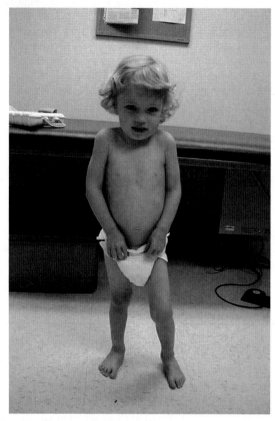

Fig. 8.1 A 2-year-old girl with arthritis of the left knee. (From Zitelli BJ, Davis HW. *Atlas of Pediatric Physical Diagnosis*. 5th ed. Philadelphia: Mosby, 2007.)

TABLE 8.1 **Rheumatic Disorders: Clinical Signs**
Pauciarticular JRA • Affects four or fewer joints • Affects large joints, most commonly the knees • Risk for iridocyclitis in subtype 1 • Affects five times as many girls as boys
Polyarticular JRA • Affects five or more joints • Affects both large joints and smaller joints • Often affects the same joint on both sides of the body • RF antibodies in subtype 1 • Affects three times as many girls as boys
Systemic JRA • High-spiking fevers • Rash on chest and thighs • Joint involvement • Internal organs can be affected • Affects girls and boys in equal numbers

JRA, juvenile rheumatoid arthritis; RF, rheumatoid factor.

result is inflammation marked by redness, heat, pain, and swelling.[2] The cause of JRA varies, and in many cases, it is unknown. It is unclear what causes the immune system to malfunction, but genetic factors and viruses have been suggested to play a role. Viral or bacterial infections are commonly seen before disease onset.

CLINICAL SIGNS

There are three types of JRA: pauciarticular, polyarticular, and systemic (Table 8.1). The type of JRA is determined and a diagnosis is made within the first 6 months of onset of symptoms.

Pauciarticular JRA

Pauciarticular JRA is the most common type and affects four or fewer joints. Pauciarticular JRA is also known as *oligoarthritis*. This type of JRA is five times more prevalent among girls than boys and is the most common JRA form, seen in about half of all children diagnosed with JRA. There are two subtypes of pauciarticular JRA:

• First subtype: Children test positive for antinuclear antibodies and have a high risk for iridocyclitis (inflammation of the eye). This subtype mainly affects young girls.
• Second subtype: It affects the spine, although possibly not until the late teens, and children may test positive for the gene identified with adult ankylosing spondylitis (rheumatoid arthritis of the adult spine). This subtype mainly affects older boys.

Pauciarticular disease usually affects large joints, most commonly the hips and knees (Fig. 8.2). It is typically asymmetric and may result in a discrepancy in leg length. Involvement of other parts of the body is unusual, with the exception of the eyes. About 20% of children affected with pauciarticular JRA also develop eye disease. While many of the children with pauciarticular disease outgrow arthritis by adulthood, eye

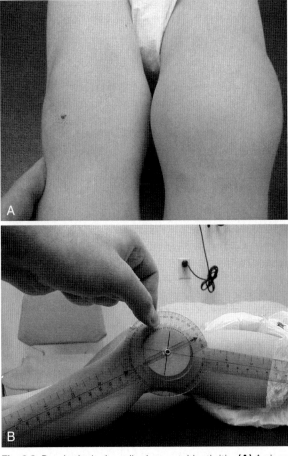

Fig. 8.2 Pauciarticular juvenile rheumatoid arthritis. **(A)** A close look at this child's knees reveals left knee swelling. **(B)** The left knee can only be extended to 35 degrees (secondary to a flexion contracture). (From Zitelli BJ, Davis HW. *Atlas of Pediatric Physical Diagnosis*. 5th ed. Philadelphia: Mosby, 2007.)

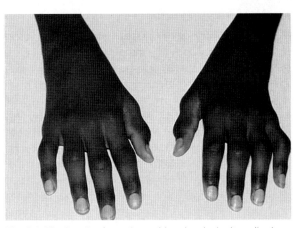

Fig. 8.3 The hands of a patient with polyarticular juvenile rheumatoid arthritis. Note the inability to fully extend the fingers. (From Zitelli BJ, Davis HW. *Atlas of Pediatric Physical Diagnosis*. 5th ed. Philadelphia: Mosby, 2007.)

problems can continue, and joint symptoms may recur in some people.

Certain children with pauciarticular JRA have special proteins in the blood called *antinuclear antibodies*. Up to 80% of those with eye disease also test positive for antinuclear antibodies, and the disease tends to develop at an earlier age in these children. To prevent serious vision and eye problems, regular eye examinations are imperative.

Polyarticular JRA

Polyarticular JRA affects about one-third of all children with JRA, with three times more girls than boys affected. In this type of JRA, five or more joints are involved. The arthritis typically involves large joints, such as knees, wrists, elbows, and ankles; however, it also affects the smaller joints of the hands and feet (Fig. 8.3). The cervical spine and temporomandibular joint may also be affected. Polyarticular JRA is often symmetric, affecting the same joint on both sides of the body. There are two subtypes of polyarticular JRA. In the first subtype, children possess a special kind of serum antibody known as *rheumatoid factor* (RF) and often have a more severe form of JRA. In the second subtype, children only experience joint involvement, which is potentially less severe than the first subtype.

Systemic JRA

The third type of JRA is known as systemic JRA. This type of JRA is characterized by high-spiking fevers off and on for weeks and a distinctive rash on the chest and thighs. Systemic JRA is also known as *Still's disease* and accounts for about 20% of cases of JRA. It is seen equally in boys and girls. Joint and muscle pain are common. A red rash over the trunk and extremities may be present. In addition to joint involvement, internal organs such as the heart, liver, spleen, and lymph nodes can be affected.

SECONDARY FACTORS

Regardless of the type, there are several secondary factors associated with JRA. Skeletal Abnormalities and opthalmic considerations are most common and will be discussed in more detail in this text.

Skeletal Abnormalities

Skeletal abnormalities may be seen in the extremity joints, spine, or jaw. Chronic hyperemia (excess blood flow) in an inflamed joint can stimulate accelerated maturation of the epiphyseal plates, which leads to skeletal overgrowth in the affected extremity. This overgrowth can result in a leg-length deformity, particularly in children with symmetric joint involvement. Associated lower-extremity involvement includes joint stiffness and limitations in hip flexion, hip abduction, and hip rotation as a result of iliopsoas and adductor spasms. Additionally, a valgus deformity in the knee may lead to resultant valgus of the hindfoot and varus of the forefoot.

In the jaw, micrognathia (abnormally small jaw), mandibular underdevelopment, and malocclusion are often related to JRA. These conditions may lead to issues in oral care and oral motor function.

In the spine, apophyseal joint disease is associated with poor development of the vertebrae and eventual fusing of the involved vertebrae. Early signs of polyarticular JRA are pain and stiffness in the cervical spine with a rapid loss of extension and rotation movements. Scoliosis is also a related pathology in children with JRA.

Ophthalmic Considerations

Regardless of the type of JRA, all children with JRA need to be followed up by an ophthalmologist for eye involvement and uveitis, also known as *iridocyclitis*, which is an inflammation of the iris and ciliary body. Children must also be followed up closely for proper nutrition to ensure that they are receiving appropriate caloric intake. Children with JRA may also have anemia. Either poor nutrition or anemia may cause increased fatigue, so children with JRA should be closely monitored for both.

INTERVENTION

Therapeutic interventions for children with JRA include a multidisciplinary team approach.[2,3] The team should include the family, a pediatric rheumatologist, pediatrician, physical therapist, occupational therapist, speech therapist, nutritionist, ophthalmologist, social worker, recreational therapist, nurses, pharmacist, and educators. All team members may not be involved in every case, however. The primary goals of treatment for JRA include relieving pain, reducing swelling, maintaining

TABLE 8.2 **Medications Used to Treat JRA**	
Drug Category	**Examples**
Nonsteroidal anti-inflammatory drugs	Ibuprofen
	Naproxen
Disease-modifying antirheumatic drugs	Gold
	Hydroxychloroquine
	Sulfasalazine
	D-penicillamine
	Methotrexate
Biologic response modifier	Etanercept
Corticosteroids	Prednisone

movement and joint mobility, and slowing the progression of the disease.

Some of the medications used to treat adult rheumatoid arthritis are used to treat JRA as well. Children may respond differently to drugs than their adult counterparts, and dosage adjustments are necessary, based on the age and weight of the child. Medications used in treating JRA can be broken into four categories (Table 8.2). Nonsteroidal anti-inflammatory drugs (NSAIDs) are the drugs of choice for treating children with JRA. Disease-modifying antirheumatic drugs (DMARDs) may be prescribed if NSAIDs fail to adequately relieve symptoms. DMARDs can slow the progression of JRA, but because they may take weeks or months to alleviate symptoms, they are often used in conjunction with an NSAID. Methotrexate is a DMARD prescribed for some children with JRA whose symptoms are not relieved by other medications. Small doses of this medication are used to relieve the arthritis symptoms. Etanercept is a biologic response modifier that works by blocking the action of tumor necrosis factor, an inflammation-promoting substance produced by the body. Etanercept is used to treat children with polyarticular JRA who have not responded sufficiently to other drug therapies. In children with very severe JRA, corticosteroids such as prednisone may be added to the treatment plan to control the child's symptoms. However, corticosteroids can interfere with a child's normal growth and cause weakened bones. Intraarticular cortisone may be used to control symptoms in individual joints. Once the medication successfully controls the more severe symptoms, the physician may reduce the dose gradually and eventually stop administering it completely.

Physical therapy interventions are important to the overall care and well-being of the child with JRA.[3]

Typically physical therapy interventions focus on pain relief, maintaining and regaining passive and active range of motion (ROM), maintaining and increasing strength and endurance, preventing secondary disorders such as deformities, improving the child's mobility and independent functioning, educating the child and family about the musculoskeletal effects of the pathology processes and secondary damage from the medications, and increasing community awareness of JRA. This may include a visit to the child's daycare center or school to provide information about the disease and any assists or precautions that may be needed for the child.

Physical therapy examination and ongoing assessment are vital for guiding the treatment of a child with JRA. Physical therapy evaluation/assessments include taking a health history, a systems review, and a hands-on physical examination. Examination of the following is of great importance:

- Pain
- Joint motion and flexibility
- Posture and body alignment
- Muscle strength and the ability to move against gravity
- Movement (motor) and functional abilities, such as floor mobility, rolling, sitting, walking, climbing, running, jumping, and transferring from a chair, car, or bed
- Endurance and fitness
- Balance
- Breathing function
- Ability to take part in activities with family and friends
- Quality of life

Physical therapy intervention for children with JRA may include activities to:

Prevent or slow the progression of muscle shortening (tightness), stiffness, and joint deformities: Intervention includes positioning, specific flexibility, and ROM exercises and recommendation for braces or splints to reshape deformed limbs or joints.

Strengthen muscles and maintain aerobic fitness: This includes strengthening exercise particularly functional strength training by focusing on functional activities.

Manage deformities and musculoskeletal problems: This includes keeping the limbs, spine, and body supported and aligned during sleep and daily activities.

Treatment may include positioning, specific flexibility and range-of-motion exercises, strengthening exercises, and recommendation for braces or splints to reshape deformed limbs or joints.

Manage fatigue, decreased fitness, and breathing complications: Intervention includes activities to improve aerobic fitness to help the child to move and stay as active as possible. Aerobic training activities may include walking, jogging, and swimming. Respiratory exercise training may be used and may include core and breathing exercises.

Maintain and improve overall movement and function: This includes improving developmental and functional skills in infants and children.

Select and use assistive devices: Therapists work with other healthcare specialists to select and modify appropriate devices to meet each person's specific needs. Therapists teach the child and caregivers how to safely use assistive devices. Assistive devices to support positioning and movement may include customized seating systems and walking devices such as canes and crutches.

Patient and family education: This may include educating the child and family about the disease process and progression and management of symptoms and home exercise programs.

Other interventions: This may include modalities such as application of cold packs or hot packs and aquatic exercise. The physical properties of water such as buoyancy are used to reduce the risk of fatigue or overworked muscles. The buoyancy and decreased gravity in water reduce weight-bearing, reducing joint stress during exercise and allowing children with JRA to move, stand, and walk more easily than they can on land.

OTHER RHEUMATIC DISEASES

In addition to JRA, several other rheumatic diseases affect children. Scleroderma is a connective tissue disease involving the skin, blood vessels, and immune system. Scleroderma is also known as *systemic sclerosis*. In its systemic form, internal organ involvement can occur. Scleroderma translates as "hard skin," and nearly everyone with the disease experiences hardening and tightening of the skin. The disorder is thought to be driven by a local inflammatory/immune response. The disease is most likely caused by a combination of many factors including genetics, dysfunction of the immune system, and environmental triggers such as exposure to certain viruses or medications. Thickening and tightening of the skin typically occur first in the hands and feet and possibly the face; the limbs, chest, and abdomen may also be affected. Thickening and tightening of the skin occur from a buildup of collagen and other natural skin proteins. Collagen, a fibrous protein made by cells, provides firmness to the skin, forms the lining of organs, and is the basic structural protein in bones, tendons, ligaments, and joints.

It is believed there are thousands of cases of juvenile scleroderma worldwide. Because it is likely that juvenile scleroderma is commonly undiagnosed or misdiagnosed, the number of children affected may be greater than suspected. There are two types of scleroderma: localized and systemic.

Localized scleroderma does not normally involve internal body systems but may affect joints, the nervous system, and the eyes. The localized type is much more common in children than adults. Children with localized scleroderma may display different types of skin involvement known as *linear morphea* or *general morphea*. Morphea is characterized by patches of thickened, waxy, ivory, or yellow-white shiny skin. Linear morphea describes markings in which the affected skin forms a line pattern down an arm or a leg. In this case, the morphea changes the skin and can interfere with the growth of a limb. Generalized morphea occurs when the lesions of morphea and linear morphea involve almost all of the skin. A distinct type of localized scleroderma is called *en coup de sabre*. In this condition, there is an indentation on the forehead or at the frontal hairline. The area of thickened skin can spread to the entire face. Atrophy of the lower part of the face is known as *Parry-Romberg syndrome*. There is no known treatment to stop the progression of atrophy. The prognosis varies; in some cases, it is limited to a cosmetic issue, whereas in other cases, the atrophy may stop before involving the entire face.[4]

Systemic juvenile scleroderma involves the internal organs and occurs less often in children than the localized version. There are two types of systemic juvenile scleroderma: limited and diffuse. The limited type is characterized by later involvement of the internal organs. It is also known as *CREST syndrome*, denoting areas of involvement (Box 8.1).

BOX 8.1   CREST

Calcinosis (calcium deposits in the skin)
Raynaud phenomenon (fingers and toes turn white, blue, red in response to cold temperatures or stress)
Esophageal dysmotility (frequent heartburn and difficulty swallowing)
Sclerodactyly (thickening of the skin of the fingers, causing contractures into flexion)
Telangiectasias (areas of red, prominent blood vessels in the skin)

Diffuse juvenile scleroderma is characterized by general skin involvement and early internal organ involvement, especially of the lungs and gastrointestinal system. This results in potential esophageal dysmotility, poor food absorption, and constipation. Additionally, Raynaud phenomenon (localized ischemia) is very common. Raynaud phenomenon results from exaggerated contraction of the small blood vessels in the fingers and toes in response to cold or emotional stress. Raynaud phenomenon involves changes to skin color of the fingers and toes to white, red, or blue. Involvement of the heart, kidneys, muscles, and joints also occurs. In any case, it is important to remember that localized juvenile scleroderma does not overlap with systemic scleroderma.

There is no known cause or cure for juvenile scleroderma. Few patients are treated at individual centers, which limits well-controlled studies. Treatment of the disease remains a dilemma, especially when determining which children should receive treatment and how the treatment should be monitored. The impact of a chronic illness on a growing child is very different from the impact of a similar disease on an adult. Children affected by scleroderma require the care of experienced pediatricians who are willing to use a skilled and coordinated approach.

Physical therapy interventions are designed to reduce pain and stiffness and prevent the development of secondary disorders such as deformities. Physical therapy interventions include managing pain, reducing joint and soft tissue inflammation, and facilitating muscle activation and movement to ensure that the child can safely perform activities of daily living (ADLs) and participate in age-appropriate activities as much as possible.

CASE STUDY OF A CHILD WITH A RHEUMATIC DISORDER

Examination

History

General demographics: Christopher is an 11-year-old Hispanic boy who is bilingual. He attends 5th grade at his neighborhood parochial school.

Social: Chris lives with his mother, father, and two younger siblings. He enjoys swimming, diving, and building things. His large extended family lives nearby and helps with child care. Chris's family travels extensively during the summer.

Growth and development: Chris is right-hand dominant. Although shorter than average in stature, he was healthy until recently. He achieved all developmental milestones at the appropriate time.

General health: Chris has been generally healthy. He had a virus 3 to 4 months ago, which may be related to current concerns.

Family history: There is no family history of JRA.

Medical history: Chris has not had any previous hospitalizations or operations.

History of current condition: Chris's mother reports he had a virus 3 to 4 months ago. On recovery, Chris complained of pain and stiffness in his joints. His physician ordered blood work and subsequently diagnosed polyarticular JRA.

Functional status and activity level: Chris had difficulty ambulating during a recent exacerbation of JRA. He also had difficulty performing ADLs. (See Tests and Measures for more detailed information.)

Medications: NSAIDs.

Lab and diagnostic tests: Blood test positive for Rh factor.

Systems Review

Cardiovascular/pulmonary: Normal
  Integumentary: See Tests and Measures
  Musculoskeletal: See Tests and Measures
  Neuromuscular: See Tests and Measures
Communication and cognition: Chris speaks fluent English and Spanish. He is studying Japanese at school. His cognition appears to be typical of a 5th grader. He does well in school and does not require additional assistance.

Tests and Measures

Endurance: Chris's endurance is within normal limits. He doesn't complain of fatigue at this point.

Anthropometric characteristics: Chris has relatively short stature for a boy his age. He has moderate bilateral swelling in his knees; wrists; and fingers 2, 3, and 4.

Assistive/adaptive devices: Chris uses a button holer and shoehorn as necessary.

Nerve integrity: All nerves are intact.

Environmental barriers: If in pain, Chris has difficulty climbing stairs. In his house there is a staircase leading to the basement.

Gait, locomotion, and balance: Chris's gait is affected by his decreased ROM. He demonstrated decreased knee extension bilaterally and diminished lateral weight shift as well. He prefers a slower cadence. His dynamic balance reactions of the lower extremities are diminished.

Integumentary: There is increased warmth and redness bilaterally in Chris's knees; wrists; and fingers 2, 3, 4.

Muscle performance

Strength: All ranges within functional limits (WFL) except:
  Bilateral knee extension: 3/5
  Bilateral knee flexion: 3/5
  Bilateral wrist flexion: 3/5
  Bilateral wrist extension: 3/5
  Bilateral radial deviation: 3/5
  Bilateral ulnar deviation: 3/5
  Bilateral grip strength: 3/5

ADLs: Prior to the current episode, Chris was independent in all instrumental ADLs and ADLs. At this time, he requires assistance with buttons and donning and doffing his shoes and socks.

Pain: Chris reports moderate to severe pain and stiffness in bilateral knees, wrists, and fingers. This may be a limiting factor in his strength testing.

Posture: Chris's postural alignment is good, and no asymmetries are noted at this time. He has slightly winging scapulae bilaterally.

ROM: All ranges within normal limits except:

Knee extension: Right -15 degrees; left -10 degrees

Knee flexion: Right -120 degrees; left -130 degrees

Wrist flexion: Right 75 degrees; left 60 degrees

Wrist extension: 0 degrees bilaterally

Wrist radial deviation: 5 degrees

Wrist ulnar deviation: 5 degrees

Finger #2: Flexion: Metacarpophalangeal joint (MCP) 15 Extension: MCP -5 right -10 left

Finger #3: Flexion: MCP 15 Extension MCP -5 right -10 left

Finger #4: Flexion MCP 15 Extension MCP -5 right -10 left

Evaluation

Christopher is an 11-year-old boy with new onset of polyarticular JRA. Joint involvement includes bilateral knees, wrists, and fingers. He is reporting pain and stiffness in these joints. He has noticeable swelling and tenderness in these joints as well. At this time, Chris is having difficulty with his ADLs and ambulation.

Continued

CASE STUDY OF A CHILD WITH A RHEUMATIC DISORDER—cont'd

Prognosis

Chris should demonstrate optimal joint mobility, ROM, and independence in ADLs.[2] He and his family will also learn how to manage his care to include pain management, joint protection, and energy conservation techniques. Expected number of visits: 18 over a 6-week period.

Interventions

Coordination, Communication, Documentation

Coordination will need to occur among Chris's teachers, pediatrician, rheumatology team, and family. At this time, he does not require any academic modifications. Communication between service providers will need to be consistent. Additionally, Chris's teachers will need to be aware of joint protection strategies and exercise/activity precautions. Chris has been given accommodations at school as needed. The family has not applied for 504 accommodations. Chris and his family will need to be in communication with the rheumatology team regarding changes in pain, swelling, and activity level.

Patient Instruction

Chris and his family received a written home exercise program (HEP) and also a recorded video of his HEP. The HEP included directions on how to gently and safely complete ROM and strength activities, energy conservation activities (don't let Chris become fatigued, provide frequent rest periods, have Chris use backpack or cart with wheels to move heavy objects), joint protection strategies (no hyperextension, proper body mechanics for bending and lifting), and pain management strategies (self-calming and visualization, medication if needed, heat at home as needed).

Direct Intervention

Therapeutic exercise: Chris's physical therapy program consisted of passive ROM (PROM) initially. As his pain symptoms subsided, ROM was advanced to include active assisted ROM and active ROM. Chris was also given a low-impact exercise program. Chris enrolled in a weekly aquatics program at the local hospital's therapeutic pool. At the pool group, he also met other children with arthritis.

Functional training: Chris learned about joint protection strategies and energy conservation techniques. He received a video of himself performing his exercise and stretching program, as well as performing activities using joint protection strategies.

Physical agents: To decrease stiffness, Chris's program included hot packs for his knees and fluidotherapy for his upper extremities. The family purchased a paraffin unit for home use.

Goals

1. Chris's ROM will return to the normal range so that he can dress himself.
2. Chris's pain will decrease so that he can play with his friends.
3. Chris and his family will learn his HEP so that he can stay healthy.
4. Chris's strength will return to normal so that he can participate in age-appropriate activities.
5. Chris will have an optometry evaluation.
6. Chris will be independent in performing his home program so that he can maintain his ROM and strength.

Re-Examination

Chris will return to rheumatology clinic in 6 weeks for a follow-up examination.

Analysis of Case Using the ICF Model

Body functions: Polyarticular JRA affecting bilateral knees, wrists, and fingers. Pain and swelling in these joints. Loss of ROM bilaterally in knees, wrists, and fingers.

Activity limitations: Decreased ambulation, decreased independence in ADLs and instrumental ADLs, decreased fine and gross motor skills.

Participation restrictions: Cannot ride on skateboard, cannot participate in age-appropriate sports as desired, difficulty changing into gym clothes at school, difficulty carrying books and supplies at school.

Environmental factors: Use backpack with wheels to manage books and schoolwork, wear gym clothes under school uniform/clothes to ease donning/doffing of gym uniform at school, add modalities to home environment.

Analysis of Case Using the Movement System Analysis

Christopher exhibits the following movement deficits: fractionated movement deficit, force production deficit.

CHAPTER DISCUSSION QUESTIONS

1. What is the disease process that causes JRA?
2. Compare and contrast pauciarticular JRA, polyarticular JRA, and systemic JRA.

	Pauciarticular	Polyarticular	Systemic
Subtypes			
Joints involved			
Gender prevalence			

3. Why is it important for a child with JRA to be followed up by an ophthalmologist?
4. What are the four medication categories for children with JRA?
5. What are the general physical therapy intervention goals for children with JRA?
6. What is CREST syndrome, and what pathology is associated with it?
7. Compare and contrast localized and systemic scleroderma.
8. What is the translation for *scleroderma*?

REFERENCES

1. Kumar N, Ramphul K, Ramphul Y, et al. Children hospitalized for juvenile arthritis in the United States. *Reumatologia*. 2021;59(4):270–272.
2. Bosques G, Singh MP. Juvenile idiopathic arthritis. Updated July 28, 2020. Accessed June 16, 2022. https://now.aapmr.org/juvenile-idiopathic-arthritis/.
3. Kuntze G, Nesbitt C, Whittaker JL, et al. Exercise therapy in juvenile idiopathic arthritis: a systematic review and meta-analysis. *Arch Phys Med Rehabil*. 2018;99(1):178–193.e1.
4. Adrovic A, Sahin S, Barut K, Kasapcopur O. Juvenile scleroderma-what has changed in the meantime? *Curr Rheumatol Rev*. 2018;14(3):219–225.

RESOURCES

Arthritis Foundation
https://www.arthritis.org/juvenile-arthritis.
Juvenile Arthritis Research
https://www.jarproject.org/about-jia?gclid=Cj0KCQjwn4qWBhCvARIsAFNAMigaB9G4o0dPaWLe_Sd9yq6OLSLzq8QjTr7N8NFOV1rJIcMGqs6XKOwaApHFEALw_wcB.
Arthritis Foundation
https://www.arthritis.org/diseases/juvenile-scleroderma.
American College of Rheumatology
https://www.rheumatology.org/I-Am-A/Patient-Caregiver/Diseases-Conditions/Localized-Scleroderma-Juvenile.

Congenital Muscular Torticollis

Margaret Mizera, PT, DPT, PCS

LEARNING OBJECTIVES

At the end of the chapter, the reader should be able to do the following:

1. Identify the three types of congenital muscular torticollis (CMT).
2. Recognize health and environmental risk factors for CMT.
3. Understand the impact of the Back to Sleep program on infant mortality, as well as on muscle development, cranial symmetry, and motor skill acquisition.
4. Recognize co-existing diagnoses, including the three types of cranial deformity.
5. Understand the unique multisystem examination of the infant with CMT.
6. Understand the severity grades for CMT and their implications for prognosis and duration of treatment.
7. Identify the five evidence-based interventions for CMT.
8. Identify reasons to refer a patient back to the physician and alternative strategies and interventions for an infant with more severe CMT.
9. Understand reasons and timelines for reassessment after discontinuation of direct physical therapy services.

CHAPTER OUTLINE

KEY TERMS

Asymmetry
Brachycephaly

Cranial deformation
Plagiocephaly

Scaphocephaly

CMT is a musculoskeletal condition in infants that involves shortening of a unilateral sternocleidomastoid muscle (SCM). Studies show it is present in 3.9% to 16% of infants,[1,2] making it the third most common congenital defect in infants. Incidence is higher in boys. It can occur in isolation or as part of other congenital syndromes and deformities.

CLINICAL SIGNS

CMT is detected at birth or within the first few months of life. The infant with CMT presents with lateral neck flexion on the shortened SCM side and rotation to the opposite side. There are three types of CMT[3]:

1. Postural, in which there is asymmetric posturing but no loss of range of motion (ROM)
2. Muscular, in which there is shortening of the muscle and loss of passive neck ROM
3. Sternocleidomastoid mass, in which an actual mass is present in the SCM (Fig. 9.1)

Infants younger than 1 year should have 100 to 110 degrees of cervical rotation and 65 or more degrees of lateral flexion.[4] Any loss of ROM or asymmetry of posturing can result in adaptive changes in the superficial and deep muscles of the neck as well as in the skeletal alignment of the cervical and thoracic spine and extremities, if untreated. These changes can affect motor development, feeding, and postural alignment in the growing child.

ETIOLOGY AND PATHOLOGY

There are several suspected mechanisms for development of CMT. Risk factors for CMT include male sex, breech presentation, difficult birth, multiple parity, and increased birthweight. Any of these can cause confinement in the womb and the potential for compression or damage to the SCM. Trauma to the SCM can occur during a difficult delivery as well.

The initial compression or injury causes ischemia and edema within the muscle belly of the involved SCM. Fibrosis occurs in the muscle itself, with eventual shortening, loss of range, and atrophy. Ultrasonography can be helpful in detecting the extent of fibrosis in the muscle.[3]

Increases in postural torticollis and plagiocephaly have been noted in recent years in the United States. These increases are attributed largely to the Safe to Sleep Program. Initiated in 1994 as the Back to Sleep program, it successfully reduced the incidence of sudden infant death syndrome (SIDS) by 50%.[5] This program mandates supine positioning for all sleeping infants and includes recommendations on bedding, use of pacifiers, avoidance of environmental smoke exposure and maternal alcohol use, and daily awake time in the prone position. Studies have found that the Safe to Sleep program has negatively impacted the amount of awake prone time for babies,[6,7] and thus has greatly impacted motor skill development. Lower Alberta Infant Motor Scale (AIMS) scores have been found at 2, 4, 6, and 10 months of age in infants with torticollis, which is strongly associated with time spent in prone.[8] Awake time in prone gives the infant opportunities to develop antigravity head control, which can be beneficial in correcting any congenital muscle imbalances.

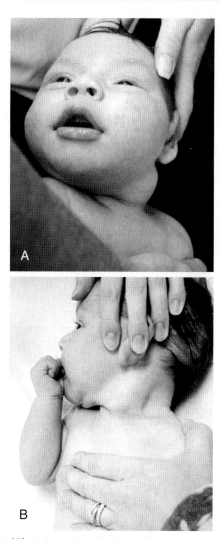

Fig. 9.1 **(A)** A 2-month-old infant with a fibrotic nodule in the left sternocleidomastoid muscle that involves the whole muscle. **(B)** Same infant at 3 months of age. From: Kaplan SL, Sargent B, Coulter C. Congenital muscular torticollis. In Palisano RJ, Orlin MN, Schreiber J, editors: Campbell's physical therapy for children Expert Consult, St. Louis, 2016, Elsevier – Health Sciences Division.

COEXISTING DIAGNOSES AND CONDITIONS

Several coexisting disorders are seen with CMT (see Table 9.1). Craniofacial asymmetry is present in up to 90.1% of infants with CMT.[3] Cranial deformity can be present in the form of plagiocephaly (flattening of the occiput on one side of the head, with frontal bossing or

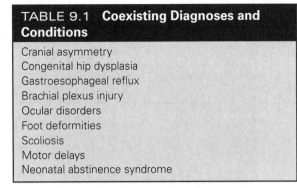

TABLE 9.1   Coexisting Diagnoses and Conditions

Cranial asymmetry
Congenital hip dysplasia
Gastroesophageal reflux
Brachial plexus injury
Ocular disorders
Foot deformities
Scoliosis
Motor delays
Neonatal abstinence syndrome

bulging on the same side of the head), brachycephaly (flattening on the back of the head), scaphocephaly (head is long and narrow), or a combination of any of these.[1] Facial asymmetries can be present including eye asymmetry and preference; frontal prominence (bossing); and ear, cheek, or jaw asymmetry. Incidence of deformational plagiocephaly has also increased dramatically since the initiation of the Back to Sleep program,[9] attributed to the increased time with weight on the back of the infant's head in supine and in positioning devices. Many of these asymmetries can be diminished by means of positioning changes and physical therapy alone. More aggressive treatment, through use of a cranial orthosis or helmet, should be initiated by 4 to 6 months of age for best results.

Congenital hip dysplasia can be present, with incidence ranging from 1% to 29% according to the literature. Gastroesophageal reflux disease (GERD) can also be present. Bercik and colleagues[10] found that 27.9% of infants with CMT also had a diagnosis of GERD.

Vision deficits can be caused by abnormal head posture or can be the cause of an abnormal head tilt or torticollis.[11,12] For this reason, all children with abnormal head posture should be seen by an ophthalmologist. Brachial plexus injury,[11] foot deformities,[11] and neonatal abstinence syndrome[13] are also associated with CMT.

Longer-term sequelae of untreated CMT can include visual changes, dental malocclusions, temporomandibular joint problems, and scoliosis.[14] Delayed developmental milestones have also been associated with CMT, exacerbated by lack of time in prone.[8] Asymmetries and lack of postural control in prone can result in difficulties with shoulder mobility, postural control, and feeding.

Early detection and referral for physical therapy are critical for best outcomes for infants with CMT. The Congenital Muscular Torticollis Clinical Practice Guideline was updated in 2018 by the American Physical Therapy Association (APTA)[15] and can serve as a template for assessments and interventions for infants with CMT.

The roles of the physical therapist in treatment of the infant with CMT include examination/re-examination, intervention, and education.

EXAMINATION/RE-EXAMINATION

A thorough review of pregnancy, birth, and all medical history should be documented. Systems review should include musculoskeletal (screening for symmetry in the head, face, shoulders, neck, spine, hips, and ribs, as well as symmetry of passive ROM at each area), neurologic (tone, reflexes, signs of nerve injury, vision), integumentary (skin folds at neck and hips), and gastrointestinal (signs of reflux or constipation). Head position preferences, any skull or facial asymmetries, and developmental milestones since birth should be noted.

Examinations should include observation of posture in all developmental positions, and passive and active ROM. Strength of the neck (including the Muscle Function scale), shoulders, and hips should be formally assessed. Pain can be assessed using the Faces, Legs, Activity, Cry, Consolability Scale (FLACC scale), and skin should be assessed for irritations, discolorations, and symmetry of skin folds (gluteal and neck). Cranial deformities should be assessed using the Argenta scale.[16] This scale classifies plagiocephaly into five types, with increasing deformation and facial asymmetry in the higher grades (Table 9.2). All facial asymmetries should be noted. These should include eye and ear asymmetry, jaw or perioral malalignments, and frontal bossing, a bulging of the forehead on the same side as the flattening on the back of the head. Red flags for referral to the primary care physician include cranial or facial asymmetry, abnormal tone, onset of torticollis at 6 months of age or older, acute onset at any time, vision deficits, suspected developmental hip dysplasia, persistent SCM mass past 7 months of age, and asymmetry persisting beyond 12 months and not responding to intervention (Table 9.3).

TABLE 9.2 Argenta Clinical Classification of Deformational Plagiocephaly	
Types	Definition
Type I	Cranial deformation limited to posterior skull
Type II	Adds displacement of the ipsilateral ear forward or downward
Type III	Adds ipsilateral frontal bone protrusion
Type IV	Adds ipsilateral facial asymmetry due to excessive fatty tissue and, less frequently, hyperplasia of the ipsilateral zygoma
Type V	Adds temporal bulging or abnormal vertical growth of the posterior skull

From Argenta L. Clinical classification of positional plagiocephaly. *J Craniofac Surg.* 2004;15:368–372. Illustrations copyright Technology in Motion Ltd.

TABLE 9.3 Red Flags for Referral to Primary Care Physician
Cranial or facial asymmetry
Abnormal muscle tone
Onset of torticollis at 6 months of age or older
Acute onset at any time
Vision deficits
Suspected developmental hip dysplasia
Persistent sternocleidomastoid muscle mass in infants aged 7 months and older
Asymmetry persisting beyond 12 months, not responding to intervention

Based on history and presentation, severity grade can be determined, using the clinical practice guidelines for CMT.[15] Lower grades are assigned for infants diagnosed earlier, with smaller asymmetries of rotation. Higher grades are assigned for infants diagnosed later, with an SCM mass and larger asymmetries of rotation (Table 9.4).

Functional outcome measurements determine activity and developmental levels for children. Developmental assessments include the Bayley Scales of Infant Development, Peabody Developmental Motor Scales II (PDMS II), and the Alberta Infant Motor Scale (AIMS), and these assessments will help determine the impact of the torticollis on motor skills. These assessments are discussed in detail in Chapter 2. Participation status should be assessed by noting positioning while patient is awake and asleep, time spent in awake prone each day, and time spent in positioning devices each day.

INTERVENTION

Intervention should include all five evidence-based interventions cited in the *2018 Clinical Practice Guideline for Congenital Muscular Torticollis*[15] as follows:

1. Neck passive ROM: This should be pain free, performed as part of daily routines such as diapering and dressing, so that it is easily and regularly performed multiple times throughout the day (Fig. 9.2).
2. Neck and trunk active ROM: Active use and strengthening of the neck and trunk muscles can be elicited through head and body righting reactions, therapeutic handling, and weight shifts within and between developmentally appropriate positions. Prone active play ("tummy time") should be a fun, engaging time for caregiver and infant. Play in this position should begin at birth and increase to 30 to 60 minutes per day (Fig. 9.3).[17,18]
3. Development of symmetric movement: Symmetry should be emphasized in all positions, motor skills, and play. This will afford functional carryover of optimal cervical muscle length to daily play, care, and positioning. It can be reinforced with sensory exploration, such as hand to knees or feet or reaching to caregiver's face.
4. Environmental adaptations: How the infant is carried, fed, and positioned can greatly support active and functional muscle activation. New carrying positions can be taught (football hold, side lying and prone carries, prone play alternatives). Alternating positions during feeding and sleeping (direction in the crib) can discourage positional preferences of the infant (see Fig. 9.4a,b). Overuse of containers or postural supports should be discouraged.

TABLE 9.4 **Grades of CMT Severity**
Grade 1—Early mild: Infants between 0 and 6 months of age with only postural preference or a difference between sides in passive cervical rotation of less than 15 degrees
Grade 2—Early moderate: Infants between 0 and 6 months of age with a difference between sides in passive cervical rotation of 15 to 30 degrees
Grade 3—Early severe: Infants between 0 and 6 months of age with a difference between sides in passive cervical rotation of more than 30 degrees or a sternocleidomastoid muscle mass
Grade 4—Later mild: Infants between 7 and 9 months of age with only postural preference or a difference between sides in passive cervical rotation of less than 15 degrees
Grade 5—Later moderate: Infants between 10 and 12 months of age with only postural preference or a difference between sides in passive cervical rotation of less than 15 degrees
Grade 6—Later severe: Infants between 7 and 9 months of age with a difference between sides in passive cervical rotation of more than 15 degrees or between 10 and 12 months of age with a difference of 15 to 30 degrees
Grade 7—Later extreme: Infants between 7 and 12 months with a sternocleidomastoid muscle mass or between 10 and 12 months of age with a difference between sides in passive cervical rotation of more than 30 degrees
Grade 8—Very late: Infants and children older than 12 months of age with any asymmetry, including postural preference, any difference between sides in passive cervical rotation, or a sternocleidomastoid muscle mass[16]

From Kaplan SL, Coulter C, Sargent B. Physical Therapy Management of Cobgenital Muscular Torticollis: A 2018 Evidence-Based Clinical Practice Guideline from the APTA Academy of Pediatric Physical Therapy. *Pediatr Phys Ther.* 2018;30(4):240–290.

5. Parent/caregiver education: The importance of "Back to Sleep, Tummy to Play"[18] should be emphasized to all parents and caregivers, along with information on the motor benefits of prone play. They should also be told that increases in tummy time can decrease the odds of cranial asymmetry.[19]

The home exercise program should incorporate all five components of intervention into the family's daily routines. The family should learn how changes in positioning and handling, and especially prone positioning, can help the infant work out muscle imbalances naturally. Parents should be empowered and supported because their handling of the infant can have the strongest effect on successful treatment of CMT.

Additional interventions can be added to supplement therapy programs. Use of kinesiotape, soft tissue massage, manual therapy, and microcurrent show promising results in the newer literature.[20-24] Any infant whose condition is not resolving with treatment should be referred back to their primary care physician. Pharmacologic (botulinum toxin) and surgical options are available for the patient with persistent or unresponsive asymmetries, especially those causing further musculoskeletal and motor development issues.

Treatment should be continued until full active and passive ROM are achieved. Parents should be informed that setbacks in posturing and range may occur during times of illness, growth spurts, and stress. For this reason, reassessment should be performed 3 to 12 months after services have been discontinued. Additional rechecks may be warranted as academic and motor demands increase.

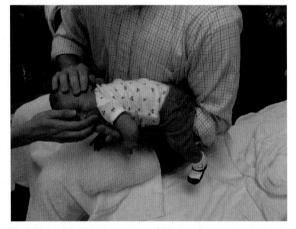

Fig. 9.2 Football style support with head turned toward the shortened side.

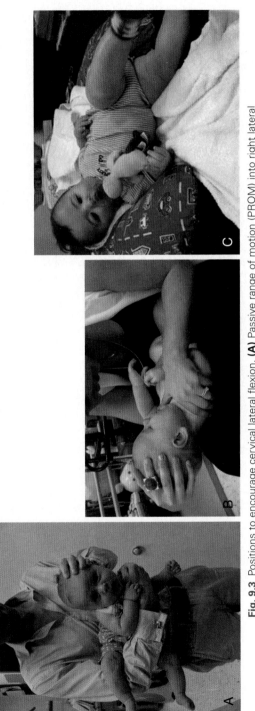
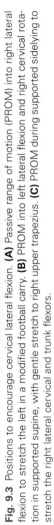

Fig. 9.3 Positions to encourage cervical lateral flexion. **(A)** Passive range of motion (PROM) into right lateral flexion to stretch the left in a modified football carry. **(B)** PROM into left lateral flexion and right cervical rotation in supported supine, with gentle stretch to right upper trapezius. **(C)** PROM during supported sidelying to stretch the right lateral cervical and trunk flexors.

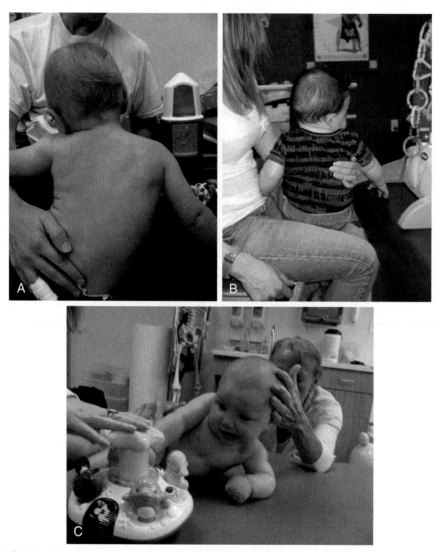

Fig. 9.4 Positions for active range of motion, strengthening, and midline orientation. **(A)** Sitting on parent's lap using weight shifting on right to encourage active left cervical and trunk lateral flexion via righting reactions. **(B)** Sitting on parent's lap to encourage active right cervical rotation to interact with toys. Notice the parent stabilizing the trunk. **(C)** Facilitated sidelying play with intermittent manual assist to encourage prolonged antigravity activation of right cervical lateral flexors.

CASE STUDY

Tommy was initially referred as a 4-month, 14-day-old infant, diagnosed with CMT. He was delivered at term by cesarean section after 38 hours of labor and weighed 8 lb, 13 oz. He weighed 16.1 lb at his initial evaluation. His mother reported that Tommy never liked to stay on his tummy. She placed him in his car seat and sometimes in an exersaucer after meals because she felt this prevented him from spitting up. She also reported that Tommy spits up regularly for up to 30 minutes after a feeding. When bottle-feeding was observed, Tommy showed good coordination of suck, swallow, and breathing, but he did gasp for air at times and then abruptly begin to cough. He showed minimal spillage or fluid loss during the feeding. Tommy produced one big dry burp at the end of his feeding and then several small milk-tinged sprays of spittle. He constantly keeps his hands in his mouth, and while this is an age-appropriate motor skill, it can sometimes be an attempt to manage fluids in the oral cavity.

Tommy showed mild flattening of the right parieto-occipital area and right frontal bossing. His right ear appeared more forward than the left, and his left eye appeared less open than the right.

Tommy showed normal tone in his trunk and all extremities. The asymmetric tonic neck reflex (ATNR) was present but not mandatory; however, Tommy strongly extended his back, neck, and legs when he was held vertically with weight on his feet.

In all developmental positions, Tommy showed a mild left sidebend and neck rotation to the right with extension. This caused a compensatory shortening on the left side of his trunk, especially in prone. His shoulders and ribcage were elevated and tense in all positions, and his left shoulder was closer to his left ear.

The following limitations and asymmetries of ROM were noted:

	Left	Right
Lateral neck flexion	0–20 degrees	0 degrees
Neck rotation	0–90 degrees	0–70 degrees

His hip flexion and abduction appeared symmetric, and no hip clicks or clunks were heard. His neck creases were asymmetric and red, and his thigh folds were symmetric. Hip ROM was symmetric. Results of Barlow and Galleazzi tests were negative. He showed significant tightness in his left SCM and bilateral upper trapezius muscles, but no SCM mass could be palpated.

Tommy initially appeared symmetric in supine, with his hands to the sides or in midline on his chest, but his shoulders were tightly elevated, with his left shoulder closer to his left ear. He could flex his hips and knees but could not yet reach his hands toward a toy or to his knees. As he stayed in supine longer, increasing shoulder elevation and left lateral neck flexion were observed, along with neck rotation to the right with extension. He used this extension to roll partially to his side in supine.

Once placed in prone, Tommy lifted his head and upper chest quickly off the mat. His hands were fisted, and he pushed up onto his forearms. He preferred to keep most of his weight on his left arm, keeping his right arm extended. He arched his neck and back and turned his head to the right. He could lift his upper chest up partially but could not roll or push up higher. He became agitated when left in this position for more than a few seconds.

Once placed in sitting, his shoulders were elevated, and upper extremities were flexed. He could not bend forward to prop himself on his hands.

Tommy loved supported standing, keeping his legs and trunk fully stiffened and extended. His hands were not free for play in this position, as they were in "high guard position," with shoulder elevation and tight elbow flexion/fisting.

The AIMS was performed to assess the effect of Tommy's torticollis on his motor skills. He performed at the 5th percentile for his age, with his weakest skills in prone. Tommy is large for his age, so he has more weight and longer lever arms to move against gravity in each position, which could make future gross motor skills increasingly difficult if his asymmetries are not addressed.

Tommy was assessed as having a Grade II torticollis. His prognosis appeared good for full correction of neck asymmetries in that he was referred early and had only a 20-degree difference in cervical rotation to each side.

Intervention began with discussion of repositioning Tommy in the crib and avoiding prolonged use of the car seat, while discontinuing use of the exersaucer. Mom was shown several Tummy Time alternative positions, face to face on Mom's chest, on his tummy over her lap, and being carried on his tummy over her arm—each of which Tommy seemed to tolerate and enjoy. She was then shown how to massage his neck and perform gentle neck stretches after each diaper change. She was shown how to pick him up by rolling him to his side slowly and then bringing him up slowly into supported sitting, waiting for him to participate and engage his own neck and tummy muscles. The therapist then used toys strategically placed in midline in various developmental positions to encourage midline head control, symmetric upper extremity (UE) weight-bearing, and active neck ROM.

Continued

CASE STUDY—cont'd

A neurodevelopmental treatment approach was used, incorporating facilitation of movement through functional play.

Therapy frequency was initially set at two times per week for 2 weeks, then dropped to once per week, with Mom performing handling and stretching at home daily. Tommy was referred back to his pediatrician because of his cranial and facial asymmetries for consideration of referral for helmeting. It was recommended that Mom also discuss Tommy's spitting up because his oral-motor behaviors and emesis could be signs of gastroesophageal reflux. Persistent reflux and discomfort with feeding could possibly slow the progression of his ROM and motor skills. Referral to an ophthalmologist was also recommended because of Tommy's asymmetric eye opening and inability to track smoothly in full ROM.

Therapy Goals

1. Tommy will achieve full neck, shoulder, and thoracic ROM for independent play, reach, and weight-bearing in all developmental positions.
2. Tommy will demonstrate active head lifting and turning in all directions in prone.

3. Tommy will push up symmetrically on his forearms in prone to view and reach for a toy.
4. Tommy will right his head to the vertical when lifted to sitting and sustain midline head control to reach for his legs or the bed in supported sitting.

Analysis of Case Using the ICF Model

Health Condition: Torticollis

Body Functions and Structure: Decreased and asymmetric neck ROM, tightness of SCM and upper trapezius muscles, muscle imbalance, plagiocephaly

Activity Limitations: Restricted neck motion and visual tracking, unable to sustain play on his tummy, unable to roll from his tummy to his back, unable to hold toys in midline with both hands

Participation Restrictions: Decreased tolerance for play in prone, possible preference for bottle-feeding to one side, potential motor delays

Environmental Factors: Use of positioning equipment, ability to change position in his crib

Personal Factors: Mother involved and invested in his care

Movement System Assessment: Tommy has force production of the contralateral SCM and upper trapezius

CHAPTER DISCUSSION QUESTIONS

1. What birth events could have contributed to Tommy's torticollis?
2. What health conditions and environmental factors could have contributed to his torticollis and plagiocephaly?
3. What type of CMT do you think he has?
4. What criteria would you use for discontinuation of Tommy's therapy?

REFERENCES

1. Chen MM, Chang HC, Hsieh CF, Yen MF, Chen TH. Predictive model for congenital muscular torticollis: analysis of 1021 infants with sonography. *Arch Phys Med Rehabil.* 2005;86(11):2199–2203.
2. Stellwagen L, Hubbard E, Chambers C, Jones KL. Torticollis, facial asymmetry and plagiocephaly in normal newborns. *Arch Dis Child.* 2008;93(10):827–831.
3. Cheng JCY, Tang SP, Chen TMK, Wong MWN, Wong EMC. The clinical presentation and outcome of treatment of congenital muscular torticollis in infants—a study of 1,086 cases. *J Pediatr Surg.* 2000;35(7):1091–1096.
4. Öhman AM, Beckung ER. Reference values for range of motion and muscle function of the neck in infants. *Pediatr Phys Ther.* 2008;20(1):53–58.
5. US Department of Health and Human Services. National Institutes of Health: About SIDS and safe infant sleep, Accessed August 24, 2023. https://safetosleep.nichd.nih.gov/safesleepbasics/about.
6. Mildred J, Beard K, Dallwitz A, Unwin J. Play position is influenced by knowledge of SIDS sleep position recommendations. *J Pediatr Child Health.* 1995;31(6):499–502.
7. Davis BE, Moon RY, Sachs HC, Ottolini MC. Effects of sleep position on infant motor development. *Pediatrics.* 1998;102(5):1135–1140.
8. Öhman A, Nilsson S, Lagerkvist AL, Beckung E. Are infants with torticollis at risk of a delay in early motor milestones compared with a control group of healthy infants? *Dev Med Child Neurol.* 2009;51(7):545–550.

9. Branch LG, Kesty K, Krebs E, Wright L, Leger S, David LR. Deformational plagiocephaly and craniosynostosis: trends in diagnosis and treatment after the "Back to Sleep" campaign. *J Craniofac Surg.* 2015;26(1):147–150.

10. Bercik D, Diemer S, Westrick S, Worley S, Suder R. Relationship between torticollis and gastroesophageal reflux disorder in infants. *Pediatr Phys Ther.* 2019;31(2):142–147.

11. Ballock RT, Song KM. The prevalence of nonmuscular causes of torticollis in children. *J Pediatr Orthop.* 1996;16(4):500–504.

12. Boricean ID, Bărar A. Understanding ocular torticollis in children. *Opthalmologia.* 2011;55(1):10–26.

13. McAllister JM, Hall ES, Hertenstein GER, Merhar SL, Uebel PL, Wexelblatt SL. Torticollis in infants with a history of neonatal abstinence syndrome. *J Pediatr.* 2018;196:305–308.

14. Kim JH, Yum TH, Shim JS. Secondary cervicothoracic scoliosis in congenital muscular torticollis. *Clin Orthop Surg.* 2019;11:344–351.

15. Kaplan SL, Coulter C, Sargent B. Physical therapy management of congenital muscular torticollis: a 2018 evidence-based clinical practice guideline from the APTA Academy of Pediatric Physical Therapy. *Pediatr Phys Ther.* 2018;30(4):240–290.

16. Argenta L. Clinical classification of positional plagiocephaly. *J Craniofac Surg.* 2004;15(3):368–372.

17. Dudek-Shriber L, Zelazny S. The effects of prone positioning on the quality and acquisition of developmental milestones in four-month old infants. *Pediatr Phys Ther.* 2007;9(1):48–55.

18. American Academy of Pediatrics Website. https://publications.aap.org/patiented/article-abstract/doi/10.1542/peo_document285/80192/Back-to-Sleep-Tummy-to-Play?redirectedFrom=fulltext.

19. Zachry AH, Nolan VG, Hand SB, Klemm SA. Infant positioning, baby gear use, and cranial asymmetry. *Matern Child Health J.* 2017;21:2229–2236.

20. Öhman AM. The immediate effect of kinesiology taping on muscular imbalance for infants with congenital muscular torticollis. *PM R.* 2012;4:504–508.

21. Keklicek H, Uygur F. A randomized controlled study on the efficiency of soft tissue mobilization in babies with congenital muscular torticollis. *J Back Musculoskelet Rehabil.* 2018;31(2):315–321.

22. Pastor-Pons I, Hidalgo-García C, Lucha-López MO, et al. Effectiveness of pediatric integrative manual therapy in cervical movement limitation in infants with positional plagiocephaly: a randomized controlled trial. *Ital J Pediatr.* 2021;47(1):41.

23. Kwon DR, Park GY. Efficacy of microcurrent therapy in infants with congenital muscular torticollis involving the entire sternocleidomastoid muscle: a randomized placebo-controlled trial. *Clin Rehabil.* 2014;28(10):983–991.

24. Thompson R, Kaplan SL. Frequency-specific microcurrent for treatment of longstanding congenital muscular torticollis. *Pediatr Phys Ther.* 2019;31(2):E8–E15.

RESOURCES

Academy of Pediatric Physical Therapy
2018 CMT CPG Resources
https://pediatricapta.org/clinical-practice-guidelines/
American Academy of Pediatrics Safe Sleep Website
https://www.aap.org/en/patient-care/safe-sleep/
Pathways.org Website
https://pathways.org/search/?query=torticollis

Developmental Dysplasia of the Hip

Roberta Kuchler O'Shea, PT, DPT, PhD

LEARNING OBJECTIVES

At the end of the chapter, the reader will be able to do the following:

1. Understand the etiology of developmental dysplasia of the hip.
2. Recognize the orthotic options for treatment of DDH.
3. Recognize the difference between the Galeazzi and Ortolani positive sign. Understand the difference between a subluxed hip and a dislocated hip.

CHAPTER OUTLINE

KEY TERMS

Acetabulum
Subluxation

Dislocation
Pavlik harness

Galeazzi sign
Ortolani sign

WHAT IS DEVELOPMENTAL DYSPLASIA OF THE HIP?

This chapter introduces the reader to developmental dysplasia of the hip (DDH) as well as the impact of DDH on a child's development of functional skills and participation. DDH replaces a previous term for this condition, *congenital dislocation of the hip*. This new term includes a variety of congenital hip pathologies: dysplasia, subluxation, and dislocation. This term is preferred because it can be applied to infants with normal physical examination findings at birth who are later found to have a subluxed or dislocated hip, in addition to those who are immediately identified as having hip pathologies.[1,2]

Risk factors for DDH can be categorized in three ways: mechanical, physiologic, and environmental. Mechanical risk factors are small intrauterine space, breech position, or positioning of the fetus's hips on the mother's sacrum.[1-3]

Physiologic risk factors include the impact of estrogen and relaxin on the female fetus.[1-3] Environmental risk factors that increase the occurrence of DDH include swaddling and positioning and carrying methods used for child (N. Mensah, Personal written communication, Jan 7, 2023).[4] More than 75% of affected infants are female. Also, certain ethnic groups have a higher rate of occurrence than others.

The risk of dysplasia increases with any type of intrauterine malpositioning that leads to extreme flexion and adduction at the hip. This occurs more commonly during first pregnancies if and when tightness of maternal abdominal or uterine musculature is present, when the infant is quite large, or when insufficient amniotic fluid restricts intrauterine motion. A higher incidence of DDH is also found among newborns with other musculoskeletal abnormalities including torticollis, metatarsus varus, clubfoot, and other unusual syndromes.[1]

DDH can be unilateral or bilateral and occurs in three forms of varying severity: (1) unstable hip dysplasia, in which the hip is positioned normally but can be dislocated by manipulation; (2) subluxation or incomplete dislocation, in which the femoral head remains in contact with the acetabulum but the head of the femur is partially displaced or uncovered; and (3) complete dislocation, in which the femoral head is totally outside the acetabulum. In unilateral occurrences, the left hip is involved three times more often than the right hip.[2]

At birth, the acetabulum is quite shallow, covering less than half of the femoral head. In addition, the joint capsule is loose and elastic. These two factors make the neonatal hip relatively unstable and susceptible to subluxation and dislocation. In the first year of life, normal development of the hip joint puts pressure and force on the femoral head and acetabulum during movement. When subluxation or dislocation is present, modeling of the acetabulum and femoral head may be affected. The most common clinical sign of DDH is limitation in hip

abduction. On clinical examination, a "click" (Ortolani sign) is felt when upward pressure is applied at the level of the greater trochanter on the newborn's or infant's flexed and abducted hip (Fig. 10.1), indicating that a dislocated hip has been manually reduced (N. Mensah. Personal written communication, Jan 7, 2023).[1] Clinical manifestations of DDH vary with age. Up through 12 months of age, any observed physical asymmetries in range of motion (no matter how small), asymmetry in the buttocks or gluteal folds (which will be higher on the affected side), extra thigh skin folds, or supine with hips flexed thigh-length discrepancies (Galeazzi sign) warrant further medical evaluation and potential imaging.[2]

The goal of orthotic management for infants with DDH is to achieve optimal positioning of the femoral head within the acetabulum while allowing typical kicking movements to occur and assist shaping of the acetabulum and femoral head for stability of the hip joint. This is best achieved if the child is consistently positioned in flexion and abduction at the hip. The Pavlik Harness (Fig. 10.2) is designed to maintain the infant's hips in good alignment. If DDH is recognized early and appropriate intervention is initiated, the hip joint is likely to develop normally. If DDH is unrecognized and untreated, it often leads to significant deformity of the hip as the child grows, resulting in functional limitations that may lead to decreased participation.[3]

In the ambulating child, uncorrected bilateral dysplasia may cause a characteristic gait pattern known as a *compensated Trendelenburg gait*. As the child sways the torso from side to side to compensate for an ineffective gluteus medius, the child assumes a waddling gait

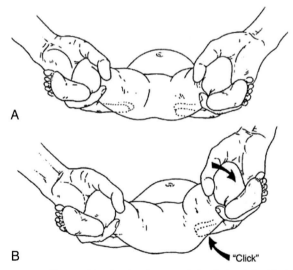

Fig. 10.1 Test position for developmental dysplasia of the hip in the newborn. **(A)** The hip is moved into flexion, adduction, and internal rotation. **(B)** A "click" when upward pressure is applied at the greater trochanter suggests that the dislocation has been reduced. (From Magee DJ. *Orthopedic Physical Assessment*. 3rd ed. Philadelphia: Saunders; 1997: p. 477.)

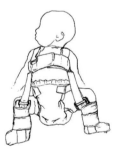

Fig. 10.2 A Pavlik harness positions the infant's lower extremities in hip flexion and abduction in an effort to position the femoral head optimally within the acetabulum, assisting normal bony development of the hip joint. The anterior leg straps allow hip flexion but limit hip extension; the posterior flaps allow abduction but limit adduction. (From Lusardi M, Jorge M, Nielsen C. *Orthotics and Prosthetics in Rehabilitation*. 3rd ed. Philadelphia: Saunders Publishers; 2013.)

pattern.[3] DDH is best treated during infancy. Residual dysplasia is a major cause of disability and should be corrected surgically at an early age.

NONSURGICAL INTERVENTIONS

The infant congenital hip dysplasia may benefit from orthopedic interventions early on.[6] For children with DDH, hip orthoses are the primary intervention for prevention of future deformity and disability.[1]

The Pavlik harness has become widely accepted as a mainstay for the initial treatment for the unstable hip in neonates from birth to 6 months of age.[1]

In a correctly fitted orthosis, the lower extremity is positioned in 100 to 120 degrees of hip flexion, as indicated by the physician's evaluation and recommendation. The limbs are also positioned in 30 to 40 degrees of hip abduction. The distance between the infant's thighs (when the hips are moved passively into adduction) should be no more than 8 to 10 cm. In a well-fitting orthosis, extension and adduction are limited, whereas flexion and abduction are freely permitted. The infant is able to kick actively within this restricted range while wearing the orthosis. This position and movement encourage elongation of adductor tightness, which, in turn, assists in the reduction of the hip and enhances acetabular development.[1,2]

SURGICAL INTERVENTIONS

Surgical correction of idiopathic DDH is one of the most challenging problems in pediatric orthopedic surgery. The treatment goal is to achieve a stable, congruent, and concentric hip joint as early as possible, which, in turn, will preclude or postpone the development of degenerative osteoarthritis of the hip.[3]

For older infants and toddlers (6–18 months) whose DDH was unrecognized or inadequately managed early in infancy, intervention is often much more aggressive and may include an abduction brace, traction, open or closed reduction, and hip spica casting.[2]

For the child being treated between the of ages 6 months and 2 years, a closed reduction is used, often with an adductor release and psoas tenotomy. An arthrogram is used to confirm the reduction followed by 3 to 5 months in a hip spica cast. Treatment after the age of 18 months requires surgical reduction, often with both femoral varus derotational osteotomy and

pelvic osteotomies in order to augment the acetabulum. Depending on the clinical presentation, tenotomy of the contracted muscles may also be required.[2] Children 3 to 8 years old are usually treated with an acetabular reshaping osteotomy.[5]

In older children with DDH, the tendency for chronic superior and posterior dislocation of the femoral head with respect to the true acetabulum exists. This induces soft tissue remodeling with muscle contracture and atrophy, particularly of the abductors muscles, and leads to secondary osteoarthritis with severe motor dysfunction, pain, and disability. Patients with osteoarthritis secondary to hip dysplasia are typically young and active with greater functional expectations than patients with primary osteoarthritis.[7] The best surgical procedure to optimize the lever arm of the hip abduction is to increase the femoral offset. However, residual gait abnormalities in patients with hip prosthesis and DDH have largely been attributed to the difficulty in correcting the weakness of those abductor muscles that have not worked properly for a long time because of loss of tension. This results in atrophy and loss of proprioception.[7,8] In addition to standard rehabilitation, a rehabilitation program for strengthening the hip abductors (especially the gluteus medius) in patients with DDH who underwent total hip reduction resulted in an increase in muscle strength that improved functional performance and patient satisfaction.[7,8]

PROGNOSIS

Outcome is directly related to the child's age at initiation of treatment. If the dislocation is corrected in the first few weeks of life, the dysplasia is completely reversible, and a normal hip can develop, with rates of success as high as 95%. If surgical reduction is required, 86% have a satisfactory outcome with rates of long-term osteoarthritis of 25% in those individuals who required a closed reduction and 49% in those who required an open reduction. When the condition is untreated, long-term problems can include degenerative joint disease, hip pain, antalgic gait, scoliosis, back pain, and the need for total hip replacement.[2]

TREATMENT

The goal of treatment for DDH is to ensure stability of the femoral head in the acetabulum, thereby encouraging the development of a normally shaped socket and femoral head. This is accomplished by re-placing the head of the femur into the acetabulum with no intervening soft tissue. The proper position then must be maintained for a period long enough for the bony and cartilaginous structures to develop sufficient stability so that the hip does not subluxate or dislocate with normal movement. Lack of contact of the femoral head with the acetabulum will allow the persistence of acetabular dysplasia. Treatment depends on the age of the child and the severity and duration of the dysplasia.[2]

PHYSICAL THERAPY

Physical therapy is often a vital part of the rehabilitation process both before and after surgery. Preoperative intervention may include lower extremity and trunk strengthening and parent/caregiver education. Positioning and handling techniques are an important aspect of the child's care both before and after surgery. After surgery, the therapist reviews cast care (or traction/orthotic care) with the child's family/caregivers.[2] A thorough assessment includes range-of-motion measurements, documentation of hip and soft tissue asymmetries, and notation of any apparent shortening of the femur/thigh length, which is also known as *the Galeazzi sign*. Hip clicks may be insignificant.[4]

CONCLUSION

It is imperative to recognize DDH early in infancy. However, DDH may be noted after the child starts to ambulate using a pathologic gait that includes waddling and pain in the hip. If DDH is caught early on, a hip orthosis worn regularly can help to hold the femoral head in the acetabulum. Weight-bearing through the hip is also of great importance. If DDH is recognized in the child between 6 months and 2 years of age, positioning,

along with soft tissue surgery, is typically warranted. The child older than 2 years typically requires bony surgery to help reposition and remodel the femoral head to be well seated in the acetabulum. After surgery, it is imperative to work on gluteal strengthening with the goal of improving patient capacity and performance, thus increasing participation.

CHAPTER DISCUSSION QUESTIONS

1. What are the common signs and symptoms of DDH?
2. Why might a diagnosis of DDH be delayed?
3. What should physical therapy interventions focus on?

REFERENCES

1. Chui KC, Milagros J, Sheng-Che Y, Lusardi M. *Orthotics and Prosthetics in Rehabilitation*. 4th ed. Philadelphia: Saunders Publishers; 2020.
2. Goodman CC, Fuller KS. *Pathology Implications for the Physical Therapist*. 4th ed. Philadelphia: Saunders Publishers; 2014.
3. Humphry S, Hall T, Hall-Craggs MA, Roposch A. Predictors of hip dysplasia at 4 years in children with perinatal risk factors. *JB JS Open Access*. 2021;6(1):e20.00108.
4. Mensah N: Written lecture notes from Orthopedic Conditions Part 1. January 7, 2023.
5. Wenger D, Bomar J. Human hip dysplasia: evolution of current treatment concepts. *J Orthop Sci*. 2003;8: 264–271.
6. Cech DJ, Martin ST. *Functional Movement Development Across the Lifespan*. Philadelphia: Saunders Publishers; 2021.
7. Rethlefsen SA, Mueske NM, Nazareth A, et al. Hip dysplasia is not more common in W-sitters. *Clin Pediatr*. 2020;59(12):1074–1079. doi:10.1177/0009922820940810.
8. LaPrade MD, Melugin HP, Hale RF, et al. Incidence of hip dysplasia diagnosis in young patients with hip pain: a geographic population cohort analysis. *Orthop J Sports Med*. 2021;9(3). doi:10.1177/2325967121989087.

Clubfoot

Leann Kerr, PT, DHS, CBIS

LEARNING OBJECTIVES

At the end of the chapter, the reader should be able to do the following:

1. Describe the different characteristics of clubfoot.
2. Formulate an appropriate treatment plan for a child with clubfoot.
3. Advocate for assistive technology for a child with clubfoot.

CHAPTER OUTLINE

KEY TERMS

Clubfoot

Ponseti method

Talipes equinus

This chapter describes the clubfoot deformity in children and associated impairments. Intervention options, surgical and nonsurgical, are reviewed. A case study helps bring the diagnosis to life for the reader.

DEFINITION

Clubfoot, or congenital talipes, is characterized by abnormal bone formation in the foot. One or both feet are twisted into an abnormal position at the time of birth (Fig. 11.1). The ratio of males to females with this diagnosis is 2.5 to 1. In the United States, one in every 1000 live births may present with the abnormalities associated with clubfoot.[1] The exact cause of clubfoot is not completely understood; however, it is considered to be a combination of multifactorial genetic traits and environmental factors. Both duplication and deletion of the chromosome 17q23 region result in clubfoot.[2,3] Linked environmental factors include cigarette smoking, early amniocentesis, viral infections, smaller intrauterine space, and multiparity.[2,3]

DIAGNOSIS

Clubfoot can be detected during a prenatal sonogram by 13 weeks' gestation using transvaginal ultrasonography. It is further diagnosed by clinical observation, typically at the time of birth. An orthopedic surgeon will confirm the diagnosis, screen for associated conditions, and facilitate arrangements for ongoing care. The baby's spine, upper extremities, and hips should be examined with both passive and active ranges of motion to detect any other abnormalities.[3] The number and severity of the deformities can be a predictor of clinical outcomes. The severity of deformity can be assessed using the Pirani scoring system and/or the Dimeglio scoring scale

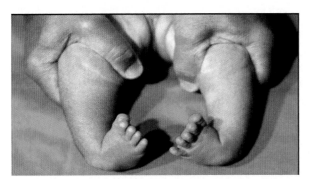

Fig. 11.1 Clubfoot, or congenital talipes equinovarus. (From Pisani G. "Coxa Pedis" today. *Foot Ankle Surg.* 2016;22:78–84.)

(Figs. 11.2 and 11.3). The Pirani scoring system is a 0- to 6-point scale; the higher the score, the more severe the deformity. The Dimeglio scoring scale is a 0- to 20-point scale comprising range-of–movement measures and four observational features: the higher the score, the more severe the deformity.[1,4,5]

PATHOLOGY

Clubfoot consists of bone deformity and soft tissue contractures. Histologic anomalies have been identified in muscles, nerves, blood vessels, tendons, ligaments, and fascia.[1,6] Four components of clubfoot that are often present are as follows: "CAVE" (C) cavus, which is a fixed plantar flexion deformity of the forefoot on the hind foot; (A) adductus, a fixed medial deviation deformity of the midfoot on the hindfoot; (V) varus, a fixed medial deviation deformity of the hind foot; (E) equinus, a fixed plantar flexion deformity of the ankle. In addition to these four classic deformities, a shortened Achilles tendon is often present.[7,8] The following muscles are often affected: peroneus brevis, triceps surae, and tibialis posterior. Other muscles of the posterior and lateral compartments of the lower extremity can also be affected but are less common. The ligaments are typically thickened. Bony deformities are present, most notably in the talus; the clubfoot is smaller than a typical foot and has a flattened superior surface resulting in reduced talocalcaneal angle. The subtalar joint facets are misshaped, and the navicular is positioned downward and more medial than that in a typical foot. Vascular abnormalities such as hypoplasia and absence of the anterior tibial artery are most

common. There are four more common variations of clubfoot: talipes varus, talipes valgus, *talipes equinus*, and talipes calcaneus. See Fig. 11.4 for additional description and images.[9,10]

INTERVENTION

Although foot deformities are often observed in newborns, the most common are positional equinovarus, metatarsus adductus, and calcaneovalgus; they usually resolve with stretching exercises and potentially casting in more severe cases.[7] Whenever prenatal or postnatal examination reveals a possible structural foot deformity, information should be provided to the caregivers, and arrangements should be made for the child to be seen by an orthopedic surgeon. Physical therapists play a key role in the management of clubfoot deformity. They monitor for improvements, assist in the casting and bracing process, distribute stretches and strengthening exercises, facilitate developmentally appropriate progression of gross and fine motor skills, and provide education to the caregivers of the child. The caregivers are instrumental in the success of treatment strategies. They should be well informed regarding the condition and encouraged to establish supportive resources for the management of the condition. See Fig. 11.5, which outlines the role of the caregiver in the treatment process.[13]

Clubfoot deformities can be successfully corrected with conservative intervention such as serial casting. This process of intervention should be started immediately following birth. The *Ponseti method* is considered the standard approach throughout the world. In this method, casts are replaced semiweekly or weekly depending on the deformity. The Ponseti method outlines a specific sequence of positional corrections to improve alignment.[12–14] Deformities are corrected in the following order: Cavus deformities first, then rotatation of the foot under the talus, and lastly the correction of the equinus. This typically requires five to seven casts. In 90% to 95% of cases, an Achilles tenotomy will be required to lengthen the tendon to obtain dorsiflexion.[11,14] The final cast is maintained until the tendon is completely healed. Pressure should never be applied on the calcaneocuboid joint during the casting process. A foot abduction brace will be used to maintain the corrected position. The brace consists of shoe orthotics and an abduction bar. Figure 11.6 shows an example of the

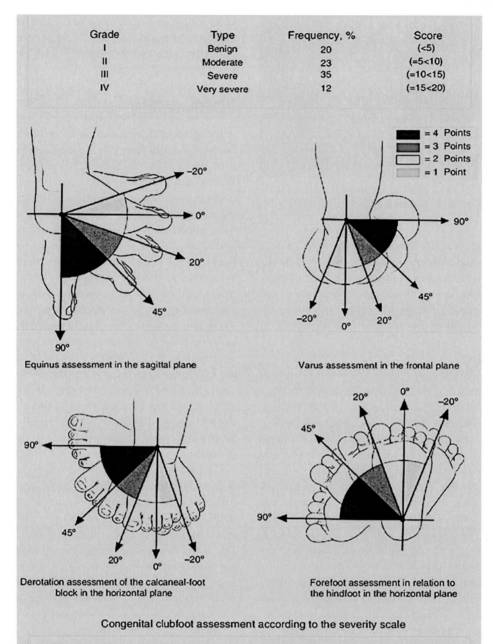

Grade	Type	Frequency, %	Score
I	Benign	20	(<5)
II	Moderate	23	(=5<10)
III	Severe	35	(=10<15)
IV	Very severe	12	(=15<20)

= 4 Points
= 3 Points
= 2 Points
= 1 Point

Equinus assessment in the sagittal plane

Varus assessment in the frontal plane

Derotation assessment of the calcaneal-foot block in the horizontal plane

Forefoot assessment in relation to the hindfoot in the horizontal plane

Congenital clubfoot assessment according to the severity scale

Features: Reproducibility	Points	Features: Other parameters	Points
90°–45°	4	Posterior fold	1
45°–20°	3	Medial fold	1
20°–0°	2	Cavus	1
<0° to –20°	1	Poor muscle condition	1

Fig. 11.2 Congenital clubfoot assessment according to the severity scale.

PIRANI SCORING OF CLUB FEET

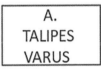

DATE																					
Side	R	L	R	L	R	L	R	L	R	L	R	L	R	L	R	L	R	L	R	L	
A Curve 1st border																					
B Medial Crease																					
C Talar Head																					
Midfoot Score																					
D Post Crease																					
E Equinus Rigidity																					
F Empty Heel																					
Hind Foot Score																					
Total Score																					
Complications Yes/No																					
Treatment																					

Treatment Code: M manipulate, C cast, T tenotomy B braces O other (describe):
Complications:

Clinical Examination (check if normal, describe if abnormal)
Head & Neck　　　Upper limbs　　　　　　　Spine　　　Lower limbs
Describe:

Consent Given: Yes　　No
Diagnosis: CTEV Syndromic TEC Positional Talipes　　Normal　　Other(describe)

Fig. 11.3 The Pirani scoring system is a 0- to 6-point scale; the higher the score, the more severe the deformity.

A. TALIPES VARUS

The foot generally turns inward so that the leg and foot look somewhat like the letter "J"

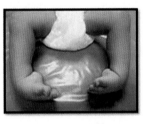

C. TALIPES EQUINUS

The foot points downward, similar to that of a pointe ballet dancer.

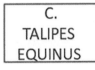

B. TALIPES VALGUS

The foot rotates outward like the letter "L"

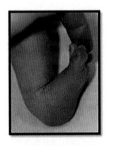

D. TALIPES CALCANEUS

The foot points upward, with the heel pointing down.

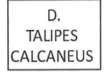

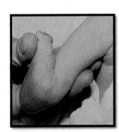

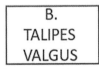

Fig. 11.4 Common variations of clubfoot presentation.

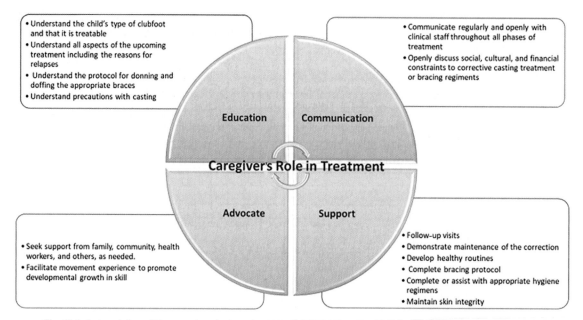

- Understand the child's type of clubfoot and that it is treatable
- Understand all aspects of the upcoming treatment including the reasons for relapses
- Understand the protocol for donning and doffing the appropriate braces
- Understand precautions with casting

- Communicate regularly and openly with clinical staff throughout all phases of treatment
- Openly discuss social, cultural, and financial constraints to corrective casting treatment or bracing regiments

Education   **Communication**

Caregiver's Role in Treatment

Advocate   **Support**

- Seek support from family, community, health workers, and others, as needed.
- Facilitate movement experience to promote developmental growth in skill

- Follow-up visits
- Demonstrate maintenance of the correction
- Develop healthy routines
- Complete bracing protocol
- Complete or assist with appropriate hygiene regimens
- Maintain skin integrity

Fig. 11.5 A description of the caregivers' role and responsibilities in the successful treatment regimen for clubfoot.

brace. The brace is worn for 3 to 4 months both day and night; the wearing schedule is gradually reduced so that the child wears it only when sleeping. The duration of intervention depends on the level of severity of the deformities and the level of adherence by caregivers. Once the deformity is corrected, the child will continue to be monitored for recurrence until skeletal maturity is achieved.

Some individuals may require an additional operation to control dynamic forefoot supination or recurrent deformity, referred to as *relapsed clubfoot*. In these cases, a tibialis anterior tendon transfer will typically be completed between 3 and 5 years of age.[13,14] The overall goal of intervention, regardless of the classification, is to correct the deformities and retain mobility and strength. Physical

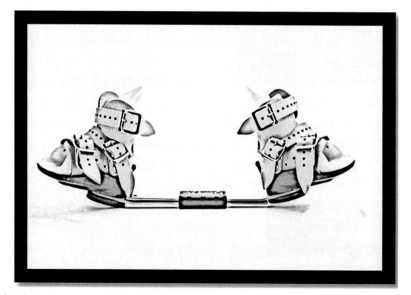

Fig. 11.6 Clubfoot shoes: Mitchell Ponseti ankle-foot orthosis (AFO) standard with Ponseti abduction bar; the Quick Clip system connects the AFO to the abduction bar.

therapists should encourage individuals to be involved in nonimpact activities such as swimming, cycling, and walking; these are recommended for the long-term exercise and care of the foot and ankle joints, especially if surgical interventions were required.[15] The foot needs to be plantigrade and must have adequate load-bearing areas to contribute to a successful functional gait.

Different types of clubfoot require different treatment options and have different prognoses. Therefore, the first step in intervention is to assess the clubfoot and then classify it into categories that will help guide effective treatment. The Ponseti method has the following five criteria for classification: (1) history of clubfoot or presence of CAVE, (2) presence of other congenital

Diagnosis and Classification of Clubfoot

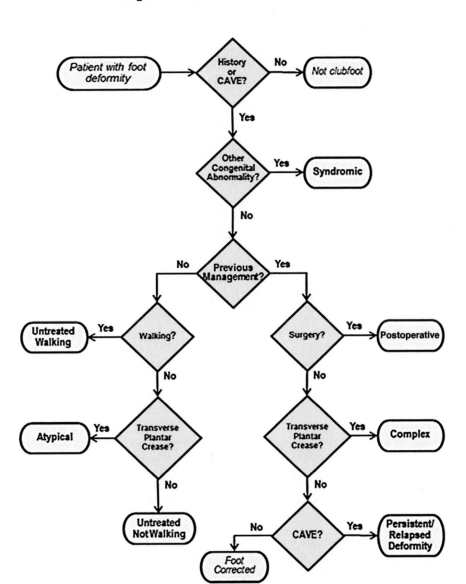

Fig. 11.7 Ponseti method algorithm for diagnosis and classification of clubfoot. *CAVE*, cavus, adductus, varus, equinus.

abnormalities, (3) evidence of previous treatment, (4) presence of a complete transverse plantar crease, and (5) patient's walking status.

Congenital anomalies can be defined as structural or functional anomalies, including metabolic disorders, which are present at the time of birth. Syndromes sometimes associated with clubfoot include amniotic band syndrome, arthrogryposis, Mobius syndrome, and spina bifida. A previously treated foot with any component of the deformity represents a residual or relapsed clubfoot. A clubfoot that has had prior surgical treatment, apart from percutaneous Achilles tenotomy, may have scarring and other deformities that may alter the underlying pathology and prognosis. The presence of a complete, deep, transverse plantar crease indicates an atypical clubfoot deformity (no previous treatment) or a complex clubfoot deformity resulting from previous unsuccessful casting. Non-weight-bearing and weight-bearing clubfeet are subject to different forces, which affect growth and pathology. Figure 11.7 shows an example of the classification algorithm from the Ponseti method.[11]

CASE STUDY OF A CHILD WITH RELAPSED CLUBFOOT

General demographics: Harper is a 5-year-old girl born with bilateral idiopathic clubfoot. She presented with forefoot adduction and hindfoot plantar flexion. She lives at home with her mother, father, paternal grandparents, and three older siblings.

General health: She was treated conservatively with the Ponseti method with excellent results. She had weekly progressive serial casting for 6 of the first 8 weeks of life. At 8 weeks, bilateral percutaneous Achilles tenotomies were performed, and she was casted for 3 weeks. At 11 weeks of age, she began wearing a foot abduction brace consisting of an adjustable-length metal bar with footplates onto which a pair of boots was attached. The wearing schedule was 23 hours per day for the first 6 weeks and decreased to 18 hours per day for an additional 6 weeks. When in the brace, her lower extremities are abducted, and the feet are externally rotated. The position helped maintain the stretch created by the serial casting and tenotomy procedure. From age 6 months to 4 years, she has worn the foot abduction brace for 10 to 12 hours each night. She was able to stand on her own by the age of 12 months and ambulated without assistance by 15 months. Six months ago, she discontinued use of foot abduction brace. Over the past 2 months, she experienced a growth spurt and has been falling more frequently.

Family history: There is no significant family history.

Growth and development:

Rolling	Met at Age-Appropriate Time	Pull to Stand	Met at 12 Months
Sitting	Met at age-appropriate time	Cruising	Met at 14 months
Supine to Sit	Met at age-appropriate time	Walking	Met at 18 months; met* complains of recent changes and increased falls
Crawling	Met at age-appropriate time	Climbing stairs	Met at 24–36 months *complains of increased difficulty with recent changes
Creeping	Delayed; met at 11 months	Running	Met at 4.5 years *currently unable to run

History of current condition: Was examined by orthopedic surgeon who believed her left foot was beginning to demonstrate clubfoot relapse. Because of decreased range of motion (ROM), the surgeon decided to serial cast and reported the following: On the left end range, dorsiflexion (DF) and forefoot abduction were limited (10 degrees shy of neutral). On the right, DF measured approximately 10 degrees, and forefoot abduction was roughly 15 degrees. The plantar surface of the left foot was "bean shaped." Today, goals are to return to activity now that serial casing is completed.

Physical therapy diagnosis: Decline in functional activities, decreased ROM, decreased strength, decreased endurance, decreased balance.

Functional status and activity level: Harper is a very happy and active child who moves around her home independently without assistive devices. She will use assistive devices when out in the community. See Tests and Measures for more detailed information.

Findings from systems review:
- Cardiovascular system: unremarkable
- Pulmonary system: unremarkable

CASE STUDY OF A CHILD WITH RELAPSED CLUBFOOT—cont'd

- Neurologic system: unremarkable
- Musculoskeletal system: left foot clubfoot relapse
- Integumentary system: healed incision lines on bilateral lower extremities, healing abrasion on left below from a recent fall
- Gastrointestinal system: unremarkable

Medications: n/a

Communication and cognition: Harper speaks fluent English, her primary language. She does not have any cognitive limitation for age-appropriate activities. Occasionally, she has difficulty solving novel complex-task problems.

Tests and Measures

Objective:

Posture: Increased lumbar lordosis, weight shift to the right in static standing

Tone: No abnormal tone noted × 4 extremities

ROM: Passive ROM in neutral limits × 4 extremities in all planes of motion, left foot resting position in 5 degrees internal rotation (IR), end range DF and forefoot abduction were limited (8 degrees shy of neutral)

Strength: Within functional limits (WFL) throughout all planes of motion

Sensation: Decreased light touch over incision lines in bilateral lower extremity (LE); otherwise, intact to light touch

Transitional movement: Sit-to-stand: noted difficulty completing without upper extremity (UE) support; required multiple attempts to complete successfully

Gait: Antalgic gait pattern with decreased stride length on the right side and decreased stand time and foot clearance in left LE

Stair management: Required bilateral UE support to climb one flight of stairs (12–14 steps)

Running: Unable to maintain balance and generate force production to vary speed of gait

Jumping: Unable to get feet off the ground; noted grimace with active attempt

Balance: Sitting: Static and dynamic sitting balance without difficulty

Standing: Static standing balance unremarkable; single leg stance (SLS), left LE unable to maintain position, right LE SLS × 10 seconds; dynamic surfaces (foam wedge) required UE support to maintain balance

Visual tracking: Unremarkable; family reported complete the visual screening for school without deficits

Fine motor skills: No deficits noted WFL

Behavior: Follows complex commands, cooperative

Standardized assessments: Timed Up and Go: 15 seconds, 5 × sit to stand 1 minute and 15 seconds

without UE support; 6-Minute Walk Test, 945 feet; required two resting breaks secondary to left LE pain and fatigue. LOB × 1 self-corrected

Assessment: Overall left LE appears to have clubfoot relapse presentation affecting the efficiency of functional gait. Patient presented with history of recent falls and abnormal gait pattern. Recommend outpatient physical therapy for appropriate exercise and gait training to reduce risk of falls and improve gross motor functional skills

Analysis of Case Using the ICF Model

Body functions and activity limitations: Decreased ROM and strength left LE, decreased overall gross motor skill performance, decreased dynamic and static balance, difficulty with single limb stance, antalgic gait pattern with decreased right stride length, decreased stand time in left LE

Participation restrictions: Limited participation in age-appropriate sporting events, decreased ability to run, increased falls with loss of balance, required bilateral UE support to climb stairs

Environmental and personal contextual factors: Excellent family support, single-story home, engaged in supportive school environment, follows complex commands, age-appropriate cognition, cooperative behavior, and recent growth spurt

Goals

Short-Term

1. Patient will be able to complete five sit-to-stands with no UE involvement to improve LE strength and balance in 4 weeks.
2. In 4 weeks, patient will be able to maintain SLS on left LE for 15 seconds to improve balance and to decrease fall risk.
3. Patient will be able to ascend and descend one flight of stairs using one UE for support to decrease fall risk in 4 weeks.

Long-Term

1. Patient will decrease TUG score from 15 seconds to 10 seconds and decrease fall risk in 8 weeks.
2. Patient will be able to perform 6MWT without any rest breaks and no LOB to improve balance and cardiovascular endurance in 8 weeks.
3. Patient will be able to run again with an appropriate symmetric gait pattern and speed to allow her to return to age-appropriate activities in 8 weeks.

Continued

CASE STUDY OF A CHILD WITH RELAPSED CLUBFOOT—cont'd

Plan

Rehabilitation potential: Patient has excellent rehabilitation potential secondary to mild complexity of diagnosis, age, and support network.

Estimated time of treatment: One time per week for 8 weeks

Treatment plan: Assess skin integrity to ensure the patient is not experiencing skin breakdown. Educate caregivers and patient about proper skin care and signs of skin breakdown. Perform mobilizations and stretches that place an emphasis on gaining dorsiflexion ROM to improve functional gait and age-appropriate play.

Re-assess ROM before and after mobilizations to ensure treatment remains appropriate. Perform static balance exercise while incorporating functional age-appropriate play to transition to dynamic balance exercises to reduce the risk of falls and injury. Perform strengthening exercises that place an emphasis on increased power of the LEs to improve functional movement and stair climbing. Educate caregivers and patient on the importance of maintaining a strict casting/bracing regimen to minimize opportunities of clubfoot relapse. Progress balance and strength training as needed to meet long-term and short-term goals.

CHAPTER DISCUSSION QUESTIONS

1. What are the identifiable deformities associated with a clubfoot diagnosis?
2. What are the examination priorities based on the medical diagnosis?
3. Identify referrals to other medical team members.
4. Based on the child's diagnosis and resources, what do you anticipate will be contributing factors to activity limitations?
5. What educational needs should be addressed for the child and the caregivers?
6. How would the intervention and plan of care change based on the age of the child?
7. What intervention do you feel would be most beneficial for this child at this time?
8. How would this child's contextual factors influence or change your patient's management?
9. Based on this patient's body function and structure impairments, what would be an appropriate outcome measure to demonstrate functional progression?

REFERENCES

1. Dyer PJ, Davis N. The role of the Pirani scoring system in the management of club foot by the Ponseti method. *J Bone Joint Surg Br.* 2006;88(8):1082–1084.
2. Ponseti I, Morcuende JA, Mosca V, et. al. *Clubfoot: Ponseti Management.* 2nd ed. Global-Help Publication; 2005.
3. Gurnett CA, Alaee F, Kruse LM, et. al. Asymmetric lower-limb malformations in individuals with homeobox *PITX1* gene mutation. *Am J Hum Genet.* 2008;83:616–622.
4. Lehman WB, Mohaideen A, Madan S, et. al. A method for the early evaluation of the Ponseti (Iowa) technique for the treatment of idiopathic clubfoot. *J Pediatr Orthop B.* 2003;12(2):133–140.
5. Alves C, Escalda C, Fernandes P, Tavares D, Neves MC. Ponseti method: does age at the beginning of treatment make a difference? *Clin Orthop Relat Res.* 2009;467:1271–1277.
6. Gray K, Pacey V, Gibbons P, Little D, Burns J. Interventions for congenital talipes equinovarus (clubfoot). *Cochrane Database Syst Rev.* 2014:CD008602.
7. Dimeglio A, Bensahel H, Souchet P, Mazeau P, Bonnet F. Classification of clubfoot. *J Pediatr Orthop B.* 1995;4(2):129–136.
8. Fan H, Liu Y, Zhao L, et. al. The correlation of Pirani and Dimeglio scoring systems for Ponseti management at different levels of deformity severity. *Sci Rep.* 2017;7(1):14578.
9. Dobbs MB, Rudzki JR, Purcell DB, Walton T, Porter KR, Gurnett CA. Factors predictive of outcome after use of the Ponseti method for the treatment of idiopathic clubfeet. *J Bone Joint Surg (Am).* 2004;86(1): 22–27.
10. Pirani S, Hodges D, Sekeramyi F. A reliable and valid method of assessing the amount of deformity in the congenital clubfoot deformity. *J Bone Joint Surg (Br) (Suppl).* 2008;90:53.
11. Gao R, Tomlinson M, Walker C. Correlation of Pirani and Dimeglio scores with number of Ponseti casts required for clubfoot correction. *J Pediatr Orthop.* 2014;34:639–642.
12. Gore AI, Spencer JP. The newborn foot. *Am Fam Phys.* 2004;69:865.
13. Graf A, Wu KW, Smith PA, et. al. Comprehensive review of the functional outcome evaluation of clubfoot treatment: a preferred methodology. *Pediatr Orthop B.* 2012;21:20.

14. Farsetti P, Caterini R, Mancini F, Potenza V, Ippolito E. Anterior tibial tendon transfer in relapsing congenital clubfoot: long-term follow-up study of two series treated with a different protocol. *J Pediatr Orthop*. 2006;26(1):83–90.

15. Epomedicine: Pirani Score and Dimeglio classification for clubfoot assessment. Epomedicine; April 13, 2022. Accessed August 26, 2022. https://epomedicine. com/medical-students/pirani-score-for-clubfoot-assessment/.

Arthrogryposis Multiplex Congenita

Roberta Kuchler O'Shea, PT, DPT, PhD
Jessica Trenkle, PT, DPT, PCs

LEARNING OBJECTIVE

At the end of the chapter, the reader will be able to do the following:
1. Describe the underlying pathology associated with arthrogryposis multiplex congenita (AMC).
2. Understand the two common forms of AMC.
3. Recognize and describe associated comorbidities.
4. Formulate a treatment plan based on clinical signs and functional impairments.

CHAPTER OUTLINE

KEY TERMS

Clubfoot deformity   Joint contractures

DEFINITION

AMC describes a nonprogressive syndrome of multiple congenital joint contractures, commonly involving a symmetric pattern in all four extremities. It is also known as *multiple congenital contractures (MCCs)*.[1,2]

PATHOLOGY

AMC has a pathology of unknown origin; it occurs in approximately 1 in 3000 live births[1] and is primarily a motor syndrome.[3] Insults seem to occur within the first trimester of fetal development.[4] Several factors are thought to contribute to atypical fetal development, including environmental, genetic, and other unknown factors. Maternal fevers, infection, vascular compromise, and limited room in the uterus or low amounts of amniotic fluid may compromise fetal development.[4] The basic pathophysiologic trigger for AMC seems to be lack of fetal movement.[5] Four causes of limited joint movement before birth have been identified[6,7]:
1. Maternal disease
2. Insufficient room within the uterus
3. Intrauterine vascular compromise
4. Atypical development of tendons, bones, joints, or joint linings

CLINICAL SIGNS

The deformities of AMC are apparent at birth and include multiple severe joint contractures, dislocations, decreased muscle strength (secondary to atrophy and sometimes absence of muscle groups), lack of normal skin creases, and diminished reflexes (although sensation may be intact).[2,8] Classically, there is much variation between children; however, extremity joints typically affected are the hands, wrists, elbows, ankles, knees, and hips (Fig. 12.1). Occasionally, a child only has a few affected joints and nearly full range of motion (ROM).[6] Typical presentation Is medially rotated/adducted shoulders, extended elbows, flexed and ulnarly deviated wrists, and clubfoot.

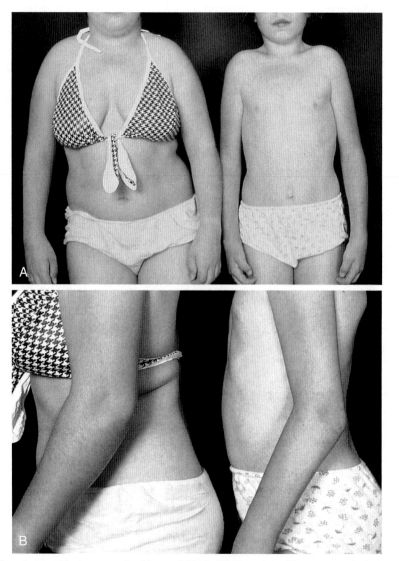

Fig. 12.1 Two sisters with the generalized form of AMC. **(A)** Note the stiff posture and tubular appearance of the limbs. Motion of all joints is limited as a result of degeneration of muscular structures or failure in their development. Their stature is short. **(B)** The lateral view highlights the flexion contractures of the elbows. (From Zitelli BJ, Davis HW. *Atlas of Pediatric Physical Diagnosis.* 5th ed. Philadelphia: Mosby; 2007.)

AMC CLINICAL SIGNS

- Multiple involvement of joints with severe contractures
- Dislocations
- Decreased muscle strength secondary to atrophy
- Possible absence of muscle groups
- Lack of normal skin creases
- Diminished reflexes, although sensation may be intact
- Extremity joints typically affected are hands, wrists, elbows, ankles, knees, and hips

INTERVENTION

A transdisciplinary team consisting of the child, family, orthopedic surgeon, physical therapist (PT), and occupational therapist should create functional goals for the child. Surgical procedures should be timed to be developmentally appropriate.

The team should discuss how and when to surgically correct the skeletal deformities and malalignments. Hence, foot alignment surgery must occur prior to the age when the child will begin standing and ambulating.

Children with AMC frequently have clubfeet. Typically, the clubfoot deformity, a condition in which the heel of the affected foot points downward and the forefoot turns markedly inward, is surgically corrected between 6 and 12 months of age.[2] Oleksak, Fernandes, and Saleh[8] found that surgical correction of the knee and foot using circular fixators (external adjustable hardware to correct bony deformities) had longer-lasting correction effects than soft tissue surgical correction alone. Children with AMC also have an increased incidence of dislocated hips. If both hips are dislocated, surgical reduction is usually not considered because the pelvis will be relatively level, but if only one hip is dislocated, surgery may be considered to balance out the pelvis and prevent scoliosis.[5] Careful assessment of the child's function and joint integrity is crucial to determining the best course of action.

Physical Therapy Assessment

Physical therapy assessment should include the following:

- Measurement of passive and active ROM of all extremities and neck and trunk
- Strength assessment of all extremities, neck, and trunk

- Evaluation of protective and equilibrium reactions forward, laterally, and backward
- Evaluation of age-appropriate gross motor skills, including transitional movements and mobility
- Evaluation of age-appropriate activities of daily living skills

Physical Therapy Intervention

The primary motor impairments for the child with AMC are limitations in joint movement and decreased strength and muscle bulk. Intensive stretching and strengthening interventions that assist in gaining and sustaining range and strength are vital. Interventions should be age appropriate and family centered.

In the upper extremities, functional independence must be at the forefront of desired treatment outcomes. Elbow flexion and extension are paramount for independence in activities of daily living skills. If bilateral extremities cannot gain motion in both flexion and extension, Tecklin[2] recommends that one arm gain in elbow flexion and the other arm gain in elbow extension, thus allowing functional tasks to be mastered unilaterally.

AMC INTERVENTIONS

- Strengthening
- Stretching
- Motor control

Infant

Intervention for an infant will incorporate techniques for the caregiver to use when holding the child and positioning the child for sleep and feeding. Effective interventions will assist the child in gaining range. Such interventions can occur as part of the family's daily routine and interactions with the child. Additionally, serial casting to treat deformities of the foot, knee flexion contractures, and wrist contractures may be implemented. Extreme care must be taken not to stretch the child's joints past end range, and then the stretch must be maintained by using splints or serial casting. Long-term splinting and orthotic use will assist in maintaining joint ROM and appropriate position. Early mobility is important and sometimes difficult. Rolling may not be optimal when lower-extremity dislocations and contractures are present. Children may learn to sit well but have difficulty transitioning into and out of this position. Many learn to scoot while sitting because quadruped mobility may be complicated by joint contractures and decreased muscle strength.

Toddler

Strengthening and stretching during the toddler years should be incorporated into play schemes. Similarly, functional tasks such as self-feeding, beginning dressing, and ambulation/mobility should be embedded into the routines of the family and not set aside as separate therapeutic activities done in isolation. For example, the child should work on object manipulation and pincer grasp to secure food while eating with the family. Range-of-motion exercise and dressing can be combined when the child is completing donning and doffing tasks throughout the day. Mobility practice can be built into the task of moving about the environment (instead of being carried). Transition from the floor to standing and standing activities can occur during play and dressing time.

An important point to remember is that the physical therapy provider can help the child's caregivers determine when a child would most likely be doing stretching or strengthening activities during the day and then embed the physical therapy intervention into the family's routines. A home exercise program is far more likely to be carried over if it harmonizes with something the family and child are already doing. To ask a family to add an isolated routine of stretching and strengthening activities to the beginning or end of their day may result in nonadherence and added family stress.

Preschool and School-Age

As the child develops, intervention, activities, and goals should reflect age-appropriate skills. Children with AMC are typically fully included in the regular education system, with adaptive physical education and therapies outlined on the individualized educational plan (IEP). Preschoolers and school-aged children need to strive to be independent in toileting, mobility, and self-care tasks.

The child should become independent in orthotic care and use of adaptive equipment during this time

as well. Orthotic intervention helps to maintain the joints in optimum alignment, and while orthotics may allow the child to be more functional, they may also contribute to a lack of strength development.[9] The team must be careful to balance the two interventions so that the child can develop optimal strength and motor control but also maintain as much independence as possible.

Strengthening should be system-wide but focused on increasing and maintaining abdominal, hip, and knee strength. Hip and quadriceps strength will be vital for ambulation, ascending and descending stairs, and moving through transitional positions. Abdominal strength is also crucial for maintaining upright positions, transitional movements, and ambulation. The PT may consider offering an intensive strengthening program to the school-aged child with AMC, meaning the child would attend therapy three to five times during the week for several hours to work intensively on stretching and strengthening activities. Research on intensive resistance training in children with neuromuscular involvement suggests that moderate intensity aerobic and strength exercise will build strength and endurance without damaging the motor units.[10] Children with AMC need to learn to strengthen and use their muscles. Often, because of weakness and lack of experience, a child will initially require motor planning and sequencing intervention to develop motor skills. After becoming familiar with the movement pattern and learning when to recruit muscle fibers and muscle groups, the child can build on this knowledge to increase strength and endurance.

Children with AMC should be able to gain ambulation skills, perhaps using orthotics in conjunction with walkers or crutches. As the child ages, decisions concerning ambulation and mobility should take into account the distance needed to be traveled, the speed necessary to be functionally mobile, and the child's energy expenditure. Often, older children and young adults will ambulate within the home or school environment but opt for wheeled mobility for longer distances in the community. The goal for all therapeutic and mobility decisions should focus on continued independence and maintaining social and work interaction with peers.

CASE STUDY OF A CHILD WITH AMG

Examination

History

Sam, the youngest of seven children, was delivered via cesarean section. His mother, Lynn, reports that at birth, his legs were "folded up and crumpled." A prenatal sonogram showed that the fetus's skeletal system had deformities. At birth, Sam was diagnosed with AMC. Sam is now 3 years, 9 months old. He lives at home with his parents, five siblings, and a dog. One sibling lives out of the home. Lynn reports that Sam is loved and well cared for by all the family, and he adores his older siblings, who love to participate in activities with him.

Current Condition

Sam has participated in several sessions of pool therapy and therapeutic horseback riding and currently receives weekly physical and occupational therapy services through his early childhood program. Sam attended a 3-week intensive transdisciplinary therapy program that included 4 hours a day, 5 days a week, of stretching, strengthening, fine and gross motor skills training, and mobility skills. The protocols also included massage and a suit therapy program to augment the aforementioned program.

Systems Review

Cardiovascular/Pulmonary: Sam does not have any pathology in his cardiac or pulmonary systems.
   Integumentary: See Tests and Measures.
   Musculoskeletal: See Tests and Measures.
   Neuromuscular: See Tests and Measures.

Functional Status

At his initial evaluation, Sam was an engaging youngster who appeared to be able to charm his way into or out of any situation. He had normal hearing and vision capabilities. He did not exhibit any sensory integration issues. His primary language is English.

Tests and Measures

Sam's skeletal build was typical of a child with AMC. He had undergone bilateral clubfoot correction in the past; the skin was well healed and intact. He had no muscle activation in his lower extremities bilaterally, and muscle atrophy was apparent in both legs. He had normal strength in his proximal upper extremities and trunk; his wrists and hands were weaker. He had intact balance reactions and protective extension of his trunk and upper extremities. His ROM was within normal limits in his trunk, neck, and upper extremities. He tended to hold his hands in an ulnar drift

pattern (hand positioned medially toward the ulna), primarily because of distal weakness. His left hip was limited in extension (–15 degrees), but he had full flexion. He had full external rotation, abduction, and adduction of the left hip. He could not achieve neutral internal rotation on the left side. His right hip had full ROM. Hip radiographs revealed well-seated hips without subluxation or dislocation. Bilaterally his knees lacked passive range. On the left, he lacked 35 degrees of full extension; on the right, he had movement between –15 degrees and 100 degrees of flexion. He could achieve 5 degrees of passive plantar flexion on the left; all other foot and ankle movement was stuck at neutral.

In order to ambulate, Sam wore bilateral KAFOs (knee, ankle, foot orthotics) with drop lock knees and bilateral anterior knee pads. He ambulated using a swing-through gait and a reverse walker at very fast speeds. With his braces on, Sam could transition from the floor to standing with minimal assistance and back again, primarily using his walker and upper extremities. Without orthotics, he was unable to maintain weight-bearing through his lower extremities. While holding onto the walker, he could maintain standing balance for a maximum of 5 to 8 seconds. If he was displaced even slightly, he would exhibit overresponsive balance reactions to maintain an upright position. He was unable to manage small perturbations quietly.

Sam could roll independently, and he assumed the prone position on hands masterfully, but he could not flex his lower extremities under him to assume a 4-point position. For floor mobility, he chose to pull himself along using his upper extremities, with the lower extremities dragging behind. He could not attain or maintain a 4-point position without assistance. He could floor-sit independently, tending to sacral-sit and use his upper extremities to change his position. He had difficulty maintaining a neutral pelvis in sitting without upper extremity support. He required maximum assistance to transition and maintain tall kneeling and to shift his weight when in tall kneeling. He complained of knee pain when in tall kneeling. He could not attain a half-kneel position.

Evaluation

Sam is a 3¾-year-old male with AMC. He has significant muscle atrophy and muscle weakness in his bilateral lower extremities. He currently ambulates with bilateral long-leg braces (KAFOs) and a reverse walker. He can move quickly using a swing-through gait. He demonstrates good balance. Sam should gain strength and more efficient mobility in an intensive therapeutic exercise program.

Continued

CASE STUDY OF A CHILD WITH AMG—cont'd

Prognosis

The prognosis for improving Sam's ambulatory functioning and increasing his strength is good.

Intervention

Coordination, Communication, Documentation

During his intensive PT training, it was important to maintain communication with Sam's physician and community- and school-based therapists.

Patient Instruction

Sam and his family received a written home exercise program (HEP) with pictures of Sam completing his exercise routine. The PTs also made a video of Sam completing all the exercise routines. Sam can use this at home while exercising. Sam's mom downloaded Pt Pal, an app to help monitor the home program and record his daily/weekly progress and be in contact with his therapy team easily.

Direct Intervention

During his 3 weeks of intensive therapy, Sam was treated with daily massage, application of hot packs, and gentle passive stretching. These warm-up activities were followed by donning the suit therapy garment. (A child receives facilitation of weak movement patterns and resistance of dominant movements when in the suit.) While in the suit, Sam completed a series of isometric exercises, including hip extension exercise when prone and dangling his legs off the end of a plinth. Sam also completed trunk extension exercises by hanging his trunk and head over the end of the plinth and attempting to complete repetitions of trunk extension. Sam required maximum stabilization to achieve one or two repetitions of these exercises. Sam practiced transitioning using typical movement patterns through the developmental sequence: sit to tall kneel, half-kneel to standing, and the reverse. He worked on isolating lower extremity muscles

so they would activate when appropriate and not randomly. He practiced improving his standing balance outside of the reverse walker and ambulating with bilateral Lofstrand crutches or with his hands held.

Goals

Sam's therapy goals for the 3-week intensive session were as follows: to achieve independent ambulation of 750 to 1000 feet with the least restrictive device; to recruit and activate appropriate muscles in lower extremities to accomplish age-appropriate tasks, such as floor sit-to-stand transitions; and to decrease the number of verbal cues needed to remind him to maintain good and safe hand position.

Termination

Sam made significant gains during his 3-week intensive session. Sam can exhibit spontaneous muscle activity in his lower extremities. He is able to transition from sit to stand using half-kneeling when verbally cued. He ambulates independently and safely with bilateral Lofstrand crutches using a reciprocal four-point gait pattern and full weight-bearing through both extremities. This case demonstrates that intensive strengthening and motor therapy can positively impact a child's life.

Analysis of Case Using the ICF Model

Body functions: Muscle atrophy and severe weakness of bilateral lower extremities; significant decreased ROM in bilateral lower extremities

Activity limitations: Ambulates with KAFOs and walker; cannot stand or ambulate without assistive technology

Participation restrictions: Cannot participate in age-appropriate community-based activities

Environmental limitations: Requires modified access to stairs at home and in the community

Movement System Analysis: Force production deficit

CHAPTER DISCUSSION QUESTIONS

1. What are the four potential causes of AMC?
2. Describe the two types of AMC.
3. Typically, who are the members of the transdisciplinary team for a child with AMC?
4. Why would intensive therapy be recommended for a child with AMC?
5. Tecklin recommends what strategy to achieve independence in activities of daily living if bilateral upper extremities cannot achieve full ROM?
6. What are two areas to work on with parents of infants with AMC?
7. What three areas should be the focus of consistent strength training?
8. When is it recommended to perform hip surgery on a child with AMC?
9. Identify three play-based activities that could be used to increase strength.
10. Identify two potential community-based activities appropriate for a child with AMC.

REFERENCES

1. Bamshad M, Van Heest AE, Pleasure D. Arthrogryposis: a review and update. *J Bone Joint Surg Am.* 2009;91(suppl 4):40–46.
2. Tecklin JS. *Pediatric Physical Therapy.* 3rd ed. Philadelphia: Lippincott Williams & Wilkins; 1999.
3. Accardo PJ, Whitman BY. *Dictionary of Developmental Disabilities Terminology.* 3rd ed. Baltimore: Paul H. Brookes; 2011.
4. Ratliffe KT. *Clinical Pediatric Physical Therapy: A Guide for the Therapy Team.* St Louis: Mosby; 1998.
5. Palisano RJ, Orlon M, Scheiber J. *Campbell's Physical Therapy for Children.* 6th ed. Philadelphia: Elsevier; 2022.
6. Akazawa H, Oda K, Mitani S. Surgical management of hip dislocation in children with arthrogryposis multiplex congenita. *J Bone Joint Surg.* 1998;80(4):436.
7. Hall JG. Arthrogryposis multiplex congenita: etiology, genetics, classification, diagnostic approach, and general aspects. *J Pediatr Orthop B.* 1997;6:159–166.
8. Oleksak M, Fernandes JA, Saleh M. The use of circular fixators for the treatment of joint deformities in arthrogryposis in children. *J Bone Joint Surg.* 2003;85:269.
9. Webster J, Murphy D. *Atlas of Orthoses and Assistive Devices.* 5th ed. Philadelphia: Elsevier; 2017.
10. Sheikh AM, Vissing J. Exercise therapy for muscle and lower motor neuron diseases. *Acta Myol.* 2019;38(4):215–232.

RESOURCE

National Organization for Rare Diseases
55 Kenosia Avenue
PO Box 1968
Danbury, CT 06813-1968
800-999-6673
203-744-01006

13

Down Syndrome

Roberta Kuchler O'Shea, PT, PhD
Jessica Trenkle, PT, DPT, PCS

LEARNING OBJECTIVES

At the end of the chapter, the reader will be able to do the following:

1. Understand the causes and developmental effects of Down syndrome.
2. Formulate an appropriate treatment plan for a child with Down syndrome.
3. Advocate services for a child with Down syndrome and the child's family.

CHAPTER OUTLINE

KEY TERMS

Atlantoaxial instability
Hypotonia

Mosaicism
Translocation

Trisomy 21

DEFINITION

Down syndrome (Fig. 13.1) was named for and originally described by John Langdon Down in 1866. The genetic error responsible for the syndrome was isolated in 1959 when Jerome Lejeune demonstrated the atypical chromosome count.[1,2]

PATHOLOGY

Three types of chromosomal abnormalities can lead to Down syndrome: (1) trisomy 21, occurring in 95% of cases; (2) translocation, making up 4% of cases; and (3) mosaicism causing 1% of cases.[1,3] Trisomy 21 results in an extra chromosome 21. Individuals with trisomy 21 have 47 chromosomes instead of the typical 46. Translocation occurs when the long arm of the extra chromosome 21 attaches to chromosome 14, 21, or 22. Individuals with mosaic trisomy display some but not all of the characteristics of the syndrome because some of the body's cells have trisomy 21, and some do not. Individuals with mosaic trisomy tend to have less significant cognitive delays than individuals with trisomy 21.[2]

In the United States, the incidence of Down syndrome is approximately 6000 per year, with increased risk associated with advanced maternal age.[4] The trisomy 21 karyotype occurs more frequently in males, while translocation occurs more frequently in females.[2]

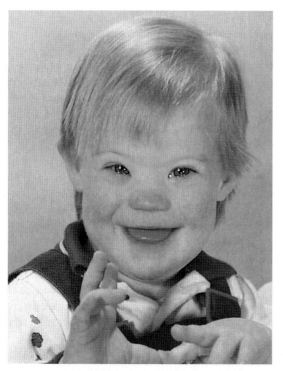

Fig. 13.1 A child with Down syndrome. Note the upward slanting palpebral fissures and epicanthal folds, flat nasal bridge, small ears, and small hands. (From Zitelli BJ, Davis HW. *Atlas of Pediatric Physical Diagnosis*. 5th ed. Philadelphia: Mosby; 2007.)

CLINICAL SIGNS

Some of the most common physical features of Down syndrome are hypotonia (low muscle tone), short stature (including short digits), flat facial profile, epicanthal folds and an upward slant to the eyes, small ears, a single transverse palmar crease, and some degree of cognitive

DOWN SYNDROME CLINICAL SIGNS

- Hypotonia
- Short stature
- Flat facial profile
- Epicanthal folds
- Upward slanting palpebral fissures
- Small ears
- A single transverse palmar crease
- Cognitive limitations
- Additional related medical conditions

limitation. Many organ systems are affected in children with Down syndrome, resulting in cardiac defects, decreased brain volume, duodenal atresia, atlantoaxial instability (excessive movement in the joint between the atlas [C1] and the axis [C2]), thyroid disorders, conductive hearing loss, Brushfield spots (speckling of the iris), and nutritional concerns.[5]

INTERVENTION

As mentioned previously, there are several related medical conditions associated with Down syndrome. Congenital heart defects occur in 66% of individuals.[6] The most common defect is an endocardial cushion defect. During normal fetal heart development, the inner cardiac tissues separate into chambers. If this process fails, holes may remain and allow mixing of oxygenated blood with deoxygenated blood. This problem is often compounded by defects in the heart valves regulating the volume of blood flow to the lungs. As a result, many individuals with Down syndrome experience a rapid decline with congestive heart failure.[7]

Individuals with Down syndrome have specific nutritional issues and are at high risk for obesity as they age.[8] Research has demonstrated that children with Down syndrome burn 15% fewer calories per day than their typically developing peers.[1,2] Rather than limit their caloric intake, it is recommended that these children be encouraged to exercise more each day, while working with a licensed dietician to maximize nutritional intake.[9] Exercise opportunities must be built into daily routines (e.g., take the stairs instead of the elevator, walk to a destination instead of driving, or get involved in a physical activity instead of watching TV). Early guidance of individuals and families of children with Down syndrome to reduce sedentary activities and improve physical fitness may help combat obesity-related complications over their lifetime

Children with Down syndrome are at risk for many orthopedic comorbidities. This may be due in large part to central hypotonia (floppiness without weakness, reduced resting muscle tone) and ligamentous laxity, which can lead to joint instability. Instability of the atlantoaxial joint must be carefully screened for and monitored because this upper spinal segment may dislocate in approximately 15% of individuals with Down syndrome; however, only 1% will experience symptoms.[2] Symptoms of subluxation include becoming easily fatigued, abnormal gait and/or difficulty ambulating, neck pain, decreased neck mobility (including torticollis), decreased hand function, sensory changes, new onset of incontinence, and clumsiness.[2] Although the American Academy of Pediatrics does not recommend routine imaging unless symptoms are present, education should be provided regarding use of caution during sports that involve heavy physical contact. Additional orthopedic concerns with a high prevalence in this population include hip dysplasia, scoliosis, and foot deformities.

Cognitive limitations are also a concern for individuals with Down syndrome. Early in life, children with Down syndrome tend to be significantly delayed in gross and fine motor skills; it takes about twice as long for independent ambulation to occur in this population. As they age and gain skills and experience, motor delays may become less significant. The cognitive delays may be more persistent and influential across the child's life span. Early intervention to address difficulties with motor, cognitive, and social skills can assist the child in learning new tasks and developing aptitudes. It is imperative that a child with Down syndrome learn the correct way to accomplish a task, be it motor or cognitive. Once the child has mastered a strategy to overcome an obstacle, strong dependence on that strategy is maintained. Children with Down syndrome have difficulty unlearning and relearning a skill or transitioning through the developmental sequence. For example, children with Down syndrome may roll as a primary means of mobility for significantly longer than their typically developing peers. Rolling is fast, energy efficient, and easily mastered. Mastery of four-point crawling is often perceived as a nuisance because it initially consumes more energy and effort than rolling. Thus, the child is less likely to transition from rolling to four-point crawling for mobility when rolling is working well. Eventually, however, the child with Down syndrome walks, runs, and masters higher-level balance activities.[10]

Research shows that 85% of children with Down syndrome have mild to moderate cognitive delays.[2] The educational program for a child with Down syndrome should provide optimal learning and stimulation for the child to grow and develop. A hybrid mix of special education and regular education classes and activities might be most appropriate. This demonstrates a great cooperative effort among educators, the family, and the child.

As individuals with Down syndrome age, screening is needed for arthritis, cardiac conditions, mental health, Alzheimer disease, and obesity-related secondary health complications.[11] Understanding of the physical and behavioral health risks throughout the life span is pivotal to caring for this population.

Physical Therapy Intervention

Physical therapy interventions should focus on assisting the child to become as independent and functional as possible. Early intervention should focus on improving the child's developmental and coordination skills. Hence, activities should promote stability at proximal joints and co-contraction of the joints. Activities that promote early development of motor skills and ambulation readiness skills following the developmental sequence are important. Short-duration treadmill training (8 min/d, 5 d/wk), initiated when a child is sitting independently, has been shown to accelerate the onset of independent walking.[12] Interventions should focus on strengthening, postural control, and endurance, with particular emphasis on activities that are meaningful to the child and family.

To improve lower extremity alignment and stability, orthotics may be considered. The rule of thumb is to provide as least restrictive orthotic intervention as possible to attain the goals. A flexible supramalleolar orthotic (SMO) is ideal for children with low tone. The SMO design uses a flexible plastic that provides stability by compressing the tissues of the foot. Thus, the foot's intrinsic muscles continue to be recruited and developed. The child is helped to develop typical balance and equilibrium reactions, which are often not fully developed when the child wears traditional orthotics. A small knee cage may be used to prevent hyperextension. The children who use it gain significant knee stability because the orthotic prevents hyperextension of the knee joints. Often, a soft dynamic orthosis such as TheraTogs, Benik, or Spio Vest can be used to help maintain good skeletal alignment and promote improved function and participation.

Early therapy should also focus on engaging and supporting the family as they adjust to having a child with a disability. This may involve locating resources for the family and giving them printed information about Down syndrome, as well as support group information. These families, like other families of children with disabilities, will need to adjust their dynamics to incorporate handling, positioning, and developmental strategies into their everyday routines. The family may need assistance with managing several coexisting medical and social service programs that often come with having a child with a disability.

DOWN SYNDROME INTERVENTIONS

- Focus on function and independence
- Promote early development of motor skills
- Engage and support family

CASE STUDY OF A TEEN WITH DOWN SYNDROME

Examination

History

Julian is a 15-year-old boy with Down syndrome diagnosed at birth. He did not have cardiac involvement and was a healthy newborn. Julian was immediately enrolled in an early intervention program for children. Three years ago, Julian was in a serious motor vehicle accident (MVA), which resulted in a perforated spleen and internal bleeding. Julian underwent emergency surgery. After a hospital stay, Julian was discharged to recover fully at home. He has no remaining issues from the MVA.

Current Condition

Julian is currently referred to physical therapy for conditioning and wellness. He is interested in playing on the high school basketball team. Julian has a stable cervical spine, based on current x-ray results.

Systems Review

Cardiovascular/pulmonary: No atypical findings
  Integumentary: No atypical findings
  Musculoskeletal: See Tests and Measures
  Neuromuscular: See Tests and Measures

Functional Status

Tests and Measures

Tone: Julian has moderate hypotonia in his trunk and all extremities. He can independently rise from the floor.
  Range of Motion: Julian has excessive range of motion in bilateral knees and elbows.
  Strength: Julian has 4/5 strength in his distal extremity musculature (wrists, ankles, knees, and elbows) and 5/5 strength in his proximal joints (hips and shoulders).
  Sensation: Julian has intact sensation to sharp/dull and light touch.
  Balance: Julian has good balance. He can maintain sitting with eyes open and closed with large perturbations. In standing, Julian can maintain static standing with eyes open with large perturbations. He is a bit more unstable in standing with eyes closed, swaying but not losing his balance with moderate perturbations. While balancing on one foot, Julian must keep his eyes open to maintain his balance. He was unable to maintain single leg stance with eyes closed for more than 5 seconds.
  Posture: Julian has erect standing and sitting posture. He can easily maintain upright against gravity.
  Gait: Julian demonstrates bilateral pronated feet and knee valgus when ambulating. He has a wide base of support but can ambulate forward without loss of balance. He has difficulty with side-to-side lateral gait. He can ambulate backward. When running, Julian has minor difficulties with tripping over his feet.
  Endurance: Julian has good endurance for day-to-day activities. He has difficulty completing 20 minutes of aerobic exercise.

Evaluation

Julian is a 15-year-old boy with Down syndrome. He currently wants to play basketball for his high school team. At this time, he demonstrates decreased strength in distal muscles, decreased exercise endurance, and decreased high-level coordination skills.

Prognosis

The prognosis for improving Julian's functioning and increasing his strength, coordination, and endurance is good.

Intervention

Coordination, Communication, Documentation

Julian was given an extensive training and conditioning program. The physical therapy staff communicated with the high school training staff prior to discharging Julian. The athletic trainer employed by the school district would monitor Julian's conditioning program.

Continued

CASE STUDY OF A TEEN WITH DOWN SYNDROME—cont'd

Patient Instruction

Julian was taught to monitor his heart rate by taking his pulse. He was taught to monitor his exertion using the perceived rate of exertion (PRE). He was to work at a PRE of 8 to 9 when exercising.

Direct Intervention

Julian participated in an outpatient exercise program with peers from school. He had a circuit training program on the weight machines that he completed two to three times per week. On alternate days, he rode the exercise bike or ran on the treadmill.

Goals

Long-term: Julian wants to be a member of his high school basketball team.

Short-term: Julian will be able to safely use the weight machines for 20 minutes.

Short-term: Julian will be able to complete aerobic activity for 20 minutes at a PRE of 9.

Short-term: Julian will be able to run four laps on a basketball court and dribble the ball with fewer than two turnovers.

Short-term: Julian will be able to shoot the basketball from the free throw line with 70% accuracy.

Termination

Julian will be re-examined in 6 weeks. At that time, his need for ongoing monitoring will be determined.

Movement System Analysis: Force production deficits

Analysis of Case Using the ICF Model

Health condition: Down syndrome

Body functions: Low tone, excessive joint play, decreased strength, overweight

Activity limitations: Decreased motor skills, limited peer interactions, decreased endurance

Participation restrictions: Cannot be successful in high school sports program, limited opportunities to be friends with peers

CHAPTER DISCUSSION QUESTIONS

1. What are some of the related medical conditions associated with Down syndrome that might interfere with exercise?
2. Because of central hypotonia associated with this syndrome, what types of positioning might be used to assist a parent with the development of head control for improved feeding?
3. Children with Down syndrome frequently have hearing impairments that interfere with learning. What types of activities might be included in an early intervention situation as you work to improve motor skills?
4. You are working in a developmental kindergarten program. A child with Down syndrome is having difficulty with activities that require one-foot standing balance because his forefoot rolls medially. What therapeutic activities might be helpful for this child?
5. As children with Down syndrome age through early childhood, what types of physical activity would you recommend to parents to improve general strength, coordination, and flexibility?
6. Families with children who have Down syndrome often seek support and information through different stages of development. What are some resources to assist families?
7. Before referring a child with Down syndrome to the local park district tumbling/gymnastics program, which musculoskeletal comorbidity should be screened for?
8. Long-term and positive participation in physical activity is the aim for all children. It is critical for this population that movement experiences be enjoyable, as well as enhance balance and motor skills. How can physical therapist assistants assist with programming so the child with Down syndrome will choose to be physically active?
9. Describe the physical characteristics of Down syndrome that may restrict participation in playground activities.
10. Susie is a 9-year-old in second grade. She has mosaic Down syndrome. One-foot standing balance is difficult for Susie, and yet the class is playing kickball during physical education/gym. What adaptations can be made so that Susie can participate in the activity?

REFERENCES

1. Accardo PJ, Whitman BY. *Dictionary of Developmental Disabilities Terminology*. 2nd ed. Baltimore: Paul H. Brookes; 2002.
2. Roizen N. Down syndrome. In: Batshaw M, ed. *Children with Disabilities*. 5th ed. Baltimore: Paul H. Brookes; 2002.
3. National Down Syndrome Society: Facts, myths & truths about Down syndrome. Accessed October 25, 2022. https://www.ndss.org/about-down-syndrome/down-syndrome-facts.
4. Mai CT, Isenburg JL, Canfield MA, et al. National population based estimates for major birth defects, 2010–2014. *Birth Defects Res*. 2019;111(18):1420–1435.
5. Pennington BF, Moon J, Edgin J, Stedron J, Nadel L. The neuropsychology of Down syndrome: evidence for hippocampal dysfunction. *Child Dev*. 2003;74:75–93.
6. Mourato FA, Villachan LRR, Mattos SDS. Prevalence and profile of congenital heart disease and pulmonary hypertension in Down syndrome in a pediatric cardiology service. *Rev Paul Pediatr*. 2014;32(2):159–163.
7. Asim A, Agarwal S. Congenital heart defects among Down's syndrome cases: an updated review from basic research to an emerging diagnostics technology and genetic counselling. *J Genet*. 2021;100:45.
8. Rimmer JH, Yamaki K, Lowry BM, Wang E, Vogel LC. Obesity and obesity-related secondary conditions in adolescents with intellectual/developmental disabilities. *J Intellect Disabil Res*. 2010;54(9):787–794.
9. Polfuss M, Sawin KJ, Papanek PE, et al. Total energy expenditure and body composition of children with developmental disabilities. *Disabil Health J*. 2018;11(3):442–446.
10. Palisano RJ, Walter SD, Russell DJ, et al. Gross motor function of children with Down syndrome: creation of motor growth curves. *Arch Phys Med Rehabil*. 2001;82(4):494–500.
11. Tsou AY, Bulova P, Capone G. Medical care of adults with Down syndrome: a clinical guideline. *JAMA*. 2020;324(15):1543–1556.
12. Ulrich DA, Ulrich BD, Angulo-Kinzler RM, Yun J. Treadmill training of infants with Down syndrome: evidence-based developmental outcomes. *Pediatrics*. 2001;108:84–91.

RESOURCES

National Down Syndrome Society
800-221-4602
www.ndss.org

National Association for Down Syndrome
PO Box 4542
Oak Brook, IL 60522
630-325-9112
www.nads.org

National Down Syndrome Congress
800-232-6372
www.ndsccenter.org

March of Dimes
1275 Mamaroneck Avenue
White Plains, NY 10605
www.marchofdimes.com

Health Care Guidelines for Individuals with Down Syndrome
https://ndss.org/resources/healthcare-guidelines

Gigi's Playhouse
https://gigisplayhouse.org/

Spina Bifida

Leann Kerr, PT, DHS, CBIS

LEARNING OBJECTIVES

At the end of the chapter, the reader will be able to do the following:
1. Describe the different types of spina bifida.
2. Formulate an appropriate treatment plan for a child with spina bifida.
3. Advocate for assistive technology for a child with spina bifida.

CHAPTER OUTLINE

KEY TERMS

Hydrocephalus
Meningocele

Myelomeningocele
Neural tube defect

Spina bifida occulta
Tethered cord syndrome

DEFINITION

Spina bifida is the most common permanently disabling birth defect in the United States.[1,2] It is a neural tube defect (NTD). The neural tube fails to develop and close properly. Normally, the neural tube forms early during pregnancy and closes by the 28th day after conception. The term *spina bifida* is Latin and means "split spine." It affects approximately 1 of every 2000 births. The symptoms of spina bifida vary significantly from person to person, depending on the type and level of involvement. There are four classification types of spina bifida: spina bifida occulta, meningocele, myelomeningocele, and a less common type called *myelodysplasia* (Fig. 14.1).

PATHOLOGY

Spina bifida can be detected prenatally using imaging diagnostic tools or laboratory tests. At approximately 18 weeks' gestation, a maternal blood test can check for the presence of alpha-fetoprotein (AFP). Elevated maternal serum AFP levels indicate potential presence of spina bifida in the fetus. Additionally, amniocentesis may be used to complete analysis of the amniotic fluid. Detection of elevated AFP levels indicates spina bifida. If acetylcholinesterase is detected, this indicates an open myelomeningocele. Diagnostic imaging looking for cranial ultrasonographic signs is used to confirm a diagnosis. The lemon sign can be viewed in a cross-section of

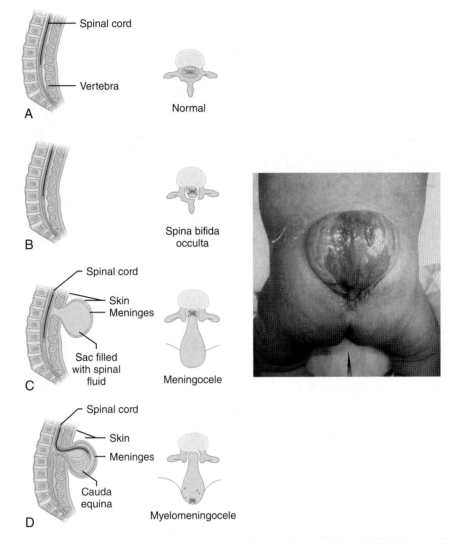

Fig. 14.1 Classification of spina bifida spinal deformities. (From Goodman CC, Fuller K. *Pathology: Implications for the Physical Therapist.* 4th ed. Saunders; 2015 and From Burg FD, Ingelfinger JR, Polin RA, and others. *Current Pediatric Therapy.* 18th ed. Philadelphia: WB Saunders; 2006.)

the brain. The lemon shape appears secondary to overlapping of the frontal bone. This is predictive of a myelomeningocele, which is seen in approximately 80% of cases. The banana sign is seen in more than 90% of cases, and it is the anterior curling and obliteration of the cisterna magna as a result of the downward displacement of the hindbrain (Fig. 14.2). Ventriculomegaly, a condition in which the brain ventricles are enlarged due to a buildup

of cerebrospinal fluid (CSF), is found in association with spina bifida in approximately 75% of cases (Fig. 14.3).

Immediate aggressive medical and surgical intervention is the current best practice. Surgical closure of the lesion will help to prevent infection and further trauma to the spinal cord and surrounding neural tissues. Surgery will not, however, repair any damage to the spinal cord or prevent paralysis.[3]

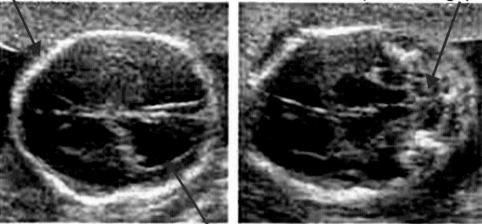

Lemon sign

Absent cisterna magna (Banana sign)

ventriculomegaly

Fig. 14.2 Brain pathology.

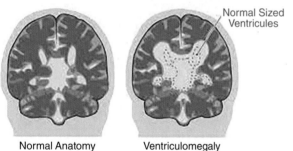

Normal Sized Ventricules

Normal Anatomy   Ventriculomegaly

Fig. 14.3 Ventriculomegaly.

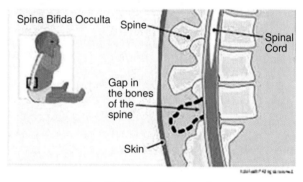

Spina Bifida Occulta   Spine

Spinal Cord

Gap in the bones of the spine

Skin

Fig. 14.4 Spina bifida occulta.

We have seen advancements in fetal neonatal surgery.[4] The National Institution of Child Health and Human Development initiated the Management of Myelomeningocele Study (MOMS) to compare prenatal and postnatal surgical closure.[5] Spina bifida is more common among White and Hispanic populations. Females are affected more often, and families who have one child diagnosed with spina bifida have a slightly higher risk for having a second child with the same condition. There are some discussions suggesting that hyperthermia and lack of folic acid in the early weeks of the pregnancy may be a contributing factor. Pre-pregnancy obesity and uncontrolled diabetes are associated with higher risk.[6]

CLINICAL SIGNS

Spina bifida occulta describes the condition in which the neural arches do not connect, but there is no neural material located outside of the spinal canal (Fig. 14.4). This is the most common form of spina bifida, characteristically involving the lower lumbar spine. It is also the most benign, with typically no resultant neurologic effects or abnormalities.[1,2] Approximately 40% of the population may have a spina bifida occulta malformation but be asymptomatic.[7]

In a meningocele, the neural arches do not connect, and the meninges (the three protective membranes covering the brain and spinal cord) protrude through the

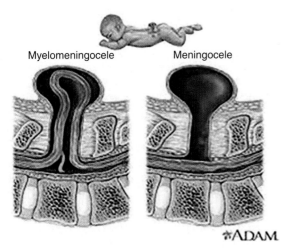

Fig. 14.5 Spina Bifida.

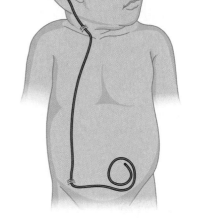

Fig. 14.6 Hydrocephalus and shunt. (From Goodman CC, Fuller K. *Pathology: Implications for the Physical Therapist.* 4th ed. Saunders; 2015.)

opening in the child's spinal column (Fig. 14.5). The spinal cord is not trapped, and these children often do not exhibit any neurologic symptoms.[1,2] The meningocele is skin covered and is intially associated with no paralysis and only contain membranes or nonfunctional nerves that end in the sac wall. Meningocele requires surgery to put the meninges back in place and close the opening in the vertebrae.

In a myelomeningocele, both the spinal cord and meninges protrude through the vertebral defect into a sac or open area in the back. It is an open spinal cord defect that usually protrudes dorsally without skin covering, and it is usually associated with spinal nerve paralysis. The spinal cord and surrounding tissues may be visible and exposed to the environment, which places the child at high risk for infection. The spinal cord is malformed, and defects may extend below the level of the primary herniation. There may be dura mater fused to the edges of the skin defect, with the sac being covered exclusively by arachnoid membrane. The child exhibits atypical development, including flaccid lower extremities and loss of sensation below the level of the myelomeningocele. The defect can occur at any spinal level but is often seen in the lumbosacral area.

Clinicians should also be aware of a related form of spina bifida, occult spinal **dysraphism** (OSD). OSD is a condition in which there is a noticeable abnormality of the child's lower back. This abnormality may be a birthmark (perhaps red), tufts of hair, a small opening in the skin, a small lump, or a sacral dimple. Babies with a sacral dimple should be further evaluated using imaging techniques to determine whether pathology is present.[1,2]

There are several other neurologic sequelae that may accompany myelomeningocele, including abnormalities of the brain, abnormal migration of neurons, hydrocephalus, and Arnold-Chiari malformation.

Hydrocephalus is found in more than 80% of children with myelomeningocele. Hydrocephalus is the enlargement of the ventricular system in the brain due to an increase in CSF.[3] The child with hydrocephalus requires immediate treatment and correction by the medical team. This correction usually takes the form of placement of a ventriculoperitoneal (VP) shunt[3] (Fig. 14.6). The shunt drains CSF out of the brain and into the gut. An extra length of tubing is typically placed in the gut to allow for growth of the child without the need to replace the shunt. Caregivers should be taught the warning signs of shunt malfunction, which include irritability, personality changes, increased sleepiness, "sunset eyes" (the child's eyes assume a downward gaze, mimicking a sunset), and headaches. The child should be brought to the physician if a shunt malfunction is suspected.

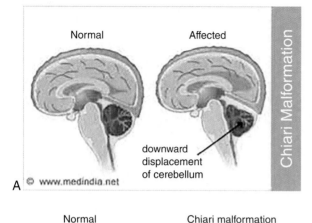

A © www.medindia.net

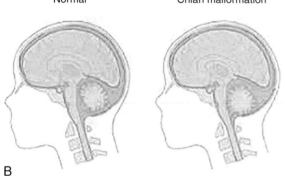

B

Fig. 14.7 Arnold-Chiari defect.

Type 2 Arnold-Chiari malformation can also be associated with myelomeningocele. An Arnold-Chiari malformation is a defect at the base of the brain (cerebellum, pons, medulla); it is elongated and protrudes into the foramen magnum (Fig. 14.7).[3]

Another impairment commonly seen in addition to spina bifida is tethered cord syndrome. This occurs when the spinal cord is fixed caudally because of pathology. The tethered spinal cord becomes stretched, distorted, and ischemic. The child with tethered cord syndrome may show atypical neurologic signs that include decreased strength, increased spasticity in the lower extremities, changing urologic patterns, back pain, and scoliosis. Surgery to free the cord is usually performed, and success of the surgery is measured by a return of neurologic function.

INTERVENTION

Physical therapy should focus on reducing secondary complications and assisting in development of independence with mobility, transfers, and recreational activities to enhance the child's ability to participate in activities with peers. The physical therapist (PT) will also assist in providing recommendations for equipment and bracing. Therapy services will take place on and off throughout the child's life span. Treatment intervention may include active stretching and strengthening of musculoskeletal tissues, increasing endurance for physical activity, developing independent transfer skills, and instruction in motor activities that improve the child's performance in everyday life routines. The complex problems encountered by children and adolescents with spina bifida require skillful collaboration between occupational therapist (OT), speech language pathologist, PT, and the patient's caregivers. Intervention will always depend on the child's lesion level, functional abilities, and age. The family should be allied with a medical and therapeutic team familiar with children with spina bifida. The family should also be referred to a relevant support group.

A child with a lumbosacral myelomeningocele may exhibit any or all of the following: flaccid paralysis, muscle weakness, muscle wasting, atypical tendon reflexes, atypical sensation, and incontinence. Comorbidities for the individual with myelomeningocele could include hydrocephalus, skin breakdown in weight-bearing areas, severe vasomotor changes, osteoporosis, soft tissue contractures, and cognitive and social delays. Additionally, there may be other congenital abnormalities related to the spinal vertebrae, cleft palate, abnormal long bone development, or skeletal malformations.[1] Interventions should address the child's functional deficits and capitalize on the child's strengths. See Tables 14.1 and 14.2 for classification of lesions and potential functional deficits.

The family must be educated in the proper care and nutrition of the infant/child with spina bifida. This will include teaching optimal positioning for the child, the importance of weight-bearing and upright positioning, reiterating shunt care and signs and symptoms of shunt malfunction, and providing information on how to safely construct the child's environment to compensate for decreased sensation. Strengthening and increasing range of motion of all extremities and the trunk are an integral portion of the child's rehabilitation program. It is easier to prevent contractures than to reverse them. Strengthening and range of motion exercises should be embedded into the family's ordinary daily routines as much as possible.

TABLE 14.1 Functional Deficits and Level of Lesion

Lowest Level Intact	Muscle Function Present	Ambulatory Status	Notes
L2	Some hip flexion (iliopsoas) may be preserved	Minimal ambulation possible with a reciprocating gait orthosis	
L3	Hip flexion and hip adduction	Some household ambulation with reciprocating gait orthosis or hip-knee-ankle-foot orthosis	Highest risk of hip instability and dislocation
L4	Knee extension (quadriceps), ankle dorsiflexion/inversion (tibialis anterior)	Household ambulation, may require ankle-foot orthosis and/or crutches	Biggest difference in mobility prognostication is between L3 and L4 levels due to quadriceps functions
L5	Hip extension and hip abduction (gluteal muscles), knee flexion (medial hamstrings), toe dorsiflexion (extensor halluces longus and extensor digitorum longus muscles)	Community ambulation, may require ankle-foot orthosis and/or crutches	Medial hamstring function helpful for community ambulation
S1	Ankle plantarflexion (gastrocnemius-soleus complex)	Community ambulation, may require ankle-foot orthosis	
S2	Toe plantar-flexion (flexor halluces longus and flexor digitorum longus muscles)	Community ambulation, may require ankle-foot orthosis	

TABLE 14.2 Walking Potential per Neurologic Level

Level	Function	Muscle	Walking Potential
Thoracic	Paraplegic		Nonwalker
L1–L2	Paraplegic, hip flexion	Psoas	Nonwalker
L3	Knee extension	Quadriceps	33% walk at 4–5 years with AFOs and crutches
L4	Knee extension	Quadriceps	100% walk at 3–4 years with AFOs and crutches
	Knee flexion	Medial hamstring	
L5	Ankle dorsiflexion	Tibialis anterior	100% walk at 2–3 years with AFOs
S1	Ankle plantar flexion	Gastrocnemius	100% walk at 1–2 years

AFOs, ankle-foot orthoses.

The child with spina bifida should be positioned in symmetric-upright posture as soon as feasibly possible. This will assist in developing strong abdominal muscles and good trunk alignment. Supported standing will also promote bone density development and good structural alignment. Practice will be needed to develop strong balance and equilibrium reactions in sitting and standing to be able to play and become independently mobile. For example, the young child with independent sitting balance is free to play on the floor with friends or sit in a chair and interact with classmates and peers. Good standing balance can enable the child to participate in more activities independently. If a child can maintain standing, then the child can participate in board activities in the classroom or sports activities at some level. The child with good static and dynamic balance will also be more mobile within his or her environment.

Orthotics play an important role in the medical management of the child with spina bifida. Ankle-foot orthoses may be needed to maintain proper foot, ankle, and knee positions during standing and ambulation. The child might also benefit from a reciprocal gait orthosis (RGO). The RGO, designed to assist in ambulation, is essentially a dynamic hip-knee-ankle-foot orthosis (HKAFO) with a trunk component incorporated into its design. When the user leans backward leading with one shoulder, the contralateral hip flexes, and that lower extremity is advanced. Typically, the child uses the RGO in conjunction with a walker or crutches to maintain balance. Many children with spina bifida will require an orthosis to support the trunk. This orthosis will be named for the body area it covers. If the orthosis encompasses the entire trunk from the inferior spine of the scapula to the pelvis, it is called a *thoracic-lumbar-sacral orthosis* (TLSO). If it only encompasses the lower back, it is referred to as a *lumbar-sacral orthosis* (LSO). Refer to Chapter 21 for more information regarding orthoses. Just-right and on-time mobility should be introduced early. A child should be referred for consultation for augmented mobility, which may allow the child to experience some level of independent mobility, which will allow the child to experience independent mobility. The team should evaluate the child for orthotics, ambulation potential, and energy expenditure with self-propelled mobility.

If it is determined that the child would benefit from wheeled mobility, a referral to an assistive technology team is worthwhile. Most children with spina bifida can propel a manual wheelchair without difficulty. Depending on the child's trunk and lower extremity strength, a contoured seating system may be needed. The child may also require a pressure relief cushion to maintain skin integrity. A complete discussion of seating and mobility equipment can be found in Chapter 22.

CASE STUDY OF A CHILD WITH SPINA BIFIDA

General demographics: Angelica (Annie) is a 3-year-old girl with spina bifida. She was diagnosed with spina bifida 8 weeks prior to birth. She lives at home with her mother, father, paternal grandparents, and three older siblings.

General health: Annie underwent surgical closure of the spina bifida lesion (at L5) when she was 2 days old. No shunt placement was necessary. Her overall health has been excellent. She has never had a bladder infection.

Family history: There is no family history of spina bifida.

Medical history: History includes postnatal surgery; all other medical history is unremarkable. Annie has received therapy services (PT, OT, and developmental therapy) through the early intervention program.

Growth and development: Annie has not determined hand dominance yet. She had delays in mastery of developmental milestones but can independently roll, sit, and transition to standing now.

History of current condition: Annie's condition was diagnosed via ultrasonography 1 week prior to birth. She was delivered at term by cesarean section and immediately transferred to the neonatal intensive care unit (NICU). After surgery, she was monitored in the NICU for several days before being discharged home.

Functional status and activity level: Annie is a very happy and active child who moves around her home independently without assistive devices. She will use assistive devices when out in the community. See Tests and Measures for more detailed information.

Medications: Annie does not take any medications. She does take nonprescription vitamins daily.

Systems Review

Cardiovascular/pulmonary: No abnormalities reported
  Integumentary: See Tests and Measures
  Musculoskeletal: See Test and Measures
  Neuromuscular: See Tests and Measures

Communication and cognition: Annie speaks fluent English, her primary language. She does have any cognitive limitations at this time, although she occasionally has difficulty solving novel complex-task problems.

Tests and Measures

Endurance: Annie experiences fatigue more quickly than her peers when walking long distances. She prefers to be carried or ride in a stroller or wagon for walks around her neighborhood. She also uses an electric toy car to play outside and keep up with her peers.

Pain: No evidence of pain or discomfort.

Integumentary: Well-healed scar on posterior lower trunk at the level of L3–L4. Callusing noted on bilateral medial and lateral foot borders. Mild redness noted at left lateral malleoli; however, this dissipated after 6 minutes.

Range of motion: Passive range of motion in all extremities and trunk. Head is held in midline, and there are no spinal asymmetries noted.

Strength: Trunk and bilateral upper extremities, 4+/5; bilateral hips in all planes, 3+/5; bilateral knee flexion and extension, 3/5; bilateral ankle strength in all planes, 3–/5; bilateral feet in all planes, 1/5.

Sensation: Decreased sensation in distal lower extremities and feet.

Environmental barriers: Annie lives in a single-story ranch house. There are no stairs inside the home. There is

CASE STUDY OF A CHILD WITH SPINA BIFIDA—cont'd

a small step at both the front entranceway and back door, which Annie can maneuver over if she concentrates.

Balance: Annie demonstrates initial self-righting responses when sitting. When standing, she uses a hip strategy but does not demonstrate an ankle strategy. When standing, Annie uses her upper extremities for support and stability.

Transitional skills: Annie independently transitions from supine to standing by progressing through half-kneeling without assistance.

Gait/locomotion: Annie ambulates with a wide stance and significant lateral sway. She maintains her upper extremities in the low guard position.

Assistive/adaptive devices: Annie does not use any assistive devices at home. If ambulating outdoors, she may choose to use Lofstrand crutches, a walker for long distances, or a powered toy for outside play. If she is feeling particularly tired, she may ask to use her walker, but that is not a typical request. She also wears bilateral hinged AFOs.

Activities of daily living: Annie can assist with donning and doffing her AFOs. She assists with dressing of the lower extremities; however, she has some difficulty donning and doffing shoes and socks. Her siblings work with her to improve her skills and speed. Annie can feed herself, comb her hair, and brush her teeth. She drinks from a cup, typically without a lid, and uses a spoon or fork to eat.

Posture: Annie sits erectly and stands with a slight lordosis.

Gross Motor Function Measure summary
- Lying and rolling: mastered all 17 items, 100%.
- Sitting: mastered all 19 items, 100%.
- Crawling and kneeling: completed 12/13 tasks, 92%. Annie had minimal difficulty with walking and tall kneeling.
- Standing: completed 10/12 tasks, 83%. Annie had minimal difficulty when attempting to stand on one foot for up to 10 seconds. She was able to maintain unilateral stance for 3 to 6 seconds.
- Walking, running, jumping: completed 20/23 tasks, 87%. Annie had difficulty stepping over a bar raised 6 to 8 inches off the floor and jumping horizontally or vertically. Annie also had minimal difficulty walking backward. She can run and ride a tricycle short distances.

Evaluation
Annie is a happy, mobile, 3-year-old preschooler. She wears bilateral hinged AFOs and typically only ambulates with Lofstrand crutches, a walker, or a power toy for long distances outdoors. She has significant weakness in her lower extremities and difficulty performing some high-level gross motor skills. Her skin is intact, and currently, there are no integumentary concerns.

Prognosis
Annie's strength and endurance should continue to improve. She is at risk for comorbidities of spina bifida as she ages, and these should be monitored. She should be able to learn and master bowel and bladder routines in the future.

Intervention
Coordination, Communication, Documentation
Coordination will need to occur between Annie's family, school therapists and teachers, clinic therapists, and physicians.

Patient Instruction
Annie and her family received a written home program for working on endurance and community ambulation skills. Annie's chores included retrieving the mail, helping to walk the family dog, or any activity that involves walking medium to long distances. Annie and her parents were shown how to check her skin after taking off the orthotics. Annie's family was encouraged to stay connected with the local support groups for spina bifida.

Direct Intervention
Therapeutic exercise: Strengthening exercises for the lower extremities using latex-free Thera-Band. Aerobic exercise, including walking on the treadmill in the clinic.

Functional training: Annie was also enrolled in a local age-appropriate swimming program to help increase her overall strength and endurance. Dynamic balance and climbing activities were offered in physical therapy to focus on higher-level gross motor skills. These included standing on a balance board and varying the balance point, walking on unstable surfaces (soft foam cushions covering the floor), jumping on a minitrampoline with a rail support, and climbing playground equipment.

Goals
1. Annie will improve lower-extremity strength by one grade so she can safely ascend and descend the school bus steps.
2. Annie will increase her endurance so she can walk two blocks to the park to play with her friends.
3. Annie will maintain good skin condition and be reevaluated for new AFOs as she grows. Annie will

Continued

CASE STUDY OF A CHILD WITH SPINA BIFIDA — cont'd

be able to dress herself with occasional assistance so she can be more independent.

Re-Examination

Annie will be reassessed in 6 months by her hospital-based clinic team.

Analysis of Case Using the ICF Model

Body functions: Spina bifida L3 level, no shunt. Significantly decreased strength in bilateral lower extremities. Decreased endurance. Decreased high-level gross motor skills. Ambulates with bilateral AFOs; uses crutches when ambulating outdoors.

Activity limitations: Difficulty playing with peers outdoors, not independent in dressing, difficulty ascending and descending stairs, tires easily.

Participation restrictions: Requires assistance for activities of daily living, requires assistance on and off the school bus, has difficulty playing at the park with peers and walking around her neighborhood.

Environmental limitations: Requires single-story home and ramps to access buildings and park equipment.

Movement System Assessment: Force production deficits

CHAPTER DISCUSSION QUESTIONS

1. Describe the warning signs of VP shunt malfunction in a toddler with spina bifida and hydrocephalus.
2. What types of assistive walking devices to be used when playing at the park might be provided for an 18-month-old toddler with spina bifida, functioning at the L4 level?
3. Juan is a 4-year-old boy with spina bifida. He uses bilateral AFOs and crutches to ambulate. His early childhood class is going on a field trip to the local firehouse. What other types of assistive devices might be used to increase his efficiency and reduce fatigue?
4. Fran is a 15-month-old girl with spina bifida, functioning at the Tl2 level. She was fitted for a vertical stander to support her in standing. Plan a program incorporating the stander into her daily routines. What types of therapeutic exercise could be encouraged with this piece of equipment?
5. Jackson attends first grade at the local public school. He is receiving physical therapy per his individualized education program (IEP). He uses AFOs and crutches for mobility. You notice a change in his gait pattern. You remove the right orthotic and note a very reddened area at the lateral calcaneus. What is your plan of action?
6. Children with spina bifida are at high risk for latex sensitivity. What type of exercise equipment might need to be modified/adapted so these children are not excluded from participating in physical education or conditioning programs?
7. Joe had surgery to lengthen soft tissue restrictions and returned to school using bilateral KAFOs (knee, ankle, foot orthotics) and a walker. Prepare a program for Joe that includes standing transfers to/from wheelchair to walker. What problems might be encountered when Joe uses a walker in a school environment?
8. Tess is a sophomore in high school. She was born with spina bifida and wears a TLSO to assist alignment for structural scoliosis. She functions at the LS motor level. Tess uses a manual wheelchair for school but will walk with bilateral AFOs and forearm crutches in the community setting. Tess is a straight-A student, president of the debate club, and class secretary. She recently fell and fractured her arm. Surgical intervention resulted in 10 weeks in an above-elbow cast with strict restrictions on weight-bearing with the fractured extremity. How can Tess achieve independent mobility at school?

REFERENCES

1. Shepard RB. *Physiotherapy in Pediatrics*. 3rd ed. Oxford: Butterworth-Heinemann; 1999.
2. Liptak GS. Neural tube defects. In: Batshaw M, ed. *Children With Disabilities*. 5th ed. Baltimore: Paul H Brookes; 2002.
3. Palisano R, Orlin M, Scheiber J. *Campbell's Physical Therapy for Children*. 6th ed. St Louis: Elsevier Publishing; 2022.
4. Columbia University Medical Center. Department of Neurological Surgery: *Spina bifida* (website): https://www.neurosurgery.columbia.edu/patient-care/conditions/spina-bifida. Accessed September 18, 2004.

5. Accardo PJ, Whitman BY. *Dictionary of Developmental Disabilities Terminology*. 3rd ed. Baltimore: Paul H Brookes; 2011.

6. Adzick NS, Thom EA, Spong CY. A randomized trial of prenatal versus postnatal repair of myelomeningocele. *N Engl J Med*. 2011;364(11):993–1004.

7. Spina Bifida Association of America. *Working to build a better and brighter future* (website): https://www.spinabifidaassociation.org/. Accessed June 1, 2022.

15

Autism Spectrum Disorder

Erin Simpson, DrOT, MOT, OTR/L

KEY TERMS

Autism   Autism spectrum disorder

DEFINITION

Autism is the most common of a series of related neurologic and developmental disorders known collectively as ASD. Autism is a neurologic disorder caused by differences in the brain and a developmental disorder because it is often diagnosed at a young age. Specific causes are not fully known; however, scientists believe that there may be a genetic component or a combination of other factors that lead to ASD. Autism, or ASD, is characterized by challenges with social communication and interaction, restricted or repetitive behavior, and difficulty with speech and nonverbal communication.

PATHOLOGY

Autism was first identified in 1943, and until the 1970s, it was generally considered a psychologic disorder caused by poor parenting. There is no known single cause for autism, but it is generally accepted that it is caused by differences in brain function or structure. Some research indicates that autism may have environmental, viral, or metabolic causes; while other research supports the theory that autism may stem from a genetic predisposition combined with certain environmental or other triggers. Whatever the cause, the number of diagnosed cases of autism has risen sharply in recent years.

According to the Centers for Disease Control and Prevention (CDC) 2020 ADDM (Autism and Developmental Disabilities Monitoring), the prevalence of autism had risen to 1 in every 36 8-year-old children, more than tripled from the 2004 rate of 1 in 125 8-year-old children.[1] The CDC estimates that 3.5 million Americans live with ASD.[2] It is unclear whether there is an actual increase in the incidence of autism or whether increased attention to and improved early identification/diagnosis of the disorder accounts for the rise in the number of cases reported.[3] The prevalence of autism is four times higher in boys than it is in girls; however, girls with ASD may not display characteristics of autism in the same way as boys and may go undiagnosed because of their different presentation.[1]

Children with autism often have one or more other disorders, including attention-deficit disorder (ADD) or attention-deficit/hyperactivity disorder (ADHD), anxiety disorder, sleep disorders, seizures, and aggression.[4] Approximately 30% of children with a diagnosis of ASD also have an intellectual disability,[4] although accurate IQ testing for children with autism can be difficult. Many children with autism do have highly developed "splinter skills," but generally not to the savant level portrayed in movies like *Rain Main* and *Mercury Rising.*

New legislation has been enacted that mandates autism-specific activities. The Autism Collaboration, Accountability, Research, Education and Support Act (Autism CARES Act) of 2019 is the primary source of federal funding for autism research, services, training, and monitoring. The focus has expanded to include the entire lifespan of people on the autism spectrum. The Autism CARES Act was originally called *The Combating Autism Act of 2006,* which enhanced research, surveillance, and education for ASDs (Box 15.1).

CLINICAL SIGNS

A medical diagnosis is made by a psychologist, developmental pediatrician, or other specialized physician based on an assessment of symptoms and results of diagnostic tests. This diagnosis is made according to the American Psychiatric Association's *Diagnostic and Statistical Manual, 5th Edition (DSM-5).* This provides standardized criteria to help diagnose ASD. To be diagnosed

> **BOX 15.1 Autism CARES Act of 2019**
>
> The Autism CARES Act requires and supports:
> - Autism prevalence monitoring
> - Training of medical professionals to detect and diagnose autism
> - Development of treatments for medical conditions associated with autism
> - The Interagency Autism Coordinating Committee (IACC) and its annual strategic plan
> - Centers of excellence in autism surveillance and epidemiology
> - Countless programs and research grants to benefit individuals with autism
>
> Because of Autism CARES, scientific developments have
> - Set a reliable diagnosis age of 18 to 24 months
> - Established that timely interventions make a lifetime of difference
> - Identified comorbidities
> - Increased understanding of biological causes of autism
> - Identified genes and possible medication targets
> - Developed early career autism researchers
>
> From Autism Speaks. Autism CARES Act. Accessed July 6, 2022. https://www.autismspeaks.org/autism-cares-act.

with ASD according to the *DSM-5,* a child must have persistent deficits in each of the three areas of social communication and interaction plus at least two of four types of restricted, repetitive behavior. For the diagnosis of autism, onset of symptoms must have occurred prior to the age of 3 years. In addition, childhood disintegrative disorder should be ruled out as a more likely cause of developmental problems before a diagnosis of autism is made.

Social Communication and Interaction Skills

Social-emotional reciprocity is an area in which children with autism generally show deficits. A child with ASD may have an abnormal social approach and be unable to participate in typical back-and-forth conversations, may have difficulty sharing interests or emotions, and may be unable to initiate or respond to social interactions.

All children must learn basic reciprocal behavior that makes social congress possible (e.g., waiting in line, taking turns, and sharing). And while such behaviors are often somewhat problematic for all young children, they are especially difficult for those with autism. The less concrete the rules for behavior are, the more problematic they are likely to be for someone with autism. For example, a child with autism might be able to learn to wait in a formal line but likely would have more difficulty dealing with the informal queuing up involved in, say, boarding a train.

Even in cases in which a child has developed language skills, there is often a marked deficit in the ability to initiate or maintain a conversation. Because of the social impairments and the attendant lack of motivation to engage in normal social exchange associated with autism, language for the child with ASD is often limited to meeting concrete wants and needs, even in cases in which the child has fluent language skills. The child might ask for something to eat but would be unlikely to tell you about his or her day. Children with autism also frequently use stereotyped or repetitive language. They often have standard rote responses to certain questions or situations or perseverate (uncontrollably repeat) a word or phrase.

The presence of deficits in nonverbal communicative behavior used for social interaction is a key diagnostic indicator for autism. Children may have poorly integrated verbal and nonverbal communication, abnormalities in eye contact and body language, or deficits in understanding and using gestures; they may also have a total lack of facial expression and nonverbal communication. Children with autism generally do not substitute mime, gesture, or other communication strategies to compensate, as would a child with a limitation such as deafness.

Individuals with autism often demonstrate poor eye contact when interacting with others. They may make no or only cursory eye contact; they may make eye contact in an unorthodox manner (such as turning their head to the side and looking obliquely at the individual with whom they are interacting); in a group, they may look at someone who is not speaking.

Individuals with autism may also demonstrate marked impairment in facial expression, body posture, and use of gestures. In contrast, children without autism learn intuitively to understand and then use appropriate facial expressions and other physical cues to reflect their own feelings and needs and to interpret nonverbal cues from others. Children with autism generally demonstrate flat affect and show marked impairment in their ability to interpret facial or gestural cues from others.

Developing, maintaining, and understanding relationships are difficult for children with ASD. Children with ASD may have difficulty in adjusting behavior to suit various social contexts and engaging in imaginative play or in making friends, or they may lack interest in peers.

Children with autism typically fail to form successful peer relationships. They often prefer to be alone and will choose activities that have no social component, such as watching videos. They will often ignore others in the area or even react negatively to attempts to "intrude" on their isolating activities. They generally do not share their interests or accomplishments. While a child without autism often wants to share an accomplishment with parents or peers ("Mommy, look at the picture I drew!"), a child with autism typically shows little or no interest in such interactions.

Individuals with autism exhibit limited or no joint attention (engaging another to interact) and frequently have difficulty shifting attention from one item or task to another. While children without autism readily learn to share attention (i.e., respond to a request or directions from a parent or peer to look at something else) or devote the communal attention necessary to complete a social task, children with autism will often resist or not even understand such requests. Children with autism will also frequently devote an inappropriate amount of attention to a particular object or activity (Fig. 15.1).

Children with autism generally do not engage in spontaneous or imitative play. While children without autism are able to generalize and abstract information, children with autism have limited abilities in these areas. Thus, they are unlikely to transfer the experience of watching an activity into imitative or spontaneous play.

Restricted or Repetitive Behaviors or Interests

A child with autism may have stereotyped or repetitive motor movements and use of objects or speech. Stereotyped motor behaviors are also common among children with autism. Examples of such behaviors include constant rocking and flapping of the hands or fingers. Such behaviors are often self-stimulatory in nature.

Insistence on sameness, inflexible adherence to routines, or ritualized patterns of verbal or nonverbal

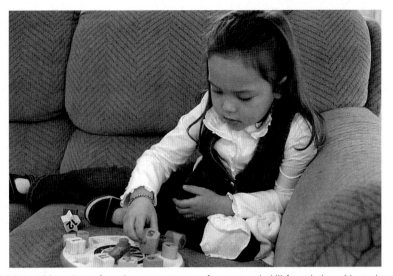

Fig. 15.1 Children with autism often demonstrate a preference and skill for relating objects in construction activities and puzzles. (Courtesy Shay McAtee.)

behavior are often seen in individuals with ASD. Children with autism often rigidly adhere to routines or rituals with no apparent functional purpose. For example, a child with autism might insist on always sitting in the same seat or always opening and closing the door to the room twice when entering. Although the purpose of the rituals is not apparent, a child with autism is likely to become upset if these routines are interrupted or interfered with.

Individuals with ASD may have highly restricted and repetitive behaviors and have fixed interests that are abnormal in intensity or focus. They may show strong attachment to or preoccupation with unusual objects. A child with autism will often demonstrate abnormally intense interest in attention to unusually narrow areas of interest. For example, you might encounter a child with autism who has memorized the entire cable television schedule and can readily tell you the date and time for any program, even those of no particular interest to the child. Another child with autism might go to a mall and want to do nothing but ride in all the elevators. This intense interest in a narrow area can manifest as an abnormal fear (e.g., a fear of elevators instead of a desire to ride in them). Children with autism may be abnormally preoccupied with certain objects—anything from pencils to paper clips to pot lids. If they encounter such an object, they may remain focused on it for hours.

Hyper- or hyporeactivity to sensory input or unusually intense responses to sensory aspects of the environment are also exhibited by those with ASD. They have an apparent indifference to pain/temperature, adverse responses to specific sounds or textures, excessive smelling or touching of objects, visual fascination with lights or movement. Odd or exaggerated responses to sensory stimuli are common in children with autism. They are often very sensitive to sound, sometimes even seeming to find normal levels of sound painful or intrusive. They may overreact to being touched or have difficulty with tags in their clothing or certain textures of cloth. Many dislike bright lights and will often choose dark, enclosed spaces. They may also have exaggerated reactions to odors or other stimuli but sometimes demonstrate an unusually high tolerance for pain.

INTERVENTION

Symptoms of autism can begin to emerge as early as 12 to 18 months and are almost always evident between 24 months and 6 years of age. Numerous studies have demonstrated that early diagnosis and treatment of autism result in substantially improved outcomes. Physical therapists work with the child, family, and the child's school. Physical therapists have training in child development and motor control. Therapists will help children with autism engage in and improve daily routines, acquire new movement skills, develop better coordination and stable posture, improve play skills, develop motor imitation skills, and increase fitness and stamina.

Physical Therapy Assessment

Autism is a developmental disability, which by its nature emerges gradually. In many cases, parents, through their intense daily experience with their child, will have noticed important but subtle issues and raise those issues with the child's healthcare provider. Pediatricians or other clinicians may dismiss parents' concerns because the signs are not readily evident during a brief visit within a clinical setting. By the time the developmental issues in question become obvious, important time has been lost, so it becomes vital that clinicians not dismiss a parent's expressed concerns out of hand.

Once diagnostic issues have been raised, the preferred option for pursuing an appropriate diagnosis is through a multidisciplinary team composed of some or all of the following disciplines: developmental pediatrician, psychiatrist, psychologist, occupational therapist, speech therapist, and physical therapist. This team can draw on a number of diagnostic instruments presently available to assist in screening and evaluating a child for autism. They include the following:

- The Ages and Stages Questionnaire, Second Edition (ASQ)
- The Autism Screening Questionnaire
- Bayley Scales II
- BRIGANCE Screen II
- Childhood Autism Rating Scale (CARS)
- The Checklist for Autism in Toddlers (CHAT)
- The Child Development Inventories
- The Parents' Evaluation of Developmental Status
- The Wechsler Preschool and Primary Scale of Intelligence, Revised Edition (WPPSI-R)

This is a representative list of some of the more commonly used instruments, but there are a variety of other instruments available. Different professionals often have different preferences.

Physical Therapy Intervention

If a diagnosis of autism is appropriate, the next step is developing a comprehensive treatment plan. There is no cure for autism, nor is there any universally adopted approach to its treatment. The treatment plan should be based on the needs of each child and must continually

---

ASD CLINICAL SIGNS

Social Communication and Interaction Skills
- Has poor eye contact
- Does not respond to his or her name
- Does not babble or coo by 12 months
- Does not gesture (point, wave, grasp) by 12 months
- Does not say single words by 16 months
- Cannot say what he or she wants
- Language is delayed
- Is not interested in other children
- Does not follow directions
- Appears deaf at times
- Seems to hear sometimes but not at others
- Used to say a few words, but now does not
- Does not smile socially
- Seems to prefer to play alone

Restricted or Repetitive Behaviors or Interests
- Lines up toys or other objects and gets upset when order is changed
- Repeats words or phrases over and over (echolalia)
- Has obsessive traits
- Must follow certain routines
- Flaps hands, rocks body, or spins self in circles
- Has unusual reactions to the way things sound, smell, taste, look, or feel
- Is oversensitive to certain textures or sounds

Other Characteristics
- Delayed language, motor, cognitive or learning skills
- Is hyperactive, uncooperative, or oppositional
- Unusual eating and sleeping habits
- Gastrointestinal issues
- Exhibits anxiety, stress, or excessive worry
- Lack of fear or more fear than expected
- Epilepsy or seizure disorder

---

be reevaluated and adjusted based on results and emerging needs. Consider too that the level of functioning varies widely among individuals with autism, and therefore, the level and direction of the treatment plan must be tailored.

An ideal treatment plan will address a wide range of issues, including communication, behavior, social skills, sensory integration, fine and gross motor skills, and activities of daily living.

An initial focus should be the development of both receptive and expressive language. Children with autism who develop verbal language skills have a significantly better prognosis than those who do not. However, many children with autism develop limited or no verbal language, and even those who do frequently also rely on various augmentative communication tools and programs. A good treatment plan will identify individual strengths and utilize those tools that play to them best.

A variety of behavioral issues, including tantrums, aggression, and lack of personal boundaries, are common to children with autism. Because most of these individuals depend on strict routines to understand and act within their environment, carefully designed and consistently followed behavior programs are an essential element of any treatment plan. Medications can also play a key role in behavior management.

Difficulties understanding and acting within appropriate social roles are a root issue. Lack of attention to or understanding of the environment also raises key personal and community safety concerns, so particular attention must be paid to helping children understand critical concepts. Role-playing exercises, guided community activities, symbol or picture scripts, and a variety of other tools and techniques can be helpful in this area.

Children with autism frequently have exaggerated or otherwise atypical reactions to vestibular, proprioceptive, auditory, visual, tactile, olfactory, or other sensory input. Those reactions can exacerbate behavioral issues, interfere with appropriate attention to the environment, leave the child in a state of under- or overarousal, or otherwise interfere with the ability to organize sensation for use. A variety of techniques have proven helpful in assisting children with autism to process and integrate sensory input and better understand and react to their environments more appropriately.

Motor skill impairments often go hand in hand with autism, so a specific evaluation of the individual's motor capabilities and a treatment plan to address impairments are vital. Interventions can include both specific stretching exercises and general exercise activity, such as horseback riding or swimming.

Helping each individual develop the highest possible level of competency with daily activities such as personal hygiene, eating, and dressing should be a key focus of any treatment plan. Special care should be taken to make the child more receptive to hygiene activities; a long-handled, soft bath brush or a mechanical toothbrush may help the child become more independent.

AUTISM AND ASD INTERVENTIONS

- Develop language skills
- Create a consistent behavior program
- Develop social skills
- Use techniques for processing and integrating sensory input
- Address motor impairments
- Develop competence in daily activities

CASE STUDY OF A CHILD WITH AUTISM SPECTRUM DISORDER

Examination

History: Nicholas is a 12-year-old boy with diagnoses of autism, ADHD, and controlled seizures. His birth history is complicated by a wrapped umbilical cord causing respiratory problems and a mother with infections in the lungs during pregnancy. He received occupational, physical, and speech therapy services through the early intervention program as a baby and continued to receive these services through the school system. He attends the local public elementary school. He has a history of generalized weakness, toe walking, and oral and tactile sensitivity. His caregivers began noticing turning in of both feet 3 months ago, and his teachers at school voiced concern about decreased function and complaints of pain in the left foot. He showed decreased ability in running and bike riding at that time. His mother reported trying an arch support insert that did not help with foot position or pain, but some improvement was noted when he was wearing high-top shoes.

Nicholas is a very mild-mannered boy who showed some difficulty following directions, requiring one or two requests, demonstration, and physical prompting. He communicated and interacted with this therapist, but with noticeably decreased attention and eye contact. He showed decreased attention to tasks and toys as well.

Nicholas's mother expressed concern about the position of his feet and would like for him to return to a more normal walking pattern and have no complaints

Continued

CASE STUDY OF A CHILD WITH AUTISM SPECTRUM DISORDER—cont'd

of pain in his foot. She would also like him to be able to return to running and bike riding so that he can keep up at school.

Systems Review
Cardiopulmonary: No concerns at this time
Musculoskeletal: Concerns
Neuromuscular: Concerns
Integumentary: No concerns at this time

Test and Measures
Range of motion: Nicholas presented with normal passive range of motion (PROM) in all joints, but bilateral dorsiflexion was limited to 0 degrees. He also showed some limited active range of motion (AROM) due to weakness and soft tissue approximation due to obesity.

Strength (manual muscle testing): These measurements may not represent Nicholas's true muscle strength, as he had difficulty following manual muscle testing directions and isolating joint motions.

	Right Lower Extremity	Left Lower Extremity
Ankle dorsiflexion	3/5	2/5
Plantar flexion	2+/5	2+/5
Hip flexion	2/5	2/5
Hip abduction	2/5	2/5
Knee flexion	3/5	3/5
Knee extension	3/5	3/5
Straight leg raise	+×1	–

Tone: Nicholas showed no increase in muscle tone with quick stretches, but decreased muscle tone throughout was suspected as evidenced by sitting and standing posture being slouched with genu valgum and bilateral foot pronation.

Pain: Nicholas had no complaints of pain during the evaluation session, but his mother reported complaints of pain in the left foot or ankle at school and at home in the evenings. She stated that Nicholas is unable to pinpoint an exact area of pain.

Endurance: Nicholas showed decreased muscle endurance with fatigue during active range of motion and manual muscle testing. Cardiovascular endurance was not tested but was suspected to be low based on his mother's report of decreased ability to walk long distances.

Gross Motor Skills/Functional Mobility
Sitting: Nicholas sat independently at the edge of a mat table with kyphotic posture and frequent use of arms for support. When reaching greater than 90 degrees, he showed decreased equilibrium reactions in the trunk as evidenced by increased trunk lean and use of opposite arm for support. He also sat independently in long sitting but showed increased kyphosis and posterior pelvic tilt.

Standing: Nicholas stood independently with kyphotic posture, genu valgum, and bilateral foot pronation with forefoot abduction causing out-toeing. He performed single leg stance (SLS) on each foot for 1 to 2 seconds for multiple trials. He required increased prompting and demonstration to complete SLS on the left foot.

Ambulation: Nicholas ambulated independently with multiple gait deviations. He showed decreased arm swing, a wide base of support, excessive lateral hip rotation, genu valgum, heel strike, and rocker motion over the lateral edge of the foot and toe off with forefoot adduction. These deviations were noted to be greater in the left foot than in the right. He ran 25 feet with decreased speed, decreased arm swing with elbows fixed into extension, minimal to no knee flexion, decreased stride length/left extremity (LE) dissociation, and minimal to no flight phase. His mother reported his running to be decreased in coordination since foot pain and deviation began.

Stairs: Nicholas went up and down four steps independently with alternating pattern and no assist of rails.

Evaluation
Prognosis
Nicholas should show improvement in functional skills with direct physical therapy to address balance and gait training, core strengthening, and a stretching program.

Intervention
Please note: This physical therapy intervention took into account Nicholas's behavioral needs secondary to his ASD. However, Nicholas also had musculoskeletal and neuromuscular impairments that required direct physical therapy services. Nicholas did not tolerate orthotics well because of his sensory issues. Nicholas required discussions and explanation of the interventions planned prior to beginning each session. He tended to have a consistent schedule of appointments and therapy routines. He did not tolerate changes in schedules or changes in routines well.

Coordination, Communication, Documentation
Coordination occurred between Nicholas's family, school therapists and teachers, clinic therapists, and physicians. Nicholas's family received education in how to enhance

CASE STUDY OF A CHILD WITH AUTISM SPECTRUM DISORDER—cont'd

his exercise program by incorporating more walking activities into the family routine, including daily walks after school.

Patient Instruction

Nicholas and his caregivers would benefit from a home program focusing on plantar flexor stretching and desensitization of both feet. It is also recommended that they be educated in the incorporation of physical exercise into their daily routine such as increased walking distances, using stairs instead of elevator, etc. His mother was educated today in the use of a mesh sponge over the medial plantar surface of the foot for desensitization.

Direct Intervention

Nicholas's program should include the following:

- High-level balance activities such as activities on a balance beam, balancing on one foot alternating with eyes open and closed, standing on a mini-trampoline while catching and throwing balls
- Jumping and hopping activities
- Core strengthening exercises including resistance training using TheraBand, Swiss ball activities
- Swimming to help increase proprioception and improve overall strength
- Lower-extremity stretching program
- Taping of soft tissues followed by application of shoe orthotics to help align Nicholas's foot position and decrease foot pain

Goals

Nicholas will ambulate without foot pain for the entire school day.

Nicholas will increase his bilateral hip muscle strength 1 muscle grade to decrease wide base of support and waddling gait deviation.

Nicholas will improve ankle strength 1 grade to improve push-off during gait.

Nicholas's overall strength and endurance will improve so that Nicholas can climb three flights of stairs and arrive to class without being late.

Nicholas will be able to ride his bike 12 miles to participate in family bike rides.

Re-Examination

Nicholas received 8 weeks of direct physical therapy services two times per week. He has begun a weekly swimming program that seems to have positively affected his endurance and overall strength. At the end of the 8-week session, Nicholas was able to ambulate at school without complaints of pain. He can ascend three flights of stairs at a faster pace but is occasionally late for class, especially at the end of the day. On observation, Nicholas achieved consistent push-off, but his mother reports that he requires verbal cueing on occasion to correct gait deviations.

Analysis of Case Using the ICF Model

Body functions: Significantly decreased strength in bilateral lower extremities, decreased endurance, decreased high-level gross motor skills, foot pain.

Activity limitations: Difficulty playing with peers outdoors, difficulty ascending and descending steps, fatigues easily.

Participation restrictions: Some of Nicholas's restrictions are secondary to his autism behaviors. However, Nicholas is also limited in participating in age-appropriate sports activities and bike riding activities with family members.

Environmental limitations: None. Nicholas's family was encouraged to have Nicholas walk more and take the elevator at school and in the community less. They were encouraged to walk short distances within the neighborhood instead of driving.

Movement System Assessment: Possible sensory selection and weighting deficit.

CHAPTER DISCUSSION QUESTIONS

1. Identify two characteristics of children with autism.
2. What legislation improved services for children with ASD?
3. What communication techniques might a child with autism use?
4. Identify varying social patterns used by children with autism.

REFERENCES

1. Autism Society of America: *The autism experience: understanding autism* (website): https://autismsociety.org/the-autism-experience/. Accessed May 25, 2022.
2. Centers for Disease Control and Prevention. *Autism spectrum disorder: latest data from the ADDM Network* (website): https://www.cdc.gov/ncbddd/autism/index.html. Accessed May 25, 2022.

3. Soke GN, Maenner MJ, Christensen D, et al. Brief report: estimated prevalence of a community diagnosis of autism spectrum disorder by age 4 years in children from selected areas in the United States in 2010: evaluation of birth cohort effects. *J Autism Dev Disord.* 2017;47(6):1917–1922.

4. Hyman SL, Levy SE, Myers SM. Council on Children with Disabilities, Section on Developmental and Behavioral Pediatrics: Identification, evaluation, and management of children with autism spectrum disorder. *Pediatrics.* 2020;145(1):e20193447.

SUGGESTED READINGS

1. American Psychiatric Association. *Diagnostic and Statistical Manual of Mental Disorders.* 5th ed. Washington, DC: American Psychiatric Association; 2013.

2. APTA Academy of Pediatric Physical Therapy. Autism: current practice resources for physical therapists. https://pediatricapta.org/includes/fact-sheets/pdfs/Fact-Sheet_AutismCurrentPracticeResources_2014.pdf.

3. Cowley G. Boys, girls and autism. *Newsweek.* September 8, 2003.

RESOURCES

Autism Society
http://www.autism-society.org

Autism Speaks Inc.
http://www.autismspeaks.org/

Centers for Disease Control and Prevention (CDC)
http://cdc.gov/actearly

First Signs
http://firstsigns.org

National Autism Association
http://www.nationalautismassociation.org/

Developmental Coordination Disorder

Margaret Mizera, PT, DPT, PCS

LEARNING OBJECTIVES

At the end of the chapter, the reader will be able to do the following:

1. Identify the four criteria that must be met for a diagnosis of developmental coordination disorder (DCD).
2. Recognize the clinical signs of DCD.
3. Identify coexisting diagnoses.
4. Understand the role of evaluation and ongoing assessment of the child with DCD.
5. Identify appropriate treatment strategies and use of equipment to address goals for the child with DCD.

CHAPTER OUTLINE

KEY TERMS

Coordination

Dyspraxia

Executive functioning

Developmental Coordination Disorder (DCD) is a neurodevelopmental disorder affecting motor and academic performance in children. DCD has been recognized for almost a century under many names such as *clumsy child syndrome, developmental disorder of motor function, sensory integrative dysfunction*, and *dyspraxia*.[1] Its present name was recognized in 1994, and it is now listed and further defined in the *Diagnostic and Statistical Manual of Mental Disorders*, 5th edition (*DSM-5*).[2]

DCD occurs in 5% to 6% of children and reportedly is 1.7 to 2.8 times more likely in boys than girls.[1] Incidence is higher among children born prematurely (<32 weeks' gestation) and those with low birthweight (<1500 g). DCD can cause delayed gross and fine motor skills, resulting in difficulty with ball skills and balance. This can also greatly impact activities of daily living (e.g., eating and dressing) and academic performance because of the impact on manual dexterity needed for handwriting.

The diagnosis of DCD is usually considered when there is no known neurologic or medical reason for developmental delays. Established in 2013 in the *DSM-5*, the following four criteria must each be met for a diagnosis of DCD (see Table 16.1).

Diagnosis is typically made near 5 years of age, despite parents' reports of symptoms much earlier.

CLINICAL SIGNS

Children with DCD stand out from their peers in many ways.[1,3] They usually appear weaker, with poor balance and coordination. They appear awkward or clumsy, and fall more frequently than peers. These fine motor

TABLE 16.1   **Four Critical Criteria for a Diagnosis of DCD**
1. Motor skills and coordination are below what is expected for chronological age and experience
2. Motor difficulties are impacting daily living skills, school performance, leisure, and play
3. Symptoms begin in the developmental period
4. Symptoms cannot be explained by other intellectual, vision, neurologic, or motor impairments[3]

difficulties or dyspraxia can cause difficulty with hand-writing, dressing, and tying shoes, and may impact school performance. Children with DCD may have delays in meeting developmental milestones.

Children with DCD are less physically active and may have sensorimotor deficits and difficulty with social interactions. They may even present with mental health concerns, such as low self-esteem or anxiety. Secondary effects of the sedentary life of children with DCD can include increased risks for heart disease, obesity, and musculoskeletal disorders. Recent studies show additional difficulties with executive functioning, those skills needed to plan, perform and adapt behaviors and strategies to a particular task. Difficulties with executive functioning can impact visuospatial and verbal working memory, inhibitory control, and tasks requiring cognitive flexibility.[4]

Symptoms of DCD can persist well into adolescence and adulthood, with adults experiencing more difficulties with executive functioning and attention and more anxiety. These symptoms can, in turn, further impact employment options, independent living, and general quality of life.

PATHOLOGY

While an exact structural cause of DCD has not been found, involvement of the prefrontal cortex, posterior superior temporal gyrus, and especially the cerebellum, is strongly suspected.[5-7] It is the cerebellum that largely impacts timing, grading, motor control, motor learning, and spatial and error processing, and thus, impacts the quality of gross and fine motor skills and activities of daily living (ADLs). Associated conditions can include hypotonia, joint laxity, balance deficits, and obesity.

COEXISTING DIAGNOSES

Children with DCD often have one or more coexisting diagnoses. In addition to the diagnosis of DCD, they may be diagnosed with attention-deficit/hyperactivity

TABLE 16.2   **Common Coexisting Disorders in Children With DCD**
Attention-deficit/hyperactivity disorder
Autism spectrum disorder
Learning disabilities
Speech/language deficits
Executive functioning deficits
Sensorimotor impairments
Cognitive impairments

disorder (ADHD), autism spectrum disorder (ASD), learning difficulties, sensory issues, and speech difficulties.[1] They may also have cognitive or psychologic conditions, including depression and anxiety, executive functioning deficits,[4] decreased social interactions, and diminished quality of life. It is now believed that these motor and psychologic difficulties can continue throughout the lifespan, impacting physical, academic, social, and vocational performance[8] (Table 16.2).

Physical therapists (PTs) and physical therapist assistants (PTAs) play an integral role in the detection, referral, and treatment of children with DCD. Because of their presence in diverse settings (schools, hospitals, clinics, home health, and early intervention programs), PTs and PTAs are likely to be the first professionals to observe and assess the motor, academic, and social deficits that are paramount to a diagnosis of DCD. Early detection and treatment can help improve motor performance as well as offset the long-term emotional, social, and health consequences of DCD.

Multiple systematic reviews of assessments and interventions for DCD have been published, with the result being development of clinical practice guidelines by many medical and professional organizations. The American Physical Therapy Association (APTA) published its own clinical practice guidelines for DCD in 2020,[3] basing its examination and intervention recommendations on levels of evidence from research studies and expert opinion.

ASSESSMENT/REASSESSMENT

Physical therapy assessment and subsequent reassessments of children with DCD include history, systems review, clinical observations, and formal testing.

History and systems review include a thorough medical, birth, and developmental history; family history, child's educational history, and history of participation in the home (including ADLs and social, physical, and recreational activities). A thorough systems review should be completed to determine those symptoms affecting the child, as well as those needing immediate physician referral. The systems reviewed should include musculoskeletal (height, weight, range of motion [ROM], strength, skeletal abnormalities or asymmetries), neuromuscular (muscle tone, soft neurologic signs, history of falls, balance issues, headaches, toe-walking), integumentary (bruising and other signs of injury, pigmentation differences, nail bed color), cardiopulmonary (heart rate, respiratory rate, endurance, activity level), cognitive/behavioral (attention, communication, ability to follow instructions, academic and social performance, behavioral regulation), and vision.

Referral to the primary care physician should be made if DCD is suspected, if other medical or developmental diagnoses are suspected, and if any red flags are present. Red flags requiring immediate referral to the primary care physician include history of head injury or trauma, headaches or blurred vision, deterioration in gait or motor or cognitive skills, and abnormal muscle tone (low, high, fluctuating, or asymmetric). Referral to other healthcare providers (e.g., speech and language pathologist, occupational therapist, psychologist, behavioral health specialist) should also be initiated at this time (Table 16.3).

Clinical observations should include movement analysis of functional activities and transitional movements. Balance and posture in sitting, sit-to-stand, standing, gait, and advanced motor skills (balance on one foot, jumping, hopping, running, skipping, catching and throwing a ball) should be observed. Coordination, fluidity of movement and mid-range control during these activities should be thoroughly assessed (Table 16.4).

Functional outcome measures help to determine participation limitations, activity limitations, motor performance, and impairments in body functions and structures. Chapter 2 provides a more detailed description of some of the tests and measures listed below. Choice of functional outcome measures used is often determined by availability of the test materials, cost, and time constraints. *Participation* in the family, home, school, and community can be assessed using the Canadian Occupational Performance Measure (COPM), the Goal Attainment Scale (GAS), the Perceived Efficacy and Goal Setting (PEGS) Program, the Children's Assessment of Participation and Enjoyment (CAPE), or the Preferences for Activities for Children (PAC). *Activity limitations* can be assessed using the Developmental Coordination Disorder Questionnaire (DCDQ'07), the Little DCDQ-CA, the Movement Assessment Battery for Children (MABC-2-C), or the School Function Assessment (SFA). Standardized measures of *motor performance* include the MABC-2-C, the Bruininks-Oseretsky Test of Motor Proficiency (BOT-2), and the Test of Gross Motor Development (TGMD-2). Evaluations of *impairments of body functions and structures* include assessments of balance, endurance, fitness, and strength. Some appropriate tools include the 6-Minute Walk Test (6 MWT), the 20-meter shuttle run test (20 m SRT), the Progressive Aerobic Cardiovascular Endurance Run (PACER) test, manual muscle testing (MMT), and ROM.

TABLE 16.3 Red Flags Requiring Immediate Referral to Primary Care Physician

History of head injury or trauma
Headaches or blurred vision
Deterioration in gait or motor or cognitive skills
Abnormal muscle tone (low, high, fluctuating, or asymmetric)

TABLE 16.4 Clinical Signs of DCD

Poor strength
Poor coordination
Awkwardness, clumsiness
Frequent falls or "accidents"
Poor balance
Delayed gross motor skills
Weak grasp, poor handwriting skills, difficulty with shoe tying and buttons
Difficulty with motor and visual sequencing tasks
Weakness of hand muscles and delayed fine motor skills
Difficulty with printing and handwriting
Sensory and perceptual deficits
Often frustrated
Poor self-esteem
Obesity

TABLE 16.5   Guidelines for Physical Activity and Sleep

Children aged 3 to 4 years:
- At least 180 minutes of physical activity daily, of which at least 60 minutes is moderate to vigorous intensity
- 10 to 13 hours of sleep per day, distributed between naps and uninterrupted nighttime sleep

Children and adolescents aged 5 to 12 years:
- At least 60 minutes of moderate to vigorous intensity exercise per day and vigorous intensity aerobic or strengthening activities at least three times per week
- 9 to 12 hours of sleep

Children and adolescents aged 13 to 17 years:
- At least 60 minutes of moderate to vigorous intensity exercise per day and vigorous intensity aerobic or strengthening activities at least three times per week
- 8 to 10 hours of sleep

INTERVENTIONS

According to the APTA Clinical Practice Guideline for Developmental Coordination Disorder,[3] task-oriented interventions, combined with body function and structure-focused intervention programs, are the first-choice intervention for children with DCD. Specific functional motor skills or neuromotor tasks should be included, combining strength, balance, coordination and sensorimotor feedback. Alternate strategies or additional time may be helpful for the child to succeed with new tasks. It may also be important to lessen distractions during teaching of a new skill, as sensorimotor input can be interpreted differently by the child with DCD. Core stability, cardiorespiratory training, and power training can be incorporated into skilled therapy programs.

These interventions can be provided via individual or small group sessions. Supplemental community activities should be recommended to augment first-choice interventions. These would include community-based or individualized soccer, Tae Kwon Do, swimming, basketball, and other sports.

Education and home exercise programs should be given to both parents and children to support and reinforce the chosen interventions. A schedule of direct physical therapy interventions, home programs, and community-based activities should be created. Guidelines for physical activity and sleep, set by the World Health Organization[9] and the Centers for Disease Control and Prevention,[10,11] should be explained to caregivers and teachers as well as the children (Table 16.5).

SUMMARY

DCD is a complex, under-identified neuromotor condition. It affects participation and functioning in daily life skills, including fine and gross motor skills, coordination, and balance. This secondarily affects academic and sports performance, and associated executive functioning deficits can impact academic and employment performance. Psychosocial development can be impacted, as secondary health and socioemotional problems arise including obesity, depression, problems with time management, and difficulty with organization.

Early diagnosis and intervention can improve developmental motor skills and performance in the home, school, and community. Skilled physical therapy can prevent the secondary and long-term effects of DCD, which include obesity, low self-esteem, difficulties with academic achievement, and diminished quality of life.

CASE STUDY

Peter is an 8-year-old boy initially referred to physical therapy for left knee pain and recurrent patellar subluxation. He is big for his age, being 4'7" and weighing 95 lb. He does not like to participate in gym or sports because he cannot keep up with peers. He prefers to play alone or with younger children and has frequent falls. He is a bright boy but has difficulty with handwriting and organization of schoolwork. His mother states that his hands get tired when he is doing extensive handwriting or schoolwork, and he has difficulty tying his shoes. He enjoys basketball, but he has difficulty dribbling, passing, and throwing the ball. He responds by overshooting or using excessive force. Peter fatigues easily. He has not learned to ride a bike without training wheels. His footsteps are very loud when he walks. He often toe-walks.

His left knee pain and knee subluxation from a recent fall are further limiting his ability to play with peers. He now shows diminished strength and ROM at both hips, both knees, and both ankles. He shows mild effusion on

CASE STUDY—cont'd

the left knee in response to palpation, but it is not warm or extensive. He cannot jump, run, hop, or play without pain and extreme fatigue.

Further history and a systems review reveal significant trunk, hip, knee, and ankle weakness. He has ROM limitations at his hips and ankles and poor eccentric control at his hips and knees. He has been diagnosed with sickle cell disease. He attended school virtually for 2 years because of the global pandemic. He received direct physical therapy services as an outpatient 4 years ago for similar knee pain. He did not receive school-based physical therapy.

Observational Movement Analysis

Peter stands with a strong lordosis and bilateral hip flexion. His left knee hyperextends, and his right knee is in more neutral alignment. He has a very hypotonic and inactive trunk. He will only squat to 45 degrees of hip and knee flexion. If he squats further and then attempts to stand up, his knees will snap into hyperextension and his patellae will subluxate laterally. He can pick up a toy from the floor but keeps knees extended, reaching instead by rounding his back and bending his hips minimally.

Peter ambulates independently with a narrow base of support. He takes short strides and shows no arm swing in gait at his low speed. He fatigues quickly after any "burst" of movement, as in running 10 feet.

He can jump in place but complains of left knee pain after ten jumps. He can stand on either leg for 8 to 10 seconds, but marked upper extremity (UE) flailing occurs during weight-bearing on only his left leg. He can hop on either foot, but on the left, he needs to jump in circle and flail his arms to balance. He can walk on a straight line but cannot stand and balance in tandem on line.

Formal testing should assess strength and ROM. Ideal outcome measures for him would be the BOT-2 and the DCDQ'07. Other measures could be performed in subsequent treatments, as time allows.

Treatment will need to address his primary concern of knee pain and instability but also his underlying coordination and performance issues.

Plan of Care: Peter will be seen for outpatient physical therapy twice weekly for eight visits.

Goals
1. Peter will attain pain-free knee stability in standing and gait.
2. Peter will be able to bend his hips and knees as he dribbles a ball in place using alternating hands, 20 times in a row.

3. Peter will be able to run 50 feet without knee pain or breathlessness to follow his team and the ball down the court.

Interventions

Multiple diverse exercises, activities, and equipment will be used. Isolated hip and knee muscle strengthening will be done in supine and sidelying, progressing to standing and eccentric work.

Grading of quads will be practiced in double and single leg stance, avoiding range in which he subluxates. His left knee will be taped and a patellar stabilizing orthosis will be ordered and used to promote stability during exercise and play. A glider swing will be used for fun work on strength, timing, balance, and coordination. Treadmill training and use of an elliptical can be performed for targeted strengthening and endurance work. Basketball skill training will include running and dribbling drills and free throw practice.

Analysis of Case Using the ICF Model

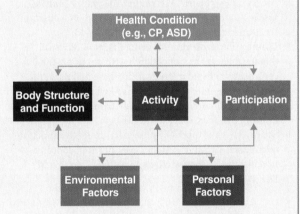

Body functions: Weakness, incoordination, balance, pain
Activity limitations: Difficulty running, dribbling and throwing a ball, early fatigue with motor activities, cannot ride a bike
Participation restrictions: Difficulty with participation in gym at school, limited opportunities to play with friends
Environmental limitations: No access to home exercise equipment, requires school gym restrictions, isolation and limited peer play due to COVID restrictions

Movement System Approach

Peter could be assigned different categories, and this would drive the intervention direction.
Force production deficit: Weakness in lower extremities and trunk leading to pain and dysfunction
Movement pattern coordination disorder: Difficulty with dribbling basketball and with handwriting

CHAPTER DISCUSSION QUESTIONS

1. Identify the four criteria that must be met for a diagnosis of DCD.
2. What are the clinical signs of DCD?
3. What other diagnoses may be present in the child with DCD that will impact motor and academic performance?
4. Explain the role of evaluation and ongoing assessment for the child with DCD.
5. Identify four treatment strategies to address the goals of the child with DCD, including the equipment you could use to make therapy fun and functional.

REFERENCES

1. Harris SR, Mickelson ECR, Zwicker JG. Diagnosis and management of developmental coordination disorder. *CMAJ.* 2015;187(9):659–665.
2. American Psychiatric Association. *Diagnostic and Statistical Manual of Mental Disorders.* 5th ed. Washington DC: American Psychiatric Association; 2013.
3. Dannemiller L, Mueller M, Leitner A, et al. Physical therapy management of children with developmental coordination disorder: an evidence-based clinical practice guideline from the Academy of Pediatric Physical Therapy of the American Physical Therapy Association. *Pediatr Phys Ther.* 2020;32:278–313.
4. Sartori RF, Valentini NC, Fonseca RP. Executive function in children with and without developmental coordination disorder: a comparative study. *Child Care Health Dev.* 2020;46:294–302.
5. Wilson PH, Ruddock S, Smits-Engelsman B, et al. Understanding performance deficits in developmental coordination disorder: a meta-analysis of recent research. *Dev Med Child Neurol.* 2013;55(3):217–228.
6. Zwicker JG, Missiuna C, Harris SR, et al. Developmental coordination disorder: a review and update. *Eur J Paediatr Neurol.* 2012;16(6):573–581.
7. Deng S, Li WG, Ding J, et al. Understanding the mechanisms of cognitive impairments in developmental coordination disorder. *Pediatr Res.* 2014;75(1–2):210–216.
8. Kirby A, Sugden D, Purcell C. Diagnosing developmental coordination disorders. *Arch Dis Child.* 2014;99(3):292–296.
9. World Health Organization. *To grow up healthy, children need to sit less and play more: new WHO guidelines on physical activity, sedentary behaviour and sleep for children under 5 years of age.* News release. April 24, 2019. https://www.who.int/news/item/24-04-2019-to-grow-up-healthy-children-need-to-sit-less-and-play-more. Accessed June 8, 2023.
10. Centers for Disease Control and Prevention: *Physical activity: how much physical activity do children need?* (website): https://www.cdc.gov/physicalactivity/basics/children/index.htm. Last updated June 3, 2022.
11. Centers for Disease Control and Prevention, National Center for Chronic Disease Prevention and Health Promotion (NCCDPHP): *Do your children get enough sleep?* (website): https://www.cdc.gov/chronicdisease/resources/infographic/children-sleep.htm. Last updated March 15, 2021.

RESOURCE

CanChild Website

https://canchild.ca/en/diagnoses/developmental-coordination-disorder

Pediatric Burns

Roberta Kuchler O'Shea, PT, DPT, PhD
Alison Garlock Small, MS, OTR/L, BT-C

LEARNING OBJECTIVES

After reading this chapter, the reader will be able to do the following:

1. Differentiate between the various thicknesses of burns.
2. Identify medical complications that occur after a burn injury.
3. Formulate treatment activities appropriate for the patient's degree of burn and stage of recovery.
4. Differentiate acid burns from alkali burns.
5. Discuss what burns are most common in given pediatric age groups.
6. Describe how to measure total surface burn area for children and adults.

CHAPTER OUTLINE

KEY TERMS

Chemical burn
Electrical burn
Escharotomy
Full-thickness burns

Hypertrophic scar
Partial-thickness burns
Rule of nines

Superficial burns
Thermal burn
Total body surface area

This chapter introduces the reader to pediatric burn care including mechanisms of injury, demographics, and the management and treatment of burn injuries in children. Children have very different reactions to burns than adults, and children may have more difficulty during their recovery. Because of the often-disfiguring effects of burns and anticipated growth, many of these children will undergo burn, skin, and scar management as a lifelong process fraught with very difficult and sometimes painful procedures.[1a] Additionally, impairments may develop as a child ages. Understanding all the potential mechanisms and outcomes of burns is vital to the successful rehabilitation of these children and education of their families.

Burn care is a highly specialized area of care, and clinicians interested in pediatric burn care should receive advanced training.

Burn injuries in infants and children can be quite devastating and are caused by a myriad of mechanisms and methods (Fig. 17.1). Burns, especially those visible to others, can be extremely distressing to both the child and the family, including siblings, parents, and caregivers. Depending on the severity of the burns, the social and physical implications for a particular child can be quite dramatic

DEFINITION

Statistics show that burn-related injuries are the leading cause of accidental death among children younger than 2 years and the second leading cause of death among children younger than 14 years.[1] According to the American Burn Association, approximately 1.2 million people in the United States seek treatment for burns each year. Of those, 30% to 40% are children.[2] Over the past 20 years, the incidence of burns among children has decreased.[2a] Nearly 24,000 children are treated in hospital emergency departments each year for scald burn injuries,[3] and approximately 4000 children experience electrical injuries.[4] Between 25,000 and 100,000 chemical burns are reported each year,

but specific statistics for children in this group are lacking.[5] The median length of inpatient stay has slightly increased for children with burns covering more than 20% of total body surface area (TBSA) but decreased for children with burns covering less than 20% of TBSA.[2a]

The majority of burn accidents occur during the first 4 years of life.[2a,6] In this time period, the mechanism of injury is most often related to abuse and neglect.[7] The prevalence of scald burn injuries from hot liquids is extremely high among children (nearly 50% of all reported burns).

Survival prognosis following burns in children is directly related to the percentage of skin affected by the burn, the skin thickness affected by the burn, the prevalence of infection, and the ability of medical personnel to provide adequate fluid replacement. Most children (59%) ultimately have a minor loss of function; however, children with moderate loss of function have about 28% of reported burn injuries.[2a] The mortality of children has decreased In recent years, with the majority of children with burns covering 20% of TBSA or more having the highest mortality.[2a]

PATHOLOGY

Burn injuries occur when energy is shifted from a heat source to the body. If the heat is not dissipated at a rate greater than it is absorbed, then the cellular temperature increases beyond the point at which cells can survive. This causes cell death and a myriad of other cellular-level

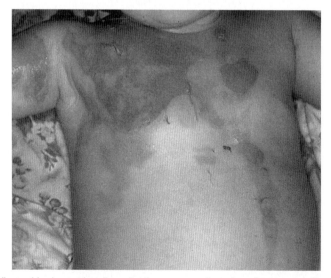

Fig. 17.1 This toddler grabbed a pot handle projecting out over the edge of a stove, spilling hot soup over her chest and shoulder. (From Zitelli BJ, Davis HW. *Atlas of Pediatric Physical Diagnosis.* 5th ed. Philadelphia: Mosby; 2007.)

destructions. The temperature to which the skin is exposed and the length of time the skin is exposed to the heat source determine the depth of the injury.[8] Burns are classically divided into four types: *thermal, chemical, electrical,* and *radiation* burns. For purposes of this chapter, radiation burns will not be discussed; they are extremely rare, especially in children.

Burn injuries are further classified as *superficial, partial-thickness,* or *full-thickness,* with full-thickness burns extending into the deeper tissues (Fig. 17.2). Because the

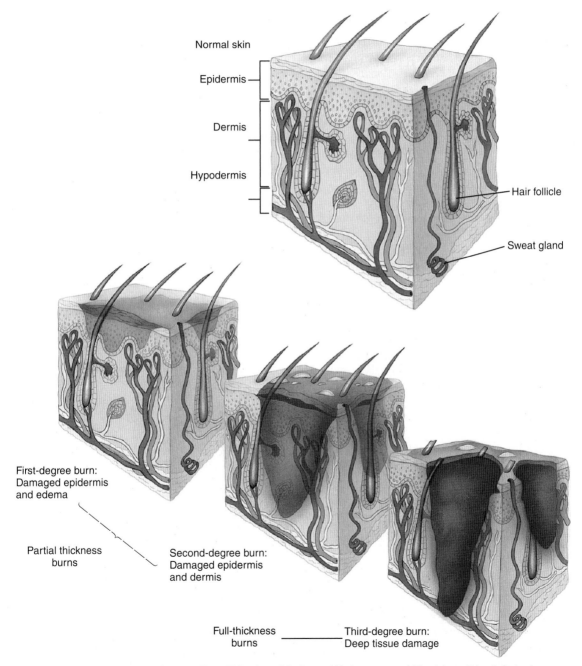

Normal skin

Epidermis

Dermis

Hypodermis

Hair follicle

Sweat gland

First-degree burn: Damaged epidermis and edema

Partial thickness burns

Second-degree burn: Damaged epidermis and dermis

Full-thickness burns

Third-degree burn: Deep tissue damage

Fig. 17.2 Classification of burns. (From Thibodeau GA, Patton KT. *Anatomy and Physiology.* 5th ed. St Louis: Mosby; 2003.)

surface area of a 6-month-old infant differs considerably from that of an 8-year-old child, the infant will have deeper burns from heat of the same intensity that might cause only partial-thickness injuries in the older child.

CLINICAL SIGNS

Superficial burns are limited to the epidermis. The most common type of superficial burn is sunburn; it is painful but self-limiting. Superficial burns tend not to lead to scarring. Partial-thickness burns are typically divided into superficial and deep partial-thickness burns. Superficial partial-thickness burns entail damage to the epidermis and a small part of the dermal layer of the skin. These burns exhibit increased sensitivity to pain and temperature, with noted redness and large, thick-walled blisters. Involvement of the epidermis and a deeper portion of the dermal layer of the skin characterizes deep partial-thickness burns. Increased sensitivity to pain and temperature, a marbled-white edematous appearance, and large, thick-walled blisters that typically increase in size are also features of deep partial-thickness burns. Full-thickness burns entail total destruction of the epidermis and dermis, which

may include deeper tissues, such as fascia, muscle, or subcutaneous fat. Temperature and pain sensation are not intact because of the destruction of the epidermal and dermal layers, which contain sensory nerve endings. The skin will have a white, brown-black, or charred appearance and a leathery texture. Blistering does not typically occur.[4,5]

The measurement of the extent of a burn injury can be estimated by using the rule of nines, although this is highly unreliable for children younger than 15 years because it overestimates the extent of burns to the legs and underestimates the extent of burns to the head and face.[9] This method divides the body surface into areas, each of which is considered to be 9% or a multiple of 9% of the TBSA. In children, the head and neck are considered to be 18%, and the lower extremities, 14%. Another method of burn surface area estimation, although less accurate, is to use the palm of the child's hand, which is roughly equivalent to 1% of the child's TBSA.[3] This is not recommended for use with large burns because of its limited accuracy. The most accurate and time-consuming method of burn surface area estimation is the Lund-Browder chart, which subdivides the extremities into segments (Fig. 17.3). The healthcare provider has

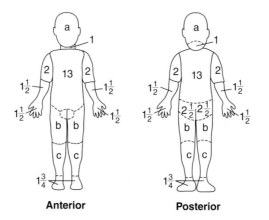

Anterior   **Posterior**

Relative percentage of body surface area (% BSA) affected by growth

Body Part	Age				
	0 yr	1 yr	5 yr	10 yr	15 yr
a = ½ of head	9½	8½	6½	5½	4½
b = ½ of 1 thigh	2¾	3¼	4	4¼	4½
c = ½ of 1 lower leg	2½	2½	2¾	3	3¼

Fig. 17.3 Lund-Browder chart for children for estimating the extent of burns. (Redrawn from Artz CP, Moncrief JA. *The Treatment of Burns*. 2nd ed. Philadelphia: Saunders; 1969.)

an anterior and posterior diagram of the child (available for different age groups) on which the clinician colors in both the anterior and posterior burned regions of the child's body. The sum of the colored areas is the TBSA involved.[3] When the Lund -Bower chart is used in evaluation of infants, for instance, the head and neck are 21 % each, the trunk and back are 13% each, the buttocks and genital area are 6.5%, the lower extremities are 13.5%, and the upper extremities are 10% each. Most burn units follow the American Burn Association guidelines for assessment and treatment of burns. Infants and children with burn injuries should be referred to and followed up by a specialized burn unit.

BURNS CLINICAL SIGNS

Superficial Burns
Damage to epidermis

Superficial Partial-Thickness Burns
Damage to epidermis and small part of dermal layer
Increased sensitivity to pain and temperature
Red skin and large, thick-walled blisters

Deep Partial-Thickness Burns
Damage to epidermis and deeper portion of dermal layer
Increased sensitivity to pain and temperature
Marbled-white edematous appearance and large, thick-
   walled blisters that will increase in size

Full-Thickness Burns
Total destruction of epidermis and dermis
No temperature or pain sensation because of damaged
   sensory nerve endings
Leathery skin with a white, brown-black, or charred
   appearance

Thermal Burns

Thermal burn injuries are the most likely category to affect infants and children. The most common types of thermal burn injuries are scald and flame burn injuries.[2a]

Scald burn injuries are extremely common among young children and can occur from spilled food and beverages (including grease), hot tap water, clothes irons, hair curling irons, space heaters, and ovens/ranges.[2] When assessing burns, especially in a child younger than 4 years, there are prototypical locations for abuse-related burns. Burns on the feet, perineum, and back of the buttocks, but not on the posterior knees or anterior hip regions, are often indicators of a child being dipped into a tub of scalding water.[10] Approximately 100,000 scald burn injuries result from spilled food or beverages; the injuries occur quite commonly when a child pulls on a hanging cord or tablecloth while walking or using a baby walker. The incidence of burn injuries to children using baby walkers is quite high, despite safety warnings placed on the walkers.[11] Five thousand children are scalded by hot water every year; scald burn injuries commonly occur when an unattended child in the bathroom either turns on the hot water tap or falls into a full tub of hot water. Often, apartment building water heaters are set at higher temperatures to accommodate the increased volume of use, and this can lead to accidental scald burns. Contact thermal burns result from contact with hot objects such as clothes irons, curling irons, ranges, or ovens, which often cause hand burns. Space heaters are a common cause of house fires, especially in the winter months in cold climates. Each year, approximately 60,000 children are burned by contact with a hot surface.[2] At 52°C (126°F), it takes 2 minutes to cause full-thickness burns, compared with only 5 seconds of immersion at 60°C (140°F).[3]

Flame burns are a common cause of burn-related injuries among older children. These commonly occur in house fires, which often start at night and escape early detection because no one in the home is awake. During the winter months, space heaters, electrical failures, and oven heating are often to blame. A secondary injury that can occur with flame burns, especially during a house fire, is smoke inhalation injury. Smoke inhalation injury, if severe enough, can cause brain damage as a result of the increased carbon dioxide and decreased oxygen in the blood.

In colder climates, frostbite is also a risk for children. However, ice packs applied incorrectly without a protective barrier can also cause localized frostbite. Frostbite occurs when ice crystals form in the cells after prolonged exposure to subzero temperatures. Ischemia and inflammation may also occur in response to the necrotic cell death. Frostbite is characterized similar to burns in stages: first-degree, second-degree, third-degree, and fourth-degree frostbite injury.[12]

Chemical Burns

Chemical burn injuries are divided primarily into two groups: acid and alkali. Several industrial-strength products are available to the general public, and these are often responsible for chemical burn injuries among children. To successfully assess and treat the presenting chemical burn injury, the physician requires a complete description of the offending agent, including its composition and concentration, whether it is an acid or an alkali, the type of exposure (e.g., inhalation, cutaneous, ocular, or gastrointestinal), duration of exposure, and other events or injuries associated with the burn, such as an explosion, fall, or trauma.[4,5]

Acids produce coagulation necrosis by denaturing proteins on contact with tissue, and the development of this area of coagulation limits any extension of the injury. Common types of acids are toilet bowl and drain cleaners, tile cleaners, battery acid, and engraving solution.

Alkalis cause a liquefaction necrosis, meaning the tissue is liquefied by the presentation of the alkali and then necroses as a result. These burns are potentially more dangerous than acid burns. In contrast to acid burns, alkali burns continue to penetrate to much deeper tissue levels.[4,5] Typically, younger children are exposed to these types of injuries accidentally because of inadequate childproofing.[5] Older children and young adults may experience exposure because of impetuous behaviors or experimentation. Often, these are ingestion burns.[4,5] Common types of alkalis are drain and oven cleaners, ammonia-based cleaners and detergents, household bleach, and dishwashing and clothing detergents.

Electrical Burns

Electrical burn injuries comprise a variety of mechanisms. Injuries range from the very mild, as seen with low-voltage household current, to the truly devastating, as seen with high-tension electrical injuries. No reliable statistics are available on the prevalence of lightning-strike injury to children. Electrical burn injuries affect approximately 4000 children every year, and the most common mechanism is low-voltage contact. Electricity involves the flow of energy along the path of least resistance toward a natural ground. All objects are either resistors or conductors. The skin acts as a natural resistor to flow. Standard household current in the United States and Canada is 110 V AC with a frequency of 60 Hz.[4,5] Skeletal muscle is stimulated into tetany by currents with frequencies of 40 to 110 Hz. Because most low- and high-tension electric currents are AC, AC produces tetany and the "locked-on" phenomenon.[4,5] As a result, an individual's grasp is uncontrollably locked onto the object, which can increase the length of time the current passes through the body and may result in greater injury.[4,5] Low-voltage injuries have very low morbidity and mortality. Both morbidity and mortality increase proportionally as voltage increases. Low-voltage injuries among toddlers often result from chewing on electrical cords or sticking objects into outlets; these injuries are most common in boys.[4,5] Overall, prognosis for patients with low-voltage electrical burn injuries is quite good. Unfortunately, neurologic sequelae may be present following electrical burns. The neurologic impairments may not be observed near the time of the injury but may appear weeks to months following the injury.[13]

MEDICAL TREATMENT

The burn unit functions as a very different sort of trauma unit compared with other acute care units. Typically, a strong multidisciplinary approach is taken in most pediatric burn units because children with burns require that all aspects of care, development, and well-being be addressed.[1a] The pediatric burn team in the intensive care burn unit and many rehabilitation hospitals commonly includes burn-specialized surgeons/physicians, nurses, physical and occupational therapists, speech/language pathologists, infant development specialists (for children younger than 3 years), clinical dieticians/nutritionists, social workers, psychologists or psychiatrists, child life specialists, and school teachers.[1a] Other personnel are consulted as needed. They may be orthotists, prosthetists, or medical sculptors. When assessing and treating infants and children with burns, the team approach and minimizing any further trauma to the infant or child are vital considerations.

Medical treatment of burns, albeit slightly different depending on the mechanism, follows a standardized method of assessment. The initial assessment of the burn is focused on determining the extent of the burn injury, including an estimate of the TBSA involved and the child's overall condition. Immediate decisions are made about whether intubation, mechanical ventilation, and intravenous fluid therapy are required. Shock is a common aftereffect of burns and can even occur with very small burns when they are full-thickness in nature, as well as with increased TBSA.

The fluid replacement requirement is typically greater in children because they experience more evaporative water loss than adults.[13a] As a result, children have greater fluid requirements during resuscitation. As more water is lost, heat loss increases, and the ability to avoid hypothermia becomes more difficult. Fluid replacement becomes even harder to manage for infants younger than 6 months; these infants exhibit renal immaturity, which leads to increased difficulties with handling fluid overload.[4,5]

Once the pediatric patient with a burn injury is stabilized, a nasogastric tube is usually placed because the child's caloric needs for wound healing will be far greater than what the child can ingest orally. Following burn injury, there is a dramatic increase in the basal metabolic rate, which may increase to twice the baseline. As a rule, metabolic expenditures increase in proportion to the burn injury. Therefore, a child with a 60% TBSA burn will require a 60% increase in the basal level of energy ingestion.[4,5]

Escharotomy, or an incision through a burn, may be necessary to reduce the pressure within the burn caused by the ever-increasing edema during the initial stages of the burn progression. This is done to restore circulation when the tissue pressures increase beyond 40 mm Hg.[10]

Thorough and aggressive wound care is necessary to promote the development of well-granulated tissue, which then promotes healing and closure. Often, skin grafting is required for full- and partial-thickness burns and promotes wound closure and healing. Various types of grafting procedures are available, but often, with children, split-thickness skin grafts taken from the child are utilized as donor sites. Typically, donor sites never extend across joints and therefore should not cause significant range-of-motion (ROM) limitations. All areas of the body are possible donor sites, except for the face and the hands. Dressing changes are normally done daily, but after skin grafting, a period of 5 to 7 days elapses prior to the initial dressing change to allow the graft to grow into the wound bed.

Potential complications of burn injuries include heterotopic ossification, amputation, and peripheral nerve involvement. Heterotopic bone ossification is not common among smaller children, but it can occur in adolescents, typically at the elbow joint. This complication occurs in 2% to 3% of the population with burn injuries. Aggressive ROM is the treatment of choice. Amputations present a myriad of challenges for the child with a burn injury. Toleration of stump compression and weight-bearing can be quite poor because of fragility

of the newly grafted or healing skin, open wounds, and sensory impairments. Other amputations, such as of the fingers, also impact the child quite dramatically and create the need to relearn activities of daily living and play skills with the remaining digits. Peripheral nerve involvement occurs as a result of compression of the nerve tissue or compartment, edema with elevated tissue pressures, and/or nutritional deficiencies.

Scarring and musculoskeletal deformities are the two greatest limitations to successful outcomes for children who have sustained burn injuries. The body's recuperative abilities after either a minor or significant burn injury are both amazing and problematic. As the body repairs its skin, especially deep dermal injuries, it produces massive amounts of fused, highly disorganized collagen that replaces the normal dermal elastic tissue with a more inelastic substance. The microblasts begin to contract, and an inflammatory response causes increased vascularity and localized edema.[13a] The bonding of the twisted collagen and the inelastic substance, together with the contraction of the microblasts, contributes to the thickness of a hypertrophic scar. A child with darker skin exhibits a greater propensity for hypertrophic scarring.[14] The active inflammatory process of scarring typically lasts for 1½ to 2 years following burn injury. Redness, itching, irritation, and thickness are all indicators that the inflammatory process is still occurring and requires medical and pharmacologic management.

Pharmacologic management is highly varied and very physician dependent. New research is examining the effects of using topical lotions with salicylic acid (aspirin) on scars to minimize inflammation, redness, itching, and further development of scarring.

Once an infant or child is medically stable in the burn unit, determining the most appropriate next step for that child's recovery and rehabilitation will be paramount. For children with larger partial- and full-thickness burn injuries or open areas that require closure, one option for furthering recovery is transitioning the child to an inpatient rehabilitation program specializing in burn care and rehabilitation. This option offers the child the benefits of intensive, comprehensive therapies that are very important to the success of recovery. Depending on the nature and extent of the child's injuries, the length of stay for this course of treatment is quite variable. Burn rehabilitation stays can range from 3 to 16 weeks and possibly longer if a child is receiving a pharmacologic regimen requiring weaning from a narcotic or if the skin is not closing adequately.[15]

For children who have experienced less severe burns and do not require the intensive therapy of an inpatient rehabilitation program, other options include day rehabilitation programs and outpatient therapies. Day rehabilitation programs offer intensive, daily therapies in a clinic environment but allow the child to be at home at night with caregivers and family. Day rehabilitation programs are often a natural progression from inpatient rehabilitation for many children—less often for infants with burns and more often for children who require ongoing outpatient therapies. They are often appropriate for an infant or child with ongoing ROM and/or functional limitations. Early intervention programs do not ordinarily involve themselves with burn rehabilitation; they are more developmentally focused.

INTERVENTION

Physical Therapy Assessment

The physical therapy examination will typically begin immediately within the acute burn unit and again in an intensive inpatient rehabilitation program, usually in conjunction with occupational therapy. Early initiation of treatment ensures ROM, flexibility, and muscle length are maintained. The physical therapy examination should include assessment of integumentary integrity, in particular, the burn, donor, and graft sites; joint integrity and mobility; muscle performance, including strength, power, and endurance; the need for any orthotic, protective, or splinting devices; pain levels; posture in all appropriate developmental positions; sensory integrity; functional mobility; and home and environmental requirements. For young children and infants, a thorough developmental assessment should be completed and compared with their pre–burn injury status. A variety of standardized gross motor tests are available to the physical therapist (PT) for completion of this assessment.

As soon as all examinations are completed, the expected length of stay in the rehabilitation program, day rehabilitation program, or outpatient therapy program should be determined and discussed with the child and the family to anticipate the child's emotional, physical, and physiologic needs and ensure they will be met. Communication between the therapy staff and family

is essential to the success of the rehabilitation program and can make certain the family is an active member of the rehabilitation team.

Based on this thorough examination, the PT completes the evaluation, synthesizes the data, makes clinical judgments, and determines a diagnosis. The primary dysfunctions are identified and become the focus of the direct interventions. Then the plan of care is created, and through this, the functional and measurable goals and expected outcomes are determined. It is of great importance to include the goals of the family/caregivers in this process, and even the child if appropriate, to ensure their participation in the child's recovery. The family and caregivers are vital to successful rehabilitation, especially for children and infants who have sustained burn injuries.

Physical Therapy Intervention

Physical therapy interventions will begin immediately within the acute burn unit to ensure ROM, flexibility, and muscle length are maintained.[1a] Pain control is also an important focus of early rehabilitation.[1a] As the skin heals, the loss of elasticity causes it to become tight and resistive to stretch, and this can produce contractures at joints across which the burns are located. The maintenance of ROM of all joints affected by the burns, donor sites, and positional deformities, if present, is the main goal of burn rehabilitation. Restoration of function will return the child to baseline functional levels.

Several treatment interventions to address ROM limitations are active, passive, and active assistive ROM and splinting, including thermoplastic splinting and use of dynamic splinting systems, knee immobilizers, or custom-made orthotics and/or prosthetics, if required. Serial casting or splinting to increase ROM can be quite effective and can be used for both upper and lower extremity contractures. The goal of serial casting or splinting is to provide gradual realignment of the collagen in a parallel and lengthened state.[14] This is accomplished by positioning the limb near the end range of movement and casting the limb to provide a slow, constant stretch. The cast is changed frequently (every 2–4 days), and a new cast is applied until the desired ROM has returned. In the case of serial splinting, the splint is adjusted to increase the stretch until the desired ROM is achieved. Positional programs are also effective methods of improving and maintaining ROM throughout the body. An advantage to creation of a positioning program early in the rehabilitation process is that it helps to manage edema and inflammation, especially with the use of elevation.[1a] Additionally, ambulation and functional skills should be incorporated into the plan of care and the child's daily routine.

Compliance with positioning and splinting programs is often a contentious experience with children because of their difficulty in seeing the long-term implications of joint contractures and scarring. Reward programs such as sticker charts, sticker games, and point charts are often effective methods of motivation for children. These programs should be based on the child's chronological and cognitive age levels, so they provide salient motivation for the child to perform and comply with splint-wearing programs.

As children with burn injuries begin to heal, they appear very "stiff-looking." This may be a result of the child's desire to not move joints through any ROM in an attempt to prevent pain and stretching of the burned tissue. It is the role of the PT and physical therapist assistant (PTA) to engage the child in appropriate therapeutic exercises to maintain ROM, muscle strength, and functional abilities. Therapeutic exercises must have a large element of relevant "fun" for the child, and this will vary depending on the child's age and cognitive level. Allowing the child to select an activity, then using that activity to promote therapeutic goals, gives the child an increased level of control in the rehabilitation process. The advancement of the therapy interventions must be made on a daily basis to continue the progression of regaining functional skills, ROM, and overall recovery.

Pressure garments are commonly used to minimize scarring following burn injury. A variety of manufacturers create custom-made garments from highly detailed measurements obtained from the child's affected areas. Staley and Richard[16] studied why the pressure garments are beneficial during the healing process and concluded that the pressure created by the garments enhances the skin's maturation process. Because these garments are not only tight but create heat at the skin surface, initial research is exploring the role of the heat in minimizing scarring for individuals who have sustained burn injuries. Custom-made burn pressure garments are worn approximately 23 hours a day for up to 2 years following burn injury.

Fabrication of a custom-made, clear facemask can provide full facial contact to the child with extensive facial burns. Children and their parents are typically more compliant with use of the clear facemasks than they are with cloth facemasks.

As stated earlier, children who sustain burns are in need of both immediate and long-term therapy interventions to prevent the development of excessive scarring and the loss of ROM and function. Family involvement and support of the therapy program are critical to the outcome of burn rehabilitation. Working as a team, which includes the child and family, to return the child to participating in family life and school and community routines is paramount.

BURNS INTERVENTIONS

- Address ROM limitations with splinting or positioning programs
- Maintain ROM, muscle strength, and functional abilities through therapeutic exercises
- Minimize scarring with pressure garments

CASE STUDY OF A CHILD WITH BURNS

Examination

History

T.W. is a 9-month-old boy who was brought to a community hospital with significant burns over his entire body. His mother reports he was in the care of her boyfriend when she went to the store. When she returned to the hotel room in which they were living, T.W. was unresponsive and blistered over his entire body. Approximately 24 hours after the burn incident, T.W.'s mother took him to the community hospital. On initial examination in the emergency department, T.W.'s burns were estimated to involve more than 76% of his body. His face was the only area not burned, according to the initial assessment. Because of the severity of his burn injuries, he was immediately intubated and placed on mechanical ventilation. A nasogastric tube was put in place for nutrition, and intravenous fluid replacement was started. He was transferred by helicopter to a pediatric trauma center specializing in severe burn injuries.

At the trauma center, T.W. was mechanically ventilated for 4 weeks. Several times, the severity of his injuries and risk of infection led to the expectation that he would

Continued

CASE STUDY OF A CHILD WITH BURNS—cont'd

not survive. He underwent several surgical procedures for wound debridement, skin grafting, and compartment syndrome release of his left anterior-lateral compartment. After 4 weeks of intubation and mechanical ventilation, T.W. was removed from the ventilator and extubated. He remained in a medically induced coma for pain management, and plans for the rehabilitation phase of his care began. It was determined he would be transferred to an intensive inpatient rehabilitation program for further therapies and wound care. Prior to his transfer, the court granted Child Protective Services custody of T.W. after it was established that the infant had been dunked in a bathtub full of scalding water by his mother's boyfriend as a punishment for wetting his diaper. The mother's delay in seeking medical treatment for T.W. made her culpable as well. Specialized foster care placement will be required for T.W. when he is ready for discharge.

On arrival at the inpatient rehabilitation program, T.W. continued to be highly sedated and was seldom awake; this was required because of the extent of his injuries. Initial physical, occupational, and developmental therapy examinations were done, and a plan of care was determined.

No family was present at the time of the initial examination because of the removal of custody from T.W.'s mother.

Review of Systems

On initial examination of T.W., the following were noted:
1. T.W. exhibited severely impaired skin integrity throughout his body, except for his face.
2. T.W. exhibited severely impaired ROM throughout his trunk, neck, and extremities.
3. Because of the medically induced coma, T.W. was unresponsive to stimulation.
4. T.W. was unable to move his extremities actively.
5. T.W. was unable to communicate verbally.

Physical, occupational, and developmental therapies were involved in T.W.'s care from the time of admission. Once his sedative medications were decreased and he became more alert and responsive, speech therapy was to be initiated to address feeding and communication impairments.

Tests and Measures
Impairments

T.W. exhibited severely impaired skin integrity with minimal closed skin areas; the majority of his skin was still open. He had significant burned areas, and his scalp was used as a donor site. His left anterior-lateral thigh had undergone a compartment release because of the development of compartment syndrome, and as a result, had a "filleted" appearance. ROM throughout his trunk and all extremities was highly limited in all planes of movement, and he did not come with any splinting when transferred. Because of his medically induced coma, he was highly unresponsive, and no further examinations were completed at the time.

Once his medications were reduced and his alertness increased, complete functional motor skills assessment and testing would need to be completed.

Functional Limitations and Disability

T.W. initially exhibited limited responsiveness due to a medically induced coma, but once sedative medications were decreased, standardized testing with the Peabody Developmental Motor Scales, 2nd edition (PDMS-2) was completed. He displayed gross motor skills at a 2-month level for reflexes, a 2-month level for stationary skills, and a 3-month level for locomotion skills.

Diagnosis

On synthesis of the examination information, the following diagnoses were determined for T.W.: impaired arousal, attention, and cognition, most likely due to medically induced coma for pain management; impaired integumentary function; impaired ROM; impaired motor functioning; impaired sensory integration; and impaired functional mobility. Because of the seriousness of his burn injuries, T.W. exhibited severe impairments in all of the areas listed above.

Prognosis

Given the extent of T.W.'s burn injuries, he will most likely exhibit lifelong integumentary, ROM, and functional limitations, likely requiring surgical intervention to address these impairments as he grows. The psychologic implications for T.W. are currently unknown but will likely need to be addressed as he ages and begins school and socialization with peers. With the excellent care he received both at the trauma center and now at the rehabilitation center, T.W. could make excellent progress with highly intensive services.

Plan of Care

T.W.'s length of stay in the intensive rehabilitation program was estimated at the time of the examination to be approximately 24 to 28 weeks to best maximize his potential for integumentary, motor, sensory, psychologic, and cognitive recovery.

CASE STUDY OF A CHILD WITH BURNS—cont'd

The following goals and outcomes for physical therapy were determined:

Goals

1. T.W. will tolerate passive, active, and active assistive ROM for all affected joints.
2. T.W. will maintain independent sitting.
3. T.W. will tolerate prone play and will creep independently.
4. T.W. will exhibit an intact integumentary system with no open areas.
5. T.W. will use all of his extremities in play.
6. T.W. will cruise on a supportive surface.

Outcomes

1. T.W. will tolerate all skin and burn care during daily hygiene activities.
2. Once identified, T.W.'s foster parents will increase their understanding of scald burns and their effects and the anticipated goals and expected outcomes.
3. T.W. will participate in age-appropriate social interactions with modifications, as required.
4. T.W. will tolerate wearing pressure garments to minimize scarring.
5. T.W. will play with toys and interact with other children and adults.

Intervention

T.W. received extensive physical therapy services in an inpatient rehabilitation program for 26 weeks, with physical therapy services delivered two to three times a day, Monday through Friday; once daily on Saturdays; and for the first 8 weeks of his rehabilitation admission, once daily on Sundays as well. (T.W. was unable to maintain his ROM without daily intervention, so Sunday treatment was initiated.) Intervention included weekly staffing/care conferences and multidisciplinary rounds, reintegration of T.W. into child life activities once or twice daily as he became more alert, and extensive caregiver training once a specialized foster care placement was identified. A foster family was identified during week 20 of T.W.'s 26-week rehabilitation stay, and his foster parents became highly involved in his day-to-day care and therapy programs. His foster mother was a registered emergency department nurse, and his foster father was a pharmacist.

Treatment interventions focused on passive, active, and active assistive ROM, splinting, positioning for edema control, and restoration of functional mobility. As T.W.'s pharmacologic management became more simplified and narcotics began to be tapered, his alertness began to increase. Age-appropriate play activities were introduced in therapy to promote increased functional use of his hands and functional developmental mobility, including standing and using a Crawligator for prone mobility (Fig. 17.4).

The use of pressure garments was initiated once his skin no longer had open areas. Silicone gel sheets provided lubrication of his skin surfaces.

Outcome

At the time of discharge, T.W. was beginning to independently cruise along furniture for approximately 5 to 6 feet. He was able to creep independently on a level surface and was able to creep up and down four stairs with supervision. At the time that the PDMS-2 was readministered, T.W. was 16 months old and functioning at a gross motor age equivalency of 10 months for reflexes, 12 months for stationary skills, 12 months for locomotion skills, and 12 months for object manipulation skills. This indicated a great improvement in his developmental mobility since admission and also demonstrated the success of his ROM, positioning, and mobility programs. He had begun to talk and say single words. Although the use of his hands for fine-motor play was his greatest remaining impairment, he demonstrated amazing improvements during his inpatient rehabilitation stay. T.W. was discharged home with his foster parents, who lived in a rural setting on a horse farm and inquired about the appropriateness of taking T.W. horseback riding and swimming at the local indoor pool. T.W. was also going to continue intensive rehabilitation services at a day rehabilitation program near his home 5 days per week for 4 hours per day. As of 3 years after burn injury, T.W. is a very happy, ambulatory little boy who will always have integumentary impairments that require ongoing therapy services and future surgical interventions. He is also continuing to be followed up by child psychiatric services and the pediatric burn team.

Analysis of Case Using the ICF Model (at Discharge)

Body functions: Healing burns on four extremities and trunk, decreased ROM

Activity limitations: Decreased fine and gross motor skills, decreased self-care, limited play and interactions

Participation restrictions: Extended inpatient status secondary to guarded medical condition, cannot play, cannot participate in age-appropriate activities, living with a new family

Environmental factors: Extended inpatient stay at hospital transitioning to rural home setting; involved with child protection agency

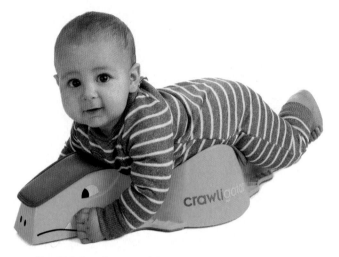

Fig. 17.4 Crawligator mobility toy. (www.crawligator.com.)

CHAPTER DISCUSSION QUESTIONS

1. Discuss why young children are more susceptible to scald burns than older children.
2. Identify the characteristics of first-, second-, and third-degree burns based on alternative labels for burn classification, physical characteristics, pain/sensation, and cause of burn.
3. Describe total burn surface area and the three ways to measure it.
4. Compare and contrast acid and alkaloid burns.
5. Identify two possible complications from a burn injury.
6. How can healing tissue cause difficulties in the rehabilitation process?
7. What are the two main goals for someone who is recovering from a burn injury?
8. Why would a family be more accepting of a clear facemask versus a cloth facemask?

REFERENCES

1. Warden GD, Lang D, Housinger TA. Management of pediatric hand burns with tendon, joint and bone injury. *Paper presented at the meeting of the American Burn Association*, Cincinnati; March 1993.
1a. Ohgi S, Gu S. Pediatric burn rehabilitation: philosophy and strategies. *Burn Trauma*. 2013;1:73–79.
2. Brigham P. *Data Compiler: Burn Foundation*, PA, American Burn Association, Chicago, Il; 1999. https://ameriburn.org/wp-content/uploads/2017/05/2016abanbr_final_42816.pdf. Accessed June 8, 2023.
2a. Armstrong M, Wheeler KK, Shi J, et al. Epidemiology and trend of US pediatric burn hospitalizations, 2003–2016. *Burns*. 2021;47(3):551–559.
3. Baradaran A. *Thermal Burns*. https://emedicine.medscape.com/article/1278244-overview. Accessed July 5, 2023.
4. Vande Ven H. *Electrical Burn Injuries*. https://emedicine.medscape.com/article/1277496-overview. Accessed July 5, 2023.
5. Cox RD. *Chemical Burns*. https://emedicine.medscape.com/article/769336-overview. Accessed July 5, 2023.
6. Feller I. Burn epidemiology: focus on youngsters and the aged. *J Burn Care Rehabil*. 1982;3:285.
7. Bennett B, Gamelli R. Profile of an abused burned child. *J Burn Care Rehabil*. 1998;19(1):88.
8. Carrougher GJ. *Burn Care and Therapy*. St Louis: Mosby; 1998.
9. Mikhail NJ. Acute burn care: an update. *J Emerg Nurs*. 1988;14(1).
10. Doane CB. Children with severe burns. In: Pratt PN, Allen AS, eds. *Occupational Therapy for Children*. St Louis: Mosby; 1989.
11. Cassell OC, Hubble M, Milling MA, et al. Baby walkers—still a major cause of infant burns. *Burns*. 1997;23(5):451.
12. Skandamis KG. Cold weather related injuries. *J Urgent Care Med* (jucm.com). 2010. https://www.jucm.com/wp-content/uploads/2021/02/2010-5311-17-Clinical-Mgmt.pdf. Accessed July 5, 2023.
13. Isao T, Masaki F, Riko N, et al. Delayed brain atrophy after electrical injury. *J Burn Care Rehabil*. 2005;26:456–458.
13a. Monafo WW. Initial management of burns. *N Engl J Med*. 1996;335(21):1581.

14. Bennett GB, Helm P, Purdue GF, et al. Serial casting: a method for treating burn contractures. *J Burn Care Rehabil.* 1989;10:543.

15. Bull JP, Squire JR. A study of mortality in a burn unit: standards for the evaluation of alternative methods of treatment. *Ann Surg.* 1949;130(2):160.

16. Staley MJ, Richard RL. Use of pressure to treat hypertrophic burn scars. *Adv Wound Care.* 1997;10(3):44.

RESOURCES

Burn Recovery Center
877-640-3200
www.burn-recovery.org

About.com: Physical Therapy
www.physicaltherapy.about.com
Burn Survivors Online
www.burnsurvivorsonline.com
Severe Burns, by Andrew M. Munster
Coping Strategies for Burn Survivors and Their Families,
by Norman R. Bernstein and others.

Limb Deficiencies

Yasser Salem, PT, PhD, NCS, PCS

LEARNING OBJECTIVES

At the end of the chapter, the reader will be able to do the following:

1. Label the amputation levels using current appropriate terminology.
2. Compare and contrast congenital and acquired amputations/limb deficiencies.
3. Design an exercise program based on level of amputation.

CHAPTER OUTLINE

KEY TERMS

Acquired limb deficiency
Amelia
Amniotic band syndrome

Congenital limb
  deficiency
Hemimelia

Prosthesis
Residual limb

DEFINITION

Limb deficiencies, also called limb differences, in children may affect the upper or lower extremities and may involve one limb or several limbs. Causes fall into one of two categories: congenital limb deficiency or acquired limb deficiency (amputation). Congenital limb deficiency is one of the most common congenital deficiencies.[1] Congenital limb deficiencies are further classified into transverse and longitudinal. Nomenclature of the acquired types has changed over the last several years, but both previously accepted labeling (above knee, below knee, above elbow, and below elbow) and current

labeling (transfemoral, transtibial, transhumeral, and transradial) continue to be used.[1] For this chapter, when appropriate, the historical system is provided in parentheses.

PATHOLOGY

Congenital

Congenital limb deficiency occurs in utero when part or all of a fetal limb does not completely form. Deficiency includes absence of a limb or limbs or loss of muscles and ligaments in limbs. Amelia refers to a case in which an entire bone/segment is missing; hemimelia refers to a longitudinal anomaly in which all or part of one bone is missing, and phocomelia refers to the congenital absence of the proximal section of a limb.[2,3] Transverse amputations occur in the transverse plane of the extremity through the shaft of the involved bone. These amputations occur in the proximal, middle, or distal third of the involved limb. Longitudinal deficiencies may be unilateral or bilateral and symmetric or asymmetric. One of the bones in the segment is missing or malformed along the long axis of the segment (e.g., the ulna or fibula may be missing). These deficiencies may cause the remaining bones in the segment to be malformed; in the case of a missing ulna, the radius may be bowed. Segments proximal or distal to the limb deficiency may be completely formed.

The etiology of congenital limb deficiency is heterogenous and includes genetic and environmental factors,[1] but causes are mostly unknown and vary from child to child. A common cause of congenital limb deficiency is amniotic band syndrome (ABS), which occurs in 1 of 1200 live births; 80% involve anomalies of the fingers and hands.[2] The entrapment of fetal parts in a fibrous amniotic band in utero is believed to cause ABS. The amnion ruptures early and entangles the fetus. This may in turn cause several varying birth defects, including deficiency of the arms, legs, and digits.[2] ABS is sporadic, not hereditary, and there is typically no risk of recurrence within families.[2] Congenital limb deficiency can be associated with other congenital abnormalities.

Acquired

Acquired amputations may be due to trauma, vascular disease, tumors, infections, or burn injuries. Amputations secondary to trauma occur twice as frequently as amputations due to disease. Partial or complete removal of a limb may be necessary following a traumatic incident.[4] Different types of amputations are described in Table 18.1.

INTERVENTION

The rehabilitation team typically includes the child and family; physicians; nurses; physical, occupational, and developmental therapists; social workers; and prosthetists. The rehabilitation team works closely to design a plan that includes residual limb shaping and desensitization, exercise and strengthening, improving endurance, and prosthetic tolerance. The child and the family play an important part in the child obtaining full independence. As the child grows and matures, he or she should be given a progressively larger role in making prosthetic decisions.

Children with congenital limb malformations or deficiencies may undergo surgery to adapt the residual limb for prosthetic wear. Surgery should be undertaken with the goal of restoring function. Typically, a multidisciplinary team, including the child and family, makes a decision regarding surgery and follow-up rehabilitation. With a traumatic amputation or disease process, surgery may be the only option, and the medical team will lead that decision. Following surgery, however, the entire rehabilitation team cooperatively creates a postoperative rehabilitation and prosthetic plan.

In the case of a baby with a congenital amputation, the parents can be initially devastated by the defect. They may feel shame and anger and want to hide the child or the affected limb. The parents may blame themselves for an incident, real or perceived, that occurred during pregnancy. It is vital for the family to be connected with a rehabilitation team as soon as possible and with a social network that includes individuals who have experienced what they are currently experiencing. These connections can help the family adjust to the child's missing limb and formulate a story to share with others. Families need time and peer assistance to put together the words that positively describe their child and acknowledge their child's disability as a secondary consideration. Other parents will share their experiences, triumphs, and pitfalls, thus easing the pain and assisting them on their journey.

LIMB DEFICIENCIES INTERVENTIONS

- Shape and desensitize residual limb
- Plan a program for exercise and strengthening
- Improve endurance
- Improve tolerance of prosthetic
- Promote age-appropriate developmental skills
- Promote functional independence

Congenital Upper Extremity Limb Deficiency

Upper extremity interventions focus on promotion of upper extremity developmental skills, functional independence, and coordination. Interventions include

TABLE 18.1 Types of Amputations

Amputation	Characteristics
Upper Extremity	
Shoulder disarticulation	Humerus and all distal structures are missing.
	Child will require prosthesis that includes a mechanical shoulder joint, elbow joint, and hand components.
Transhumeral (above elbow)	Amputation occurs through the shaft of the humerus.
	Child will require prosthesis with an elbow and hand components.
Transradial (below elbow)	Amputation occurs through the shaft of the radius and ulna.
	Elbow joint remains intact.
	Prosthesis includes a hand component.
Wrist disarticulation	Amputation occurs at wrist level.
	Prosthesis will include hand component.
Hand	Amputation includes all or part of the hand and all or part of the fingers.
	Prosthesis will include hand components.
Lower Extremity	
Hemipelvectomy	Amputation includes half of the pelvis and all anatomic structures of the ipsilateral lower extremity.
	Prosthesis will include a bucket socket to contain distal trunk structures; mechanical hip, knee, ankle, and foot components will be attached to this bucket socket.
Hip disarticulation	Amputation includes femur and all distal anatomic structures.
	Prosthesis will include hip, knee, ankle, and foot components.
Proximal femoral focal deficiency (PFFD)	A longitudinal deficiency in which the femur is malformed and shortened
	Typically, the remaining femoral segment is held in flexion, abduction, and external rotation.
	This deformity is classified into four types: Class A, B, C, or D.
	• Class A: normal hip joint with intact and well-seated femoral head and acetabulum, shortened femoral segment with subtrochanteric varus angulation
	• Class B: femoral head present, acetabulum adequate but defective, capital fragment within acetabulum
	• Class C: femoral head and acetabulum absent, short femoral fragment, no articulation between femur and acetabulum
	• Class D: femoral head and acetabulum absent, no relation between femur and acetabulum
	Several surgical intervention strategies are available to the child with PFFD, depending on the length of the remaining limb. Prosthetic components may or may not include a knee joint but will include ankle and foot components.[1]
Transfemoral (above knee)	Amputation occurs through the shaft of the femur.
	Prosthetic components include knee, ankle, and foot.
Knee disarticulation	Amputation occurs at the knee joint.
	Femur is intact; distal lower extremity is removed/missing.
	Prosthesis includes a knee joint, ankle, and foot components.
Transtibial (below knee)	Amputation occurs through the shaft of the tibia and fibula.
	Anatomic knee remains intact.
	Prosthesis includes ankle and foot components.
Syme amputation	Ankle disarticulation with intact heel pad.
	Prosthesis includes foot component.
Foot	Amputation includes all or part of the foot and all or part of the toes.
	Prosthesis includes shoe filler.

facilitation of age-appropriate developmental skills, range of motion (ROM) and flexibility exercises, functional strength training, coordination training, prosthetic training, and child and parent education.

For the child with a congenital amputation, prosthetic fittings and therapy begin at developmentally appropriate stages. Typically, the child should be evaluated as soon as possible to determine a plan of action and introduce the family to the remedial medical systems. For a child with an upper extremity limb deficiency, prosthetic wear will occur as early as 3 months of age. This will enable the child to develop age-appropriate developmental skills such as prone and bimanual skills. As the child grows, the components of the prosthesis should match the child's development. Decisions concerning passive versus dynamic hand, voluntary opening versus voluntary closing hand, and traditional versus myoelectric should be made in light of the type and extent of limb deficiencies and the child's development

and activity level. Table 18.2 lists appropriate outcomes by age for children with upper extremity amputations.

Myoelectric prosthetics use the body's power to open and close the terminal device. The child must have sufficient activation of muscle groups to be able to activate at least two directions of motion. Children can be fitted for a myoelectric prosthetic device when they can cognitively understand and motor plan a volitional muscle contraction on demand. Thus, the muscle must generate a contraction when commanded to do so and not necessarily within the framework of a functional activity. Training is crucial to develop the ability to the use the myoelectric prosthesis in daily life.[5] Myoelectric devices have many pros and cons that must be considered prior to recommending them. These devices are heavier than traditional body-powered prosthetics; they are battery operated; they require a higher level of maintenance and care; and they do not hold up well against sand, water, grime, or dirt. On the other hand, children perceive

TABLE 18.2	Intervention Outcomes for Children With Upper Extremity Deficiencies and Their Parents	
Age of Child	Intervention Outcomes for Children	Intervention Outcomes for Their Parents
Infant	Comfort with the prosthesis Tolerate wearing prosthesis Can clasp large objects using prosthesis Use the prosthesis to aid in sitting and crawling	Can apply and remove the prosthesis correctly Can care for child's skin and child's prosthesis Can recognize and report any problems with the prosthesis
Toddler	Child can control terminal device and elbow unit Child can perform bimanual prehension activities Child can use prosthesis as an assist in functional activities	Should provide toys that require bimanual prehension/manipulation Encourage child to think of the prosthesis as an assistive device Inspect skin regularly for signs of irritation
School-aged	Child has an opinion about type and function of prosthesis Child can maintain proper prosthetic fit and recognize when repairs are needed Child can grasp firm or fragile objects without dropping or crushing them Child can successfully open and close the terminal device Child can don and doff prosthesis independently Child can dress self independently	Encourage child to be independent in all activities of daily living and play

Data from Lusardi MM, Nielson CC. *Orthotics and Prosthetics in Rehabilitation*. 2nd ed. Philadelphia: Butterworth-Heinemann; 2006.

myoelectric devices as "cool." Additionally, a myoelectric device can nicely mimic a biologic hand.

Congenital Lower Extremity Limb Deficiency

As in the case of upper limb deficiency, the team should evaluate the child with a congenital lower extremity deficiency as soon as possible. Lower extremity interventions focus on promotion of upper extremity developmental skills and functional independence. Interventions include ROM and flexibility exercises; functional strength training; facilitation of age-appropriate developmental skills; gait, balance, and prosthetic training; and child and parent education. Prosthetic wear typically occurs as the child begins to develop lower extremity weight-bearing skills. These skills include assuming and maintaining four-point position, pulling to stand, cruising, and standing. Decisions concerning prosthetics will need to be made in light of the child's limb deficiency level and developmental level.

Traumatic or Surgical Amputation

For the child with a traumatic amputation, postoperative rehabilitation should begin as soon as medically feasible. Particular attention should be paid to ROM, skin condition, and the strength and shape of the residual limb. The child may also have issues of phantom pain and hypersensitivity in the residual limb. Family support is another integral part of the rehabilitation process.

Traumatic amputations and surgical amputations are equally traumatic for the family nexus. In the case of traumatic amputation, the incident that caused the child's injury may have been preventable. The parents may experience guilt and remorse, even if there is no way they could have prevented it. Similarly, families will grapple with issues surrounding surgery and limb salvage. It seems that most caregivers' and clients' initial response is to save the limb; however, as time passes, the family or child may decide that a revised limb with a prosthesis is more functional, stronger, and more cosmetically acceptable than the salvaged limb.

Families and children require peer support as well to help them journey through this process. Following amputation surgery, peers with the same-level amputation can offer support, encouragement, and direction to the family and child. Professionals should be available to visit the child's school with the parents before the child returns from amputation surgery and recovery. This visit will allow the child's school peers to ask questions, touch and feel different prostheses and components of prostheses, and talk through some of their fears and concerns about their classmate. The hope is that these sessions will help ease the transition back to school and minimize any apprehension the children and school staff may be experiencing. The child with an amputation should be encouraged to resume his or her previous activities and routines as soon as possible. Table 18.3 details appropriate outcomes by age for children with lower extremity amputations.

PROSTHETIC COMPONENTS

Although prosthetic components change and are upgraded frequently, categories of components share commonalities. These generalizations will be discussed, keeping in mind that new technology is constantly evolving. It is crucial for the comprehensive rehabilitation team to include members who have up-to-date knowledge of prosthetic technology.

Transtibial prosthetic components include the following:

- Hard socket: The hard socket is made of a rigid laminate material. It can be reinforced with carbon fiber for strength. The socket is shaped to exactly fit the child's residual limb. The socket helps to maintain the soft tissues of the residual limb in a safe and efficient position.
- Prosthetic socks: Socks come in a variety of thicknesses, typically 1-, 3-, 5-, and 10-ply. They are made of cotton or wool and must be carefully cared for. As the residual limb shrinks in size, the sock offers a mechanism to take up some of the excess room, so that the residual limb will not experience shearing or friction from pistoning. A sock also acts as a shock absorber for the residual limb.
- Soft liner: A thin, soft liner can be used in lieu of socks. It acts as a shock absorber between the residual limb and prosthesis socket. Care must be taken to ensure that the liner fits properly and is cleaned regularly.
- Suspension mechanics: When properly suspended, the prosthesis should not swivel or move on or about the residual limb. Similarly, the residual limb should not piston or move about within the prosthesis. If movement occurs or areas are not properly loaded for appropriate weight-bearing, the child could be at risk for skin breakdown, development of sores or blisters, and inefficient and unsafe gait.

TABLE 18.3 Intervention Outcomes for Children With Lower Extremity Deficiencies and Their Parents

Age of Child	Intervention Outcomes for Children	Intervention Outcomes for Their Parents
Infant	Comfort and tolerance of prosthesis Child can stand by leaning against a table Child can cruise around furniture Child can walk with or without support of an age-appropriate push toy	Parents can apply and remove the prosthesis correctly Parents can care for child's skin and child's prosthesis Parents can recognize and report any problems with the prosthesis
Toddler	Child tolerates wearing prosthesis all day Child uses prosthesis when completing age-appropriate ambulatory activities	Encourage use of the prosthesis Provide toys and equipment that require age-appropriate activities and mobility Inspect skin regularly for signs of irritation
School-aged	Child has an opinion about type and function of prosthesis Child is able to independently monitor and maintain proper prosthetic fit, including skin inspection, and recognize when repairs are needed Child can independently don and doff prosthesis, as well as dress independently Child can complete all ambulatory activities and mobility activities independently	Encourage child to be independent in all activities of daily living and play Encourage child to be active in group sporting activities

Data from Lusardi MM, Nielson CC. *Orthotics and Prosthetics in Rehabilitation.* 2nd ed. Philadelphia: Butterworth-Heinemann; 2006.

- Supracondylar suspension systems: Supracondylar suspension grips the child above the medial and lateral femoral condyles and is used with a transtibial prosthesis. The condyles provide an ideal surface area for suspension.
- Cuff: The suspension cuff is added to the distal part of the transtibial prosthesis. The cuff is tightened around the femur just proximal to the femoral condyles. This arrangement secures the prosthesis to the residual limb and prevents pistoning or movement of the residual limb.
- Suction: With suction, the air is milked out of the socket, forming a suction seal that secures the prosthesis to the residual limb. This seal should be strong enough to maintain the prosthesis securely in place during all normal activities. When the prosthesis is to be removed, the suction seal is broken.
- Sleeve: A roll-on sleeve can be used over the standard suspension mechanisms. The sleeve provides added suspension and helps minimize any remaining movement between the residual limb and the prosthesis.

Some children use the sleeve when they participate in sports or activities requiring fast movements.

Transfemoral prosthetic components include the following:

- An ischial containment socket: This type of socket contains the ischium with the posterior prosthetic wall. The femur maintains normal adduction position, thus allowing the child to use a narrower base of support. The ischial containment design allows for more optimal force distribution along the residual femoral shaft. This socket is the design of choice for most children and adults with transfemoral amputations.
- A quadrilateral socket: This socket design was used successfully for years before the advent of the ischial containment socket. It is rarely used in contemporary prostheses. In this design, the socket has a quadrilateral shape, with each wall having a different purpose. Most notably, the ischial tuberosity sits up on the posterior wall and acts as a weight-bearing surface along with the gluteal musculature. The medial wall

is relatively high to contain the adductor tissues and provide counterpressure to the lateral wall. The lateral wall provides a working support surface for the residual femur in midstance. The anterior wall blocks forward motion of the residual limb, and the medial corner of the anterior wall contains a channel for the adductor tendon.

- Prosthetic knee options: There are several pediatric knee options, ranging from a single hinge with a manual lock to those with hydraulic components. It is commonly thought that the ambulatory child should be fitted with a working knee as soon as possible. This allows the child to develop normal gait rhythm and cycle from the onset of ambulation. Infants may use a single-axis joint that when released has full flexion and when strapped or locked is maintained in extension.

Components used for both transfemoral and transtibial prosthetics include the following:
- Prosthetic foot options: Children are frequently fitted with an energy-storing foot or at least a dynamic foot as early as possible. These are accommodating and high-performance prosthetic feet, allowing children to have greater flexibility.

Prosthetic coverings include the following:
- Exoskeletal: The covering of the prosthesis is a hard laminate material. Once fabricated, it cannot be easily modified in color or shape.
- Endoskeletal: The covering of the prosthesis is a softer foam laminate with a nylon sheath covering. The shape and color of the cover can be modified, if necessary. The downside is that the cover may be damaged or torn more easily than the exoskeletal cover.

CASE STUDY OF A CHILD WITH A LIMB DEFICIENCY

Jason was born a typically developing child. At 18 months, he contracted bacterial meningitis. By the time the devastation of the disease could be arrested, Jason's four extremities were severely affected. He lost his limbs at the following levels: bilateral transfemoral, a left upper extremity transradial, and a right wrist disarticulation. He was fitted with four prostheses. The lower extremity prostheses had solid sockets with hip joints and a waist belt for suspension. The knee joints were single-axis hinges that could be locked in extension or swing loose for flexion. He used bilateral simple energy-storing feet. Primary therapy and teaching entailed maintaining skin integrity because his skin had rough scarring from the meningitis and multiple surgical procedures. Therapy also consisted of improving his strength, coordination, balance, and equilibrium reactions and helping him learn to fall safely.

As a toddler, Jason learned first to ambulate with a reverse wheeled walker. The handle grips needed to be modified so that he could grasp and control the walker easily. As he learned to balance and shift weight more easily, Jason began to ambulate around his home with bilateral Lofstrand crutches. Finally, he learned to ambulate with a single Lofstrand crutch indoors. He preferred to use a walker when ambulating outside or for long distances. If traveling a long distance, he would be pushed in a stroller. Jason used bilateral Adept terminal devices, each with a single cable to operate the hand function. The terminal device rests in the open position (this is the opposite of a traditional hook terminal device) and closes via the cable system, which is attached to a figure-eight

harness worn over the shoulders. Jason initially needed to learn how to operate the devices so he could accomplish self-help skills such as feeding and dressing. After learning to use his prostheses as assists, he then moved on to master more delicate fine motor skills such as grasping and maintaining a hold on different objects, manipulating small objects, and performing self-help and self-care activities. He also learned rather quickly that he could cause pain without feeling pain by squeezing or pinching others with his terminal devices.

At 3 years of age, Jason attended a special education program to receive physical and occupational therapy in the school. He was transitioned into the state prekindergarten classroom at the age of 4 years. He did well in school and learned to adapt to his environment to be as independent as possible. He propelled a manual wheelchair for long-distance outings. At school he carried his supplies in a backpack and used bilateral Lofstrand crutches for mobility around the school building. After 3 years of preschool and kindergarten, he left the special education system to attend first grade at a regular public school. He was independent in all his school skills, and he and his family were self-sufficient in caring for his skin and recognizing when he needed prosthetic adjustments or replacement equipment. Jason typically had growth adjustments made over the summer so that his sudden change in height would not be as obvious to school peers. Before growth adjustments, Jason was commonly shorter in stature than his classmates. After summer break, he would return with 2 years' worth of estimated

CASE STUDY OF A CHILD WITH A LIMB DEFICIENCY—cont'd

growth built into his new prostheses, making him one of the taller students in his group.

As he grew and became a more skilled prosthetic wearer, Jason considered more technically advanced prosthetic components. He preferred to use hydraulic knee joints, advanced multiaxial energy-storing feet, and suction sockets in his lower prostheses. He tried a myoelectric upper extremity device but ultimately preferred the performance and durability of manual terminal devices. He learned to ride a bike with great determination and some modifications. He credits his ability to overcome his impairments and grow into an independent young man to self-determination and a supportive family.

He was interested in the computerized componentry that would be available to him as he grew taller.

Analysis of Case Using the ICF Model
Health conditions: Status after bacterial meningitis
  Body functions: Quadrimembral amputee, scar tissue on distal residual limbs, four prostheses
  Activity limitations: None, as long as prostheses are functioning
  Participation restrictions: None, as long as prostheses are functioning
  Environmental limitations: Requires prostheses to be independent and functional

CHAPTER DISCUSSION QUESTIONS

1. What body parts are most commonly affected by ABS?
2. If a baby is born with ABS, what is the risk that future children in the family will have it?
3. What are the two categories of limb deficiency?
4. What is the current nomenclature for the following previously accepted terms for levels of amputation: above knee, below elbow?
5. What is the difference between an amelia, a hemimelia, and a phocomelia?
6. Describe a proximal femoral focal deficiency.
7. At what age would a baby be fitted with an upper extremity prosthesis?
8. At what age would a child be fitted with a lower extremity prosthetic device?
9. What design of knee joint would you recommend for a child just beginning to stand and take steps?
10. What are two desired intervention outcomes for a young child with a lower limb deficiency?

REFERENCES

1. da Rocha LA, Pires LVL, Yamamoto GL, et al. Congenital limb deficiency: genetic investigation of 44 individuals presenting mainly longitudinal defects in isolated or syndromic forms. *Clin Genet.* 2021;100(5):615–623.
2. Amniotic Band Syndrome. *Amniotic band syndrome* (website): https://amnioticbandsyndrome.com/. Access June 1, 2022.
3. Schwickert A, Dame C, Akanbi S, et al. Pränatale Diagnostik und postnatale Komplikationen im Fall einer extrem seltenen Tetraamelie [Prenatal diagnostics and postnatal complications in a case of extremely rare tetraamelia]. *Z Geburtshilfe Neonatol.* 2021;225(3):279–282.
4. Gibson TW, Westberry DE, Carpenter AM, et al. Terminal Syme amputation of the great toe in the pediatric population. *J Pediatr Orthop.* 2021;41(9):e823–e827.
5. Widehammar C, Lidström Holmqvist K, et al. Training for users of myoelectric multigrip hand prostheses: a scoping review. *Prosthet Orthot Int.* 2021;45(5):393–400.

RESOURCES

Amputee Coalition
  900 East Hill Avenue
  Suite 288
  Knoxville, TN 37905
  888-267-5669
  www.amputee-coalition.org

National Rehabilitation Information Center (NARIC)
  4200 Forbes Boulevard
  Suite 202
  Lanham, MD 20706
  800-346-2742
  www.naric.com

Association of Children's Prosthetic-Orthotic Clinics (ACPOC)
  6300 N. River Road
  Suite 727
  Rosemont, IL 60018-4226
  847-384-4226
  www.acpoc.org

Asthma

Roberta Kuchler O'Shea, PT, DPT, PhD
Renee Theiss, PhD

LEARNING OBJECTIVES

At the end of the chapter, the reader will be able to do the following:

1. Identify the warning signs of asthma.
2. Respond to a child in respiratory distress secondary to asthmatic conditions.
3. Design an appropriate exercise regimen for a child with asthma.

CHAPTER OUTLINE

KEY TERMS

Asthma management plan
Peak flow monitoring

Preventive medications
Rescue medication

Spacer

DEFINITION

Asthma is a chronic respiratory condition with inflammation of the airways; its symptoms include breathing problems such as coughing, wheezing, shortness of breath, and chest tightness.

PATHOLOGY

Asthma severity can be classified as intermittent, mild persistent, moderate persistent, and severe persistent. Asthma episode control can be classified as well controlled, not well controlled, and poorly controlled. Asthma can be fatal without appropriate treatment. Asthma triggers and the degree to which a person reacts to a trigger vary (Fig. 19.1). Often, there are triggers that cause the airways of a person with asthma to react with swelling, narrowing of the airways, and production of excess mucus. Triggers include allergens such as pollen or pet dander, irritants such as chemical fumes or tobacco smoke, pollution, respiratory viruses, cold dry air or warm humid air and physical activity.

According to the Centers for Disease Control and Prevention (CDC), 5.8% of children younger than 18 years in the United States have asthma, making it one of the most common chronic health conditions of childhood.[1,2] In 2020, of these over 4 million children, 42.7% reported having one or more asthma attacks in the past 12 months. Racial, ethnic, and economic disparities are apparent in both the number of hospital and emergency department visits attributable to asthma as well as deaths caused by asthma.[3] Asthma-related emergency department visits and hospitalizations as well as deaths from asthma have

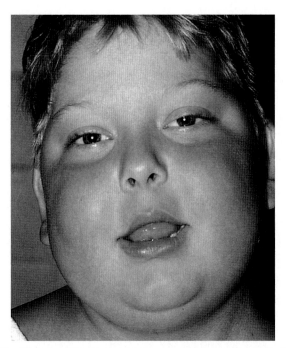

Fig. 19.1 A child with steroid-dependent asthma. (From Zitelli BJ, Davis HW. *Atlas of Pediatric Physical Diagnosis*. 5th ed. Philadelphia: Mosby; 2007.)

been shown to be more prevalent in Black and Hispanic children.[4,5]

Extensive research has established that the reasons for these differences are complex and are predominately due to structural inequalities such as segregation and policies that discriminate against children of color, as well as social inequalities such as socioeconomic status, neighborhood environment, and healthcare access, with factors such as ancestry, genes, and behaviors contributing to a smaller extent.[3] In 2010, the World Health Organization (WHO) published a paper titled "A Conceptual Framework for Action of the Social Determinants of Heath," which has been a model for organizations seeking to work at national, local, and individual levels to improve the health of individuals with asthma who are medically underserved.[3,6]

CLINICAL SIGNS

Signs and symptoms of asthma vary from person to person. Symptoms include wheezing, shortness of breath, chest tightness, and coughing. An increased respiratory rate (tachypnea) and difficulty breathing (dyspnea) may accompany an asthma attack. A child may also use accessory muscles in the ribcage to breathe; in this instance, the child may appear winded. Asthma attacks are generally recurring episodes, but airway obstruction from asthma can be reversible with appropriate intervention.[4]

CLINICAL SIGNS OF ASTHMA

Wheezing
Shortness of breath
Chest tightness
Sputum production
Coughing
Airway inflammation, obstruction, or hypersensitivity to extrinsic and intrinsic stimuli
Episodic in onset

Physical Therapy Assessment

After a review of the child's medical history, physical therapy evaluation should focus on identifying any areas of impairment, functional limitations, and activity and participation limitations.[4] Some secondary impairments related to asthma that can interfere with functional activity are listed in Table 19.1.

Physical Therapy Intervention

Physical therapy intervention for asthma comprises both short- and long-term goals. Short-term goals include addressing medical needs and musculoskeletal restrictions. Long-term goals are focused on reducing secondary impairments, usually through an established exercise regimen.[7]

In caring for children with asthma, it is imperative to have their diagnosis and asthma management plan in the charted history. Anyone involved with the child's care should be well instructed on signs and symptoms of asthma, as well as how and when to administer asthma medications or call for emergency help if needed. An individualized asthma management plan includes the child's asthma history, triggers and symptoms, ways to contact the parent/guardian and healthcare provider, physician and parent/guardian signatures, the child's target peak flow reading, and a list of current asthma medications. The plan will also include the child's treatment plan for medications based on symptoms and peak flow readings.

Peak flow monitoring can be effectively used for children aged 5 years and older. Many different peak

TABLE 19.1   Assessing Functional Limitations Associated With Asthma

Functional Activity	Secondary Problems
Breathing	Inadequate breath support and inefficient trunk muscle recruitment at rest or with activities, such that breathing or postural control are compromised
	Asthmatic triggers such as rapid air flow caused by sudden increase in physical activity, dry air, extreme temperatures, or other triggers that produce an asthmatic reaction
Coughing	Ineffective mobilization and expectoration strategies
Sleeping	Breathing difficulties, signs of obstructive or central sleep disorders
	Nocturnal reflux (GERD)
Eating	Swallowing dysfunction
	Reflux (GERD)
	Dehydration
	Poor nutrition
Talking	Inadequate lung volume and/or inadequate motor control for eccentric and concentric expiratory patterns of speech
	Poor coordination between talking (refined breath support) and moving (postural control)
Moving	Inadequate balance between ventilation and postural demands
	Breath holding with more demanding postures: use of the diaphragm as a primary postural muscle for trunk stabilization
	Inadequate lung volume to support movement
	Inadequate and/or inefficient muscle recruitment patterns for trunk/respiratory muscles, causing endurance problems or poor motor performance
	Ineffective pairing of breathing with movement, especially with higher-level activities

GERD, gastroesophageal reflux disease.
Note: These activities require adequate lung volumes and coordination of breathing with movement for optimal performance.
Typical secondary problems associated with asthma should be screened for to determine their possible contribution to the child's motor impairment or motor dysfunction.
From Campbell SK, Vander Linden DW, Palisano RJ. *Physical Therapy for Children.* 3rd ed. Philadelphia: Saunders; 2006.

flow meters are available on the market. These simple, hand-held devices measure how well air is moving out of a person's airways. Before a peak flow meter is used, the marker along the slider is moved to zero. Then the person takes a deep breath in, places their mouth on the peak flow meter, and exhales as hard and as fast as possible. This forced exhale will move the marker along a numerical line on the meter, and the number will be recorded. Usually, the steps are repeated three times to ensure accuracy. The highest number obtained with these exhalations is considered the peak flow. A person who uses peak flow monitoring as part of an asthma action plan typically has a personal best or target reading and ranges of numbers, or zones, that help determine what actions should be taken for each zone. Lower numbers may call for attention with medications and additional monitoring. Very low numbers demand emergency attention. Peak flow numbers or zones should be included in the asthma management plan. Although peak flow monitoring is quite effective,

it is only one indicator of asthma stability or problems. Other symptoms such as coughing, wheezing, complaints of shortness of breath, and chest tightness should also be considered.

Asthma may be treated and controlled with a variety of pharmacologic interventions. Many patients have at least two types of medications (Table 19.2). The first type is used as a preventive or maintenance medication. Preventive medications can be oral or inhaled and are used to help decrease the inflammation of the airways or decrease the response to triggers such as allergens. The second type is used as a rescue medication. Rescue medications are usually supplied in the form of an inhaler that contains a bronchodilator such as albuterol. Albuterol quickly helps to open the airways, enabling a person with asthma to breathe easier. It is important to distinguish between the two types of medications. A preventive inhaler will be of no help during an acute asthma attack. People with asthma should carry their rescue inhaler with them. Children with asthma should

TABLE 19.2   Current Medications for the Quick Relief and Long-Term Management of Asthma

Type of Drug	Drug Names	Function
Short-acting beta₂-agonists (SABAs), inhaled	Albuterol Levalbuterol	Reliever medications Short-acting rescue treatment of asthma attacks
Co-administered short-acting bronchodilators	Ipratropium + albuterol	
Inhaled corticosteroids (ICs)	Fluticasone Beclomethasone Budesonide Mometasone Ciclesonide	Controller medications Long-acting to manage asthma and prevent attacks
Leukotriene receptor antagonists (LTRAs), oral	Montelukast Zafirlukast	
ICs + long-acting beta₂-agonist (LABA)	Budesonide and formoterol Mometasone and formoterol Fluticasone and salmeterol	
Oral corticosteroids (OCs), systemic corticosteroids	Prednisone Prednisolone Methylprednisolone Dexamethasone	Burst therapy for severe, acute asthma exacerbations
Monoclonal antibody, injected	Omalizumab Mepolizumab	Biologic medication to control lung inflammation

Data from Lizzo JM, Cortes S. *Pediatric Asthma*. In: Abai A, and others. eds. StatPearls, Treasure Island, FL: StatPearls Publishing; 2022. Updated August 8, 2022.
Data from Chu R, Bajaj P. *Asthma Medication in Children*. In: Abai A, and others. eds. StatPearls, Treasure Island, FL: StatPearls Publishing; 2022. Updated June 23, 2022.

also keep extra rescue inhalers at school and at any caregivers' homes.

A spacer is a large chamber that is fitted to an inhaler and is useful in dispensing a dose of medication more effectively. Spacers increase the amount of medication that reaches the lungs, instead of being deposited in the mouth and throat, and can be particularly effective for children and those in distress who may have difficulty coordinating their breathing with the timing of the medication release. The medication dose is released into the spacer chamber and then can be inhaled at will by the child. In the event that the lung tidal volume is low and inhalation is difficult, the child can breathe in and out several times with the spacer and still get an effective dose. Caution must be used to avoid spraying more than one dose or "puff" at a time into the spacer. If the child's prescribed dose is two puffs, spray one and have the child inhale from the spacer, then repeat with the second puff after waiting 1 full minute.

It is vital for caregivers to be able to identify when a child is having difficulty breathing or having an acute episode. Activity should be stopped as soon as these symptoms are noticed. If a child has an asthma management plan, instructions regarding medications should be closely followed. If the child does not respond to medications or fails to improve, emergency help should be sought. Furthermore, if a child is hunched over, straining to breathe, has difficulty completing a sentence, looks ashen, or has blue lips and fingernails, immediate emergency help (i.e., a 9-1-1 call) is warranted.

Exercise-induced asthma is a special consideration. Children and caregivers can try to reduce triggers such as allergens and irritants, but exercise should not be avoided to avert an asthma attack. Rather, with medications and possibly some modifications to physical activity, the symptoms can be controlled. Often, a physician will recommend giving a dose of rescue medication prior to exercise to decrease the child's chances of having an acute asthma episode. This prophylactic approach can be very effective. A child who has had a recent asthma episode is more likely to have additional episodes; thus, the child's level of exertion should be monitored and modified as needed. The physical therapist assistant (PTA) can create an individualized exercise regimen that will improve muscle function while minimizing the risk of an asthma attack. Exercising indoors with filtered air or in a warmer environment with comfortable humidity, rather than outdoors or in a cold, dry environment, can reduce the frequency of asthma attacks.[4]

Extensive research[8] has shown that weather factors, pollen, different seasons, and global climate change have an effect on the severity of asthma symptoms. Hot and cold temperatures, high humidity, rain and thunderstorms, as well as sudden changes in weather can all increase the severity of asthma symptoms.[9] This information is important for physical therapists (PTs) and PTAs to have when designing exercise protocols for children with asthma and for PTs and PTAs who work in schools. Hot and humid days, allergy-alert days when the airborne irritant count is high, and season changes are specific times when healthcare providers must be keenly aware of the status of children with asthma.

ASTHMA INTERVENTIONS

Design an exercise protocol
Implement low-cost measures for indoor allergen avoidance
Restore, maintain, and promote optimal physical functioning

CHAPTER DISCUSSION QUESTIONS

1. Describe two triggers that may affect the ability of a child with asthma to breathe.
2. What racial and economic groups demonstrate the highest rate of childhood asthma?
3. What are the components of an asthma management plan?
4. What is the purpose of a peak flow meter?
5. Is it better to have a high reading or a low reading on a peak flow meter?
6. What is the difference between preventive medication and rescue medication?
7. What are two accommodations that may be made for children with asthma so they can participate in an exercise routine/activity?
8. What are three common signs or symptoms of an asthma attack?
9. What is the appropriate action to take if a child begins to have an asthma attack while exercising?
10. What weather-related factors seem to correlate with the severity of asthma symptoms?

REFERENCES

1. Centers for Disease Control and Prevention. Data, statistics, and surveillance: asthma surveillance data: https://www.cdc.gov/asthma/asthmadata.htm. Accessed October 9, 2022.
2. Asthma and Allergy Foundation of America. Asthma facts and figures: https://www.aafa.org/asthma-facts/. Accessed October 9, 2022.
3. Asthma and Allergy Foundation of America. Asthma disparities in America: https://www.aafa.org/asthma-disparities-burden-on-minorities.aspx. Accessed October 9, 2022.
4. Morris MJ. Asthma. In: Drugs and Diseases, Pulmonology. Medscape: https://emedicine.medscape.com/article/296301-overview. Last updated May 11, 2022.
5. Gill I, Shah A, Lee EK, et al. Community interventions for childhood asthma ED visits and hospitalizations: a systematic review. *Pediatrics*. 2022;150(4): e2021054825.
6. Solar O, Irwin A. A conceptual framework for action on the social determinants of health. *Social Determinants of Health Discussion Paper 2 (Policy and Practice)*. Printed by the World Health Organization Document Production Services, Geneva, Switzerland.
7. Campbell SK, Vander Linden DW, Palisano RJ. *Physical Therapy for Children*. 3rd ed. Philadelphia: Saunders; 2006.
8. D'Amato G, Holgate ST, Pawankar R, et al. Meteorological conditions, climate change, new emerging factors, and asthma and related allergic disorders. A statement of the World Allergy Organization. *World Allergy Organ J*. 2015;8(1):25.
9. Asthma and Allergy Foundation of America. Weather: https://www.aafa.org/weather-triggers-asthma/. Accessed October 29, 2022.

RESOURCES

Asthma and Allergy Foundation of America
  1235 South Clark Street
  Suite 305
  Arlington, VA 22202
  1-800-7-ASTHMA (1-800-727-8462)
  https://www.aafa.org/

American Academy of Allergy, Asthma, and Immunology
  555 East Wells Street
  Suite 1100
  Milwaukee, WI 53202-3823
  414-272-6071
  www.aaaai.org
US National Library of Medicine
  www.nlm.nih.gov

Pediatric Sports Injuries

Maryleen K. Jones, PT, DHS, NCS, CLT, CSRS
David Diers, EdD, MHS, PT, SCS, ATC

LEARNING OBJECTIVES

At the end of the chapter, the reader will be able to do the following:

1. Recognize the incidence and prevalence of sports-related injuries among children.
2. Identify the variances in children's sports-related injuries.
3. Describe appropriate exercise regimens for child athletes.
4. Identify the differences in anatomy between children and adults.
5. Recognize common childhood sports injuries and their etiologies.
6. Identify the signs and symptoms of concussion.
7. Compare suggested return to sport protocols for overuse and concussion injuries.

CHAPTER OUTLINE

KEY TERMS

Growth plate fracture
Osteochondritis dissecans

Scheuermann disease

Strength training

As the number of children who participate in organized sports increases, the number of children injured increases as well (Fig. 20.1). Child athletes are not smaller versions of adult athletes.[1] They have different physiologic responses to exercise and different musculoskeletal structures; thus, they are susceptible to different injuries.

INCIDENCE AND PREVALENCE

Among children aged 6 to 17 years in the United States, an estimated 54.1% participate in organized sports.[1] Of those participating in sports, more than 3.5 million are likely to sustain an injury each year, with 62% of the injuries occurring during practice versus competition.[2]

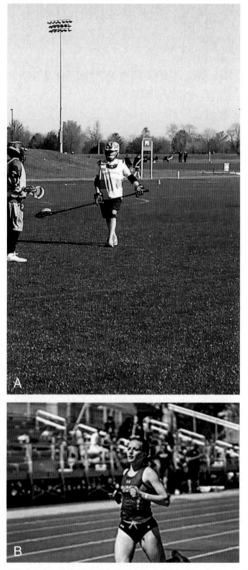

Fig. 20.1 As more children participate in organized sports, both team sports such as lacrosse **(A)** and individual sports such as track **(B)**, the incidence of injury increases.

Almost one-third of all injuries incurred in childhood are sports-related injuries resulting in loss of participation, with the most common injuries being sprains and strains.[2]

Some sports have more inherent risk of injury, such as contact sports (e.g., football) versus a noncontact sport such as swimming. However, all types of sports have the potential for injury, whether from the trauma of contact with other players or from overuse or misuse of a body part. The most serious sports-related injury is a brain injury, which can result in death. The most common recreational activities that result in a brain injury are bicycling, skateboarding, and skating.[2]

Exercise Considerations

There are many physiologic differences between the adult and the child during exercise. The child has a smaller heart than the adult; thus, there is a smaller stroke volume; in simple terms, a smaller heart pushes less blood. A child has a higher heart rate during submaximal and maximal exercise. This increased heart rate offsets some of the decreased stroke volume, but not enough to compensate for the size difference.[3] Because of these factors, a child cannot exercise as efficiently as an adult and must be monitored accordingly. Refer to Table 20.1 for normal resting heart rate ranges for children.

General recommendations for cardiovascular exercise for children aged 6 to 17 years call for 60 minutes of activity each day. Recommendations include a moderate to vigorous intensity with inclusion of activities such as walking, running, skipping, hopping, or any movement that increases the child's heart rate. Moderate to vigorous intensity can be ranked on a scale of 0 to 10, with 0 representing no effort and 10 indicating the highest level of effort.[3] Moderate intensity is represented by a ranking of 5 or 6. Rate of perceived exertion (RPE) charts may be used to effectively monitor and prescribe exercise intensity. RPE ratings may be impacted by psychologic factors such as cognitive abilities and memory, which has led to the development of simplified scales to enhance the accuracy of RPE ratings for children[3] (Figs. 20.2 and 20.3).

TABLE 20.1	Resting Heart Rate Ranges for Children
Age Range (y)	**Resting Heart Rate Range (bpm)**
1–3	90–150
3–5	80–140
5–12	70–120
12–18	60–100

From Fleming S, Thompson M, Stevens R, and others. Normal ranges of heart rate and respiratory rate in children birth to 18 years of age: a systematic review of observational studies. *Lancet.* 2011;377(9770):1011–1018.

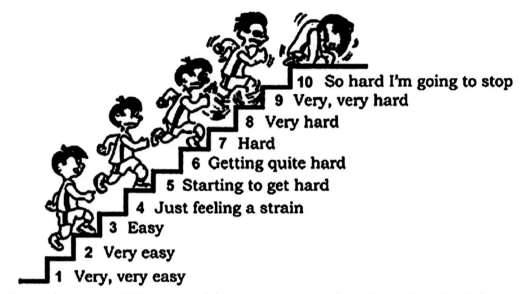

Fig. 20.2 Some younger children may benefit from using a pictural rate of perceived exertion scale to indicate their exercise intensity levels. (Yelling M, Lamb KL, Swaine IL. Validity of a pictorial perceived exertion scale for effort estimation and effort production during stepping exercise in adolescent children. *Eur Phy Educ Rev.* 2002;8(2):157–175. https://doi.org/10.1177/1356336X020082007.)

Children demonstrate different responses to strength and resistance training than their adult counterparts due to their limited muscle mass. In addition to limited muscle mass, balance and coordination are underdeveloped in children and preadolescents, which contributes to the child's susceptibility to injury with free weights. Strength training programs may use weights, machines, resistance tubing, and body-weight exercises such as pushups or squats. Adult-sized weight machines may not have properly sized lever arms for use by children, which would result in improper loading of the musculature. It has been shown that a limited amount of weightlifting improves a child's muscular strength; however, there is little gain in actual muscle mass. The strength increase is attributed to improved coordination and neuromuscular recruitment. Strength training can assist the normal muscle development occurring throughout puberty. Because of their decreased muscle mass, the recommended weightlifting program for adolescents is low weight–high repetition activity.[4] This is especially true in the beginning stages of weightlifting. Proper lifting technique is the key to avoiding injuries in the adolescent population. Single repetition maximal lifts or continuous maximal lifts are not recommended because of skeletal immaturity. For these reasons, supervision is essential for adolescent strength training. Strength training should be done 2 to 3 nonconsecutive days per week. Each session should include six to eight exercises that train major muscle groups and balance effort between flexors and extensors and the upper and lower body. Strength training programs should start with one or two sets per exercise, with two to three exercises per muscle group, with 8 to 15 repetitions.[5,6] Repetitions should be completed with some muscle fatigue but not repeated until muscle failure occurs.[4,6] Attention to rest between sets should be taken, allowing 1 to 3 minutes for recovery. There is evidence showing that there is no benefit to strength training more than four times per week.[5] Recommendations by the American Academy of Pediatrics Committee on Sports Medicine and Fitness are listed in Box 20.1.

A common question from parents is "When can a child safely begin strength training?" There is no exact chronological age when this can begin. Instead,

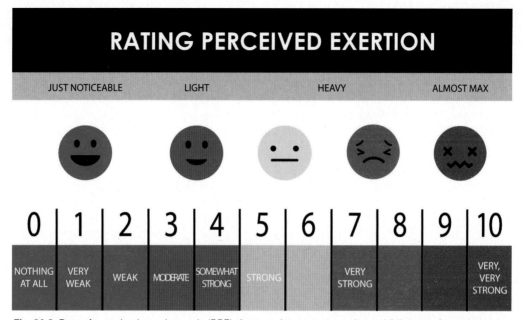

Fig. 20.3 Rate of perceived exertion scale (RPE). A convenient way to monitor a child's level of exercise intensity is by using the modified 1–10 numeric RPE scale. (Tibana AR, Frade de Sousa MN, et al., Is perceived exertion a useful indicator of the metabolic and cardiovascular responses to a metabolic conditioning session of functional fitness? *Sports.* 2019;7(7):161. https://doi.org/10.3390/sports7070161.)

strength training can begin when the child is able to understand and follow detailed instructions on proper technique and progression of the program Box 20.2.[6]

INJURY CONSIDERATIONS

Musculoskeletal

There are two general classifications of musculoskeletal differences between children and adults: bone and muscle. The differences in these structures at varying maturation stages lead to a separate set of common injury patterns. The osteology of a child varies from the adult in many ways. The bone is more porous and more susceptible to compression fractures. A greenstick fracture can also occur when there is a perpendicular force placed on a bone and the bone begins to bend. The fracture occurs on the convex side of the curve. Stress fractures are common in girls with delayed menarche or amenorrhea due to hormonal imbalances prior to and during puberty.[7] The general rehabilitation of these types of injuries involves rest,

biomechanical examination, orthotic bracing, and strengthening and stretching of the surrounding soft tissue structures. Surgery may be required if the fracture requires more support.

Another injury unique to the child is a physeal or growth plate fracture. There are many areas in the body where this can occur, and the most common ones will be discussed later in the chapter under the headings of each anatomic region. A growth plate in a long bone is most commonly found near a joint. These growth plates provide for axial and circumferential growth of bones. These areas are the weakest points around joints; thus, injuries usually occur in the growth plate, not in the joint.[8] Salter and Harris[9] described the most common way to classify the extent of the fracture. This classification separates these fractures into five categories (Table 20.2). The general rehabilitation for these types of injuries involves rest, biomechanical examination, orthotic bracing, and strengthening and stretching of the surrounding soft tissue structures. Surgery may be needed to stabilize the fracture if the fracture is too extensive or unstable.

BOX 20.1 Strength-Training Recommendations for Children

- A thorough medical examination should be completed before a strength-training program begins.
- If general health benefits are the goal, aerobic exercise should be included.
- Five to 10-minute warm-up and cool-down periods are an essential part of the strength-training regimen. Warm-up and cool-down periods should consist of aerobic activity and dynamic stretching.
- Instruction on specific strength-training exercise should be provided with no weight or load repetitions in order to focus on form and technique. Small increments of weight should be added to sets of 8 to 15 repetitions.
- All muscle groups should be included, and the activities should include full range of motion (ROM).
- Larger muscle exercises should be performed before smaller muscle exercises, complex exercises should be performed before simpler ones, and multi-joint exercises should be performed before single-joint exercises.
- If any sign of injury occurs, all activity should stop, and a thorough medical examination should be completed.

Adapted from Stricker PR, Faigenbaum AD, McCambridg TM. Council on sports medicine and fitness. In: LaBella CR Brooks MA, Canty G, Diamond AR, Hennrikus W, Logan K, Moffatt K, Nemeth BA, Pengel KB, Peterson AR, eds. Resistance Training for Children and Adolescents. *Pediatrics*. 2020;145(6):e20201011. doi:10.1542/peds.2020-1011.

BOX 20.2 Sports Injuries Interventions

Conservative rehabilitation
Rest (which is the primary factor in allowing the bone and involved tissues to heal) before initiation of a rehabilitation program
General progressive rehabilitation program that consists of strengthening and flexibility exercises for the respective area, focusing on functional activities
Surgery only when there is a loose body interfering with normal joint motion or when a displaced fracture may interfere with normal bone growth

TABLE 20.2 Salter-Harris Fracture Classification

Classification	Description
I	A fracture along the entire length of the growth plate that does not involve the surrounding osteology
II	A fracture of part of the growth plate and part of the osteology away from the joint
III	A fracture involving part of the growth plate and part of the osteology nearest the joint
IV	A fracture through the growth plate and both sides of the osteology
V	A compression fracture in the mid-substance of the growth plate

From Salter R, Harris W. Injuries involving epiphyseal plate. *J Bone Joint Surg.* 1963;45A:587.

onset.[10] The more common injury sites are the knees, hips, pelvis, and shoulders. Apophyseal fractures will be addressed later in the chapter under the headings for each anatomic region.

The general rehabilitation for a fracture to a growth plate, either a physis or an apophysis, should be conservative before surgical. Conservative intervention involves rest, biomechanical corrections, orthotic bracing, and strengthening and stretching of the surrounding soft tissue structures. Surgery may be needed to fixate the apophysis or physis if it becomes unstable. Surgical intervention is the last resort and rarely needs to occur. Caution is always the rule when these injuries are treated.[10] Growth plate injuries may lead to an alteration in normal bone growth and subsequent biomechanical problems with injuries later in life. The regional anatomy sections will detail rehabilitation programs for specific injuries.

Osteochondritis dissecans is an injury to the articular cartilage and the corresponding bone. The bone and cartilage may split from the rest of the bone and can, in some instances, separate from the bone and become loose in the joint. These injuries may be asymptomatic if no displacement occurs. The elbow, knee, and ankle are common sites for this type of injury.[11]

The general rehabilitation for these injuries is similar to the rehabilitation for physeal or apophyseal injuries: conservative before surgical. Conservative intervention

Another common injury to the bone is a fracture to an apophysis, which is growth cartilage connecting bone to tendon. In adults, this junction is ossified and not as easily injured. These injuries in children can result from a traumatic incident or overuse with an insidious should involve rest, biomechanical corrections, orthotic bracing, and strengthening and stretching of the surrounding soft tissue structures. Surgery may be necessary to fixate a partially separated injury or to remove a loose body if it is interfering with normal joint function.[11]

Muscle tissue injury causes different problems for the child. As bone growth occurs, especially during growth spurts, the muscle must adapt and lengthen. This process may take some time to occur, and during this adaptation period, the joints and growth plates have increased stress placed on them. This excess stress can lead to numerous types of injuries in any of the musculoskeletal structures.[8] General rehabilitation for these problems entails increasing the flexibility of the involved muscles and taking appropriate action for any of the other involved musculoskeletal structures.

Overuse Injuries

The National Council of Youth Sports and the Centers for Disease Control and Prevention report that more than 60 million children aged 5 to years participate in organized sports in the United States.[1] Participation in various sports carries with it the potential for injury with different etiologies. Both acute and chronic (overuse) injuries may result in loss of participation time, or at a minimum, suboptimal performance. Current literature varies in the reporting specific to overuse injuries in children. Stracciolini and colleagues[8] completed a full year review of sports-related injuries at a large academic pediatric medical center and found that a high proportion of tennis players, swimmers, dancers, track and running athletes, gymnasts, and cheerleaders experienced overuse injuries.[8] Additionally, boys participating in team sports experienced a 5.3% increase in likelihood of sustaining an overuse injury compared with boys participating in individual sports.[8] Females were found to experience more lower extremity overuse injuries; boys who experienced more upper extremity overuse injuries.[8] When encountering a child with an overuse injury, the treating physical therapist (PT) and physical therapist assistant (PTA) must consider the physical and anatomical differences between males and females with respect to their injury profile. In addition, the characteristics of the sport played must be considered. Characteristics to be considered are team versus individual, contact, and high repetitive action sports.

Participation in sports promotes both the physical and emotional well-being of children and facilitates a lifelong habit of exercise. However, in maturing children, overactivity may lead to the aforementioned overuse injuries. Overuse injuries gradually develop over time, with repeated actions resulting in insufficient recovery time between bouts of practice and play. For example, overhand pitching in baseball can be associated with injuries to the shoulder and elbow, and sports that involve running can be associated with injuries to the lower legs.

Because young athletes are still growing, they are at greater risk for injury than adults. The implications of overuse during a sport can include injuries that impair growth and may lead to long-term health problems.

If a young athlete has repeated complaints of pain, a period of rest from the sport is appropriate and necessary. If the athlete's pain continues, it is prudent to seek proper medical treatment. To ensure the best possible recovery, all parties, including the athlete, parents, trainers, therapists, and coaches must follow safe guidelines for returning to practice, play, and competition. Depending on the site of injury, treatments may include the use of orthotics or bracing to immobilize the site, anti-inflammatory medications and treatments such as ice application, stretching, and ROM exercises. A graduated reloading program of the involved tissues should be adhered to for safe return to play. Common overuse injuries are described according the relevant anatomy in the following section.

COMMON INJURY SITES

Cervical Spine

Cervical spine injuries in children need to be treated with great caution. Studies have shown that a large portion of cervical spine injuries in this age group are sports related. Any injury to the cervical spine, or any injury that causes neurologic symptoms in the upper extremity, needs thorough examination because of the possibility of long-lasting complications for the child. A three-view radiographic series consisting of lateral, anteroposterior, and oblique views is the most effective approach to diagnosing any significant problems in the cervical spine. One study found this process to be 94% sensitive for all cervical spine injuries that can lead to long-lasting deficits.[12] Once the radiographs determine the spine is stable with no osteologic, ligamentous, or neurologic deficits, examination and intervention for the musculature can continue.

The general intervention protocol will consist of a soft collar for rest, with applications of heat or ice for analgesic effect. Once the pain subsides, a progressive strengthening and stretching program should be initiated. The stretching program should begin with gentle stretching in the lateral, anterior, and posterior directions, as well as the diagonals of anterior-lateral and posterior-lateral bilaterally. The stretching program should address unilateral and bilateral rotation as well. The stretching should be pain free with no residual soreness. The strengthening program should begin with isometrics in the cardinal planes of motion and rotation and progress to the diagonals. The program should advance to active strengthening in the pain-free ROM, once the isometric exercises are no longer difficult and exhibit no residual effects. The active exercises should begin in the cardinal planes of motion and rotation, then progress to the diagonal planes. Active resistance using manual resistance by the child is a common exercise. The most important aspect of the rehabilitation program is technique. To prevent injuries, detailed instructions are very important. The child should not progress to a more difficult exercise until he or she practices the next exercise and the therapist is certain he or she can do it properly.

Thoracic Spine

Thoracic spine injuries mostly consist of osteologic injuries. The most significant difference between the mature and immature spine, as with all other bones, is the presence of growth plates. There are growth plates at each end of the vertebral body. These appear between the ages of 8 and 12 years and begin to fuse at the age of 15 years. Injuries are most common from the ages of 14 to 16 years, around the time these growth plates begin to fuse and are susceptible to fractures. The most common problem associated with these fractures is the wedging of the vertebral body. If this occurs, it will cause an increase in the kyphosis of the thoracic spine and lead to many biomechanical problems later in life.[13,14] The most common mechanisms of injury are hyperflexion with or without compression, shear forces, and distraction forces.[14]

If these fractures are stable, conservative intervention is the norm. Bed rest or a thoracolumbosacral orthosis (TLSO) allows the fracture to heal. Once the fracture has sufficiently healed, the recommended rehabilitation is a progressive stretching and strengthening program focusing on extension of the thoracic spine and scapular strengthening. A postural rehabilitation program will assist in decreasing the possibility of a habitual hyperkyphosis forming. If surgical intervention is required, the therapist should follow a physician's protocol as to when to begin the stretching and strengthening progression.[13]

Another common problem in the thoracic spine is Scheuermann's disease (Fig. 20.4). This is similar to the wedge-shaped fracture discussed previously, but it has an overuse, postural etiology.[13] The rehabilitation for this problem is similar to that for acute fractures, focusing on thoracic extension mobility, stretching of the pectoral and hamstring musculature, postural strengthening, and education to decrease the kyphosis. Scapular girdle and respiratory muscle strengthening may help, as the biomechanics and kinematics of these areas can be altered by increased kyphosis.[13,14]

Lumbar Spine

Injuries to the lumbar spine are more common than injuries to either thoracic or cervical spine injuries. Posture plays a significant role in the incidence of most injuries in this area. During periods of rapid growth, muscle and fascia may become tight and cause postural changes. These dysfunctions are common in the dorsal lumbar fascia and hamstrings.[14,15]

The child with an increased lumbar lordosis posture is more susceptible to an injury to the pars interarticularis. The pars interarticularis prevents the vertebral body from gliding anteriorly on the vertebral body inferior to it. A fracture to this area with no subsequent vertebral movement is a *spondylolysis*. If the vertebral body glides anteriorly due to this injury, it is a *spondylolisthesis*. Spondylolisthesis is classified by the distance the vertebral body translates anteriorly as confirmed by radiographs[15] (Fig. 20.5). The most common sites for this injury are L5-S1 and L4-L5. This injury is common in sports in which forced hyperextension occurs such as gymnastics or football. The rehabilitation for this injury is usually conservative. The intervention consists of trunk stabilization exercises while avoiding lumbar extension. These exercises may include back stretching and abdominal strengthening. In severe cases surgery may be required to stabilize the unstable vertebral segment.[14,15]

The child with a decreased lumbar lordosis posture is susceptible to a flexion injury of the intervertebral body

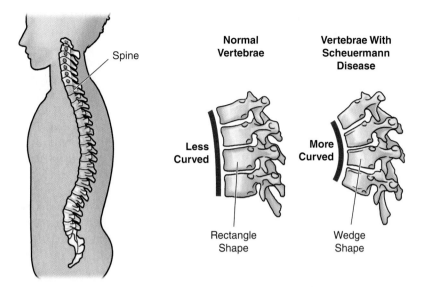

Fig. 20.4 In the immature spine of a child younger than 16 years, the vertebral growth plate may sustain a fracture and begin to wedge, resulting in an increased kyphotic posture.

or intervertebral disk. The injury to the intervertebral body is in the growth plate near the superior and inferior borders of the vertebral body. If the injury is severe enough, it can cause the wedging, as described earlier for the thoracic spine. In children, fractures in the lumbar region are more common than intervertebral disk injuries. The reason is that in the immature skeleton the disk is hydrophilic and stronger than the growth plates

in the vertebral body. Overuse repetitive trauma or acute trauma can cause either of these injuries.[15] Intervention for both injuries should include postural retraining and lumbar stabilization exercises.

Sciatica is a condition not commonly seen in children, but it can occur. Tight piriformis muscles can cause sciatica. Symptoms are similar to those associated with other lumbar spine problems.[15] Intervention

Spondylolisthesis stages

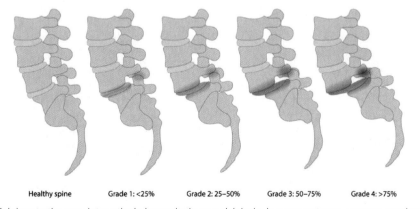

Fig. 20.5 Injury to the pars interarticularis results in spondylolysis. In severe stages, surgery may be required to stabilize the child's spine.

consists of general lumbar stabilization and flexibility exercises (Fig. 20.6) if the cause arises from the lumbar spine and piriformis flexibility exercises if the piriformis muscles are the cause.

Shoulder

The most common type of shoulder injury in the young athlete is an overuse injury. These occur most often in sports involving use of the arm overhead in activities such as throwing, racket sports, or swimming. The most commonly diagnosed injuries among throwing athletes are sprains and strains, accounting for 44% of reported injuries.[16] Sprains occur in ligaments, while strains involve muscles or tendons. Sprains and strains vary in severity from grade 1 presenting with a mild loss of ROM to grade 3, which is a complete tear of the tissue. Descriptions of the classifications of sprains and strains can be found in Table 20.3. In a study by Saper and colleagues,[17] it was estimated that overuse injuries of the shoulder and elbow for high school baseball players accounted for 71.3% and 73.9% of the cases, respectively.[17] Another common injury is a fracture of the growth plate (Fig. 20.7) and impingement of structures in the subacromial space. The repetitive stress on the growth plate (physis) leads to irregularities and a widening of the growth plate. Continued stress can lead to permanent damage of the growth plate and deformity.

For the athlete who does a great deal of throwing, prevention is the best medicine for all injuries. The primary factor responsible for the injury is the technique or biomechanics of the throwing motion. A detailed

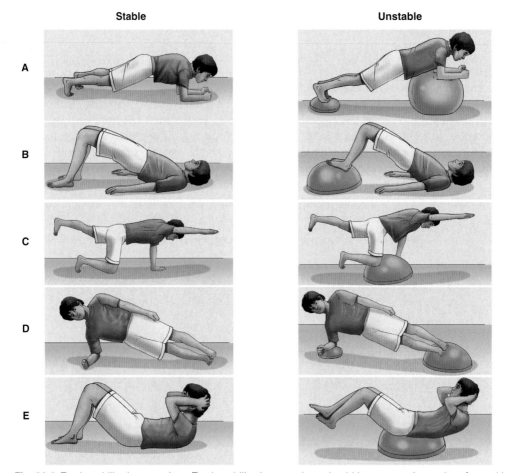

Fig. 20.6 Trunk stabilization exercises. Trunk stabilization exercises should be progressive and performed in multiple planes.

TABLE 20.3 Classifications of Sprains and Strains	
Grade 1 (Mild): **Tissue is stretched**	• Slight swelling • Mild loss of range of motion and strength 0%–25% loss • No loss of stability
Grade II (Moderate): **Involves stretching and some tearing of tissue**	• Moderate swelling • Usually includes some bruising • Moderate loss of range of motion and strength (25%–75%) • Some decrease in stability
Grade III (Severe): **Complete tearing of tissue**	• Significant swelling and bruising • Nearly complete loss of range of motion and strength (75%–100%) • Marked decrease in stability

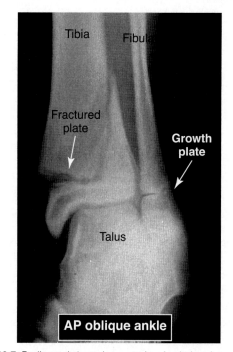

Fig. 20.7 Radiograph (anterior-posterior view) showing marked displacement of a distal femur fracture. The transverse appearance of the medial aspect of the proximal fragment suggests this is a growth plate injury. Arrow indicates the fracture. (From Lynn N. McKinnis' Fundamentals of Musculoskeletal Imaging. 4th ed. F.A. Davis Company; 2013.)

analysis of the throwing motion, with corrections and proper coaching afterward, is essential to preventing problems in the shoulder. For pitchers, the athletes who throw the most, a detailed pitch count and frequency of pitching performance are also important. Another factor for pitchers is the type of pitch thrown. Pitchers younger than 12 years should not throw breaking pitches.[16–18] Table 20.4 provides the recommended set workload limits and rest recommendations from Major League Baseball's Pitch Smart program.[19]

For racket sport athletes and swimmers, biomechanics and coaching are also important. Repetitive use of the arm overhead creates a great deal of force on the anatomical structures, and only with proper form and training can most of these problems be avoided.

One of the common overuse injuries is the proximal humeral growth plate fracture. This may be referred to as *Little Leaguer's shoulder*. Poor technique and underdeveloped musculature are the primary causes for this injury. Rehabilitation often consists of rest until the fracture has healed, usually 8 to 12 weeks, followed by a progression of rotator cuff strengthening exercises.[18] The exercises consist of scapular girdle strengthening in addition to strengthening of specific rotator cuff musculature for external rotation, internal rotation, abduction, extension, and diagonal patterns to increase the strength and stabilization of the shoulder.[17,18]

Another common injury is an impingement in the subacromial area of the shoulder. With this injury, the rotator cuff musculature is underdeveloped and is not capable of generating enough force to maintain the stability of the glenohumeral joint. The humeral head begins to glide superiorly on the glenoid fossa and impinge on the subacromial structures against the undersurface of the acromion. These structures include the rotator cuff muscles, the subacromial bursa, the glenoid labrum, and the attachment for the long head of the biceps brachii.[16–18]

Rehabilitation for impingement consists of a period of rest followed by progressive strengthening of the rotator cuff muscles to increase the stability of the joint and general strengthening of the entire shoulder complex, including the parascapular musculature. The strengthening progression starts with isometrics in the cardinal planes and the rotator cuff muscles and progresses to active strengthening in the diagonal planes, including the rotator cuff muscles. The final phase of the progression is strengthening during functional activities in the specific sport (e.g., throwing). During the functional training phase, a large part of the focus should be on technique, thus requiring closely supervised training.

Children and adolescents may also sustain acute injuries to the shoulder area. Dislocations at the glenohumeral joint can occur but are rare. Acute injuries are more common in the joints surrounding the shoulder. An acromioclavicular joint separation occurs in contact sports such as football or wrestling as a consequence of falling on the lateral aspect of the shoulder.[16–18]

Rehabilitation for dislocations consists of a period of rest to allow healing and then a progressive strengthening program for stability. At the acromioclavicular joint, there is very little musculature that crosses the joint; therefore, surrounding muscles such as the deltoid and scapular stabilizers will be the focus of the strengthening program.

A fracture of the clavicle is a common injury in children. As with acromioclavicular separation, a fall on the lateral aspect of the shoulder is typically responsible. The intervention for this injury is rest and immobilization, possibly in a figure-eight sling, to facilitate the healing of the bone in a normal alignment.

Elbow

Similar to shoulder issues, overuse injuries of the elbow occur more frequently in children than acute injuries. Most elbow problems are associated with throwing and racket sports. Proper technique and biomechanics are essential for preventing injuries to the elbow. The same guidelines that apply to the shoulder in relation to throwing apply to the elbow.

Little Leaguer's elbow is a term used for pain around the medial aspect of the elbow. A variety of injuries can cause medial elbow pain. All of these injuries are overuse injuries and most commonly seen in throwers.[18]

One of the more common injuries implicated in Little Leaguer's elbow is medial epicondylitis. This is an inflammation of the origin of the wrist flexor tendons. It is an overuse injury that occurs with "dropping the arm too low" during throwing, throwing too many pitches or too often, or throwing breaking pitches at an early age (Fig. 20.8). Rehabilitation consists of rest and gentle massage until the pain subsides, progressing to friction massage and progressive strengthening of the wrist, finger flexors, and forearm pronators. Additional training in proper throwing techniques should be incorporated into the rehabilitation program. Major League Baseball's Pitch Smart recommendations are inclusive of body weight mastery before adding external loads for strengthening exercises. Additionally, programs should be comprehensive in nature and include exercises that are aimed at maintaining joint health, function, and mobility. Exercise recommendations include flexibility, breathing, running, and conditioning as well as unilateral lower body exercises, multidirectional core, and shoulder stabilizing exercises.[19]

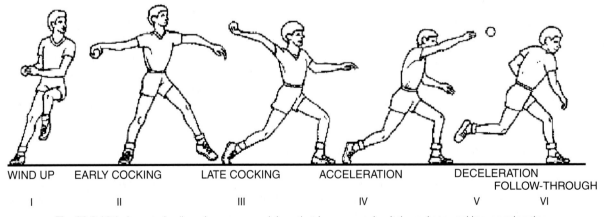

WIND UP   EARLY COCKING   LATE COCKING   ACCELERATION   DECELERATION FOLLOW-THROUGH

I   II   III   IV   V   VI

Fig. 20.8 Little Leaguer's elbow is an overuse injury that is common in pitchers. Late cocking, acceleration, deceleration, and follow-through are the phases most associated with elbow injury. (From Gerbino PG, Waters PM. Elbow injuries in the young athlete. *Oper Tech Sports Med.* 1998;6(4):259.)

TABLE 20.4 Major League Baseball's Pitch Smart Guidelines for Youth Pitchers[21]							
Age (y)	Daily Max (Pitches in Game)	0 Days Rest	1 Days Rest	2 Days Rest	3 Days Rest	4 Days Rest	5 Days Rest
7–8	50	1–20	21–35	36–50	n/a	n/a	n/a
9–10	75	1–20	21–35	36–50	51–65	66+	n/a
11–12	85	1–20	21–35	36–50	51–65	66+	n/a
13–14	95	1–20	21–35	36–50	51–65	66+	n/a
15–16	95	1–30	31–45	46–60	61–75	76+	n/a
17–18	105	1–30	31–45	46–60	61–80	81+	n/a
19–22	120	1–30	31–45	46–60	61–80	81–105	106+

© USA Baseball, https://www.mlb.com/pitch-smart/pitching-guidelines.

Another injury to the elbow is a partial or complete avulsion of the medial epicondyle from the humerus through the growth plate. The cause can be a progression from medial epicondylitis or spontaneous separation. This injury is an overuse injury that occurs when the growth plate begins to widen under repetitive stress from excessive valgus forces placed on the elbow. Rehabilitation consists of rest followed by a progressive strengthening exercise program and a structured return to throwing schedule always strictly supervised by a qualified professional (Table 20.4). Correction of a biomechanical flaw in the throwing motion, if one exists, is also necessary. If the avulsion progresses too far, surgery to stabilize the medial epicondyle is necessary for adequate healing. Primary concerns in any elbow rehabilitation are elbow stiffness and decreased ROM. Thus, active assistive movement or active ROM should begin as soon as possible.

Ulnar nerve irritation is a problem caused by any instability on the medial side of the elbow. The ulnar nerve stretches during an excessive valgus movement at the elbow, and this causes a "tingling" or "shooting" pain from the elbow to the little finger. Rehabilitation depends on the cause of the instability.

Osteochondritis dissecans (OCD) of the radial capitellum can cause lateral elbow pain. This is a condition in which there is lateral elbow pain, clicking, swelling, and loss of full elbow extension. A portion of the articular cartilage from the capitellum may be disassociated or attached. Either way, the mechanics in the elbow will be altered. Rehabilitation generally consists of rest followed by progressive strengthening of the elbow musculature. If the problem is severe enough or persists long enough,

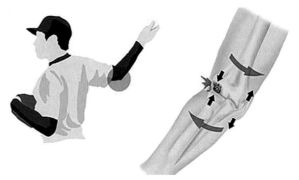

Fig. 20.9 An Osteochondritis Dissecans lesion can lead to lateral elbow pain especially in the late cocking phase to acceleration phases for the throwing athlete.

surgery may be required to remove the loose body.[19] Figure 20.9 provides a depiction of OCD.

Many elbow problems in children can cause or be caused by accelerated or delayed growth of the medial supracondylar growth plate or the superior radial growth plate. The primary cause of most of these injuries is throwing; however, upper extremity weight-bearing sports such as gymnastics or wrestling can also cause these injuries in either acute or overuse variations. Medial (ulnar) collateral ligament injuries are common in adult athletes but rare in children because before skeletal maturation occurs, the ligament is stronger than the growth plate and remains uninjured.

Wrist

Fractures are common injuries to the distal radius and wrist. Greenstick fractures are acute injuries usually sustained during a fall on an outstretched hand. These fractures typically occur in the middle to distal portion of the radius. Many of these can be treated with closed reduction and a short arm cast for approximately 4 weeks followed by flexibility and ROM exercises to regain full motion.[9]

Growth plate fractures can occur in the distal radial growth plate. The causes of these injuries can be either acute or secondary to overuse. Acute injuries commonly result from a fall on an outstretched hand. Overuse injuries are often associated with upper extremity weight-bearing sports such as gymnastics and wrestling. The rehabilitation program consists of rest with immobilization if necessary. These injuries are commonly seen in athletes involved in contact sports.[20]

Hand

Fractures of the hand are less common than those of the wrist but are similar in origin. In adults, dislocation or sprains of the fingers are common. In children, these injuries are often mistaken for phalanx growth plate injuries. These injuries may necessitate reduction and splinting for proper rest and healing. Active ROM needs to begin as soon as possible to regain full function. Ligament avulsion injuries can also occur in the fingers but are more common in the thumb. Avulsions of the ulnar collateral ligament occur at the proximal phalanx of the thumb.[20] This injury is normally treated with a cast and rest, with ROM exercises beginning as soon as possible to regain flexibility. Rehabilitation also includes restoration of joint mobility for the thumb and wrist and strengthening in all planes of motion for the wrist and thumb.

Pelvis

There are a number of muscle attachment sites throughout the pelvis where growth plate avulsion fractures commonly occur. Sites include the iliac crest, anterior superior iliac spine, anterior inferior iliac spine, the ischial tuberosity, and the pubic symphysis. Avulsions at these sites are usually the result of quick and abrupt muscle contractions. Such injuries are common in sports in which sprinting, stopping and starting, and abrupt changes of direction occur. Rehabilitation of these injuries includes rest during the early stages of recovery until the avulsion has healed. The key to a full recovery from the injury and return to full function is stretching of the muscle attached at the site of the avulsion. As with most other growth plate injuries, conservative intervention is

usually effective; however, for severe or displaced cases, surgery may be required.[8]

Hip

In children, assessing any and all hip pain should start with ruling out a growth plate injury in the femoral head. This condition is a slipped capital femoral epiphysis and can result from trauma or overuse. Intervention for this condition nearly always requires surgery followed by extensive ROM, stretching, and progressive strengthening inclusive of trunk and pelvic stabilization exercises.[8]

Fractures and dislocations of the hip in children are rare. The bone, capsule, and ligaments are stronger than the growth plates in children, so the growth plate is usually the structure that fails first under stress.[8,20]

Knee

The knee is one of the most common regions for overuse injuries in children. The sites where growth plate injuries occur in the knee are at each end of the patellar tendon. The injury when an avulsion or split of the bone occurs at the proximal end of the patellar tendon at the junction of the tendon and the patella is called *Sinding-Larsen-Johansson disease*. *Osgood-Schlatter disease* (Fig. 20.10) is an avulsion or split of the bone in which the patellar tendon attaches to the tibia. Both conditions can arise from a period of growth in which the bones have grown faster than the tendon. Children who participate in sports that involve jumping (e.g., basketball) are more vulnerable to this type of injury.[8,20] Repetitive traction on the tubercle leads to inflammation, swelling, and tenderness. The prominence of the tibial tubercle may become very pronounced. Painful symptoms are often brought on by running, jumping, and other sports-related activities. Rehabilitation consists of the application of ice for acute pain and inflammation and rest until the split has healed. The next step is an aggressive stretching program for the quadriceps and hamstrings musculature to minimize the stress on each end of the patellar tendon. After the stretching program reaches a satisfactory point, the progressive strengthening program should begin concentrating on eccentric exercises. The functional portion of the progression may include plyometrics to enhance coordination of jumping activities.

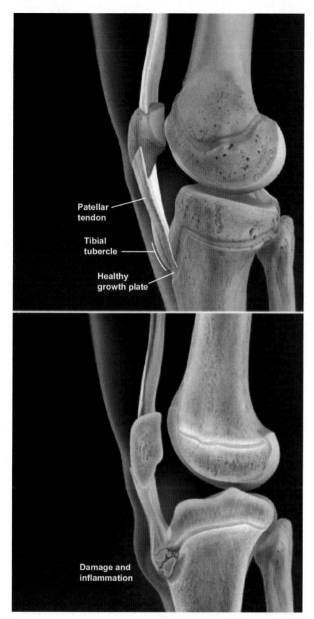

Patellar tendon

Tibial tubercle

Healthy growth plate

Damage and inflammation

Fig. 20.10 *In Osgood-Schlatter diseas* an avulsion or split of the bone in which the patellar tendon attaches to the tibia. Repetitive stress from sport activity may result in pain and swelling and subsequently cause the patella tendon to pull away from the skin bone. As a child's arms and legs have growth plates made of cartilage, which is not as strong as bone, repetitive stress from overuse may lead to serious disruption of the growth plate, resulting in a bony lump in the area where the tendon and bone join.

Jumper's knee is a term used to describe a number of different injuries that cause pain in the extensor mechanism of the knee. Two of the injuries that may be implicated in this category are Sinding-Larsen-Johansson disease and Osgood-Schlatter disease, but another common injury in this category is patellar tendonitis. This is an inflammation in the tendon generally caused by jumping or squatting, common activities in all sports. Rehabilitation for tendonitis is a gentle stretching program with ice applied for pain, followed by a progressive strengthening program focusing on eccentric activities.

Growth plate injuries of the long bones also occur in the knee region. The distal femoral epiphysis is a common site for injuries. This injury can have important consequences. If the growth plate does not heal properly, growth of the involved limb can be altered, and surgery may be required to fixate the fracture if it is unstable. Rehabilitation consists of rest until the growth plate fracture heals, followed by a general stretching and strengthening progression.

One of the most common regions for osteochondritis ossificans is the knee. Osteochondritis ossificans is a condition in which the articular cartilage and associated bone may split or detach from the rest of the bone. The injury can range from a slightly split portion of cartilage to a loose body floating in the knee joint. The condition may be asymptomatic in the mildest cases. If the cartilage detaches, surgery may be necessary to remove it.[8] Rehabilitation should begin with application of ice to control pain and edema, followed by rest until the radiographs show the split has healed. A general stretching progression follows to ensure that full motion returns.

Another musculoskeletal disorder of the knee is patellofemoral pain syndrome. The precise cause of this syndrome is not certain, but there are a few theories. One theory is that there is a malalignment between the patella and distal femur. Another theory is that the vastus medialis obliquus (VMO) may be weak and allow excess lateral movement of the patella on the femur. Excess genu valgus is another possibility for the cause of patellofemoral pain. This condition changes the mechanics of the extensor mechanism and may force the patella to slide more laterally. Rehabilitation for patellofemoral pain syndrome includes strengthening of the quadriceps muscles, particularly the VMO, and stretching of the tensor fascia lata and iliotibial band. A biomechanical examination may be needed to rule out any mechanical problem arising from the hip or ankle. The strengthening program should consist of basic strengthening and progress to functional activities, including closed kinetic chain and eccentric exercises.[4-6]

Shin splints, or medial tibial stress syndrome, is a common injury in child athletes, especially runners. This is another syndrome that may have many different causes. The primary symptom is medial tibial pain. One cause of this syndrome may be an inflammation of the connection between the posterior tibialis and soles interposes membrane and the periosteum of the tibia. Another possibility is a medial tibial stress fracture.[8] There are a few possible causes for these problems. One is a biomechanical problem in the foot, usually excessive pronation. Another common cause is repetitive eccentric contraction of the ankle dorsiflexors during gait. Rehabilitation begins with corrections in the gait pattern during walking and running; landing more toward the midfoot instead of the heel during ambulation will reduce the stress in the medial tibia. Aquatic exercises work very well as low-impact activities. The intervention should progress from ice for pain and inflammation, along with strengthening and stretching of the pretibial muscles, to functional low-impact activities. The strengthening should include eccentric activities.

Ankle

Sever disease is a growth plate injury to the posterior portion of the calcaneus near the attachment of the Achilles tendon (Fig. 20.11). Decreased flexibility of the Achilles tendon contributes to the cause of this injury. The decreased flexibility of the Achilles tendon can be a result of the bone growing faster than the muscles. As the traction force increases, the calcaneal growth plate can separate. This very rarely becomes displaced.[8] Interventions include temporary heel lifts to decrease pressure on the injury site, along with application of ice and massage, to decrease the pain and inflammation. After the injury heals, stretching of the gastrocnemius and soleus musculature is the priority. After flexibility improves, strengthening of the calf muscles is next, and this can accomplished during functional activities.

Ankle sprains are very common injuries in adults. However, in children this injury is not as common. In children the ligament structure is stronger than the bone structure, especially near growth plates. The growth plate near the distal end of the fibula can be easily injured via inversion of the ankle. This injury can have serious ramifications later in life for the child. Alterations of normal growth of the bone can occur. This may result in any number of biomechanical problems, from the lower extremity to the lumbar spine. The ankle can also become unstable, causing frequent lateral ankle injuries with only mild inversion forces in adulthood.

Rehabilitation for this injury consists of general rest until the fracture heals, followed by a strengthening program and proprioceptive progression. The strengthening program should consist of cardinal plane exercises for plantar flexion, dorsiflexion, inversion, and eversion, followed by diagonal plane strengthening. The focus of the strengthening program should be on eversion activities to strengthen the peroneal (fibularis) muscles to prevent further inversion injuries. The proprioceptive progression should include activities that begin with a good base of support and progress to minimal support. A typical progression may begin with double-leg-stance activities, progress to single-leg-stance activities, and end with activities using double- and single support on balance boards or mini-trampolines.

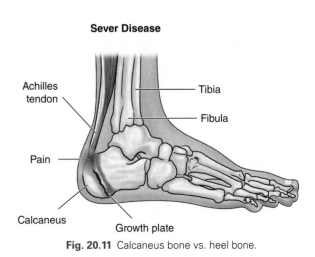

Sever Disease

Achilles tendon · Tibia · Fibula · Pain · Calcaneus · Growth plate

Fig. 20.11 Calcaneus bone vs. heel bone.

OCD can occur on the talus and cause pain, swelling, or locking of the ankle. Intervention is conservative, with rest and bracing until the bone heals. A general stretching and strengthening progression follows. If the articular cartilage becomes disassociated, surgery may be necessary to remove the loose body.

Foot

For the child athlete, stress fractures are the most common injuries seen in the foot. These are overuse injuries that occur when the force is enough to cause injury to the bone but not enough to cause it to fully fracture. These may be difficult to diagnose from normal radiographs, and a bone scan may be needed. Stress fractures are more common in girls, especially as they near puberty.[8]

Rehabilitation for these injuries will include rest until they heal and biomechanical corrections of the foot and ankle. The use of soft foot orthoses to decrease stress in the injured area is a common intervention.

Prevention

Sports-related injury burden can be significant, leading not only to missed participation in sports but also school-related absences, pain, and substantial medical costs. Participation in sports and recreational activities is important to help maintain a healthy lifestyle, inclusive of stress reduction and disease prevention.[8] Many injury prevention programs are based on neuromuscular training. Neuromuscular training (NMT) programs have been shown to be effective in improving balance, strength, and agility. Aspects of neuromuscular training are often incorporated into sports training as part of the warm-up prior to starting sports-specific drills.[8] Studies report an estimated 35% to 47% injury reduction with the incorporation of NMT into practice routines.[8] Example components of an NMT program are as follows:

Aerobic: 1 to 2 laps of side shuffles
Agility: 10 reps of single-leg jumps over a line
Strengthening: 3 reps of 30-second holds of planks
Balance: 4 reps of single-leg balance with trunk rotations

CONCUSSION

Participation in organized sports programs allows participants to benefit from teamwork, increased physical and emotional wellness, and enhanced academic performance. Sports-related concussions are estimated to be experienced by up to 3.8 million youth athletes in the United States each year.[21] Concussions, also referred to as mild traumatic brain injury (TBI), are a result of a blow to the head via a contact sport or when an athlete sustains a fall in which the head contacts either the ground or another surface. Refer to Chapter 7 for additional details on the etiology and management of TBI. Concussions may result in short-term or long-term difficulties such as headaches, visual and vestibular disturbances, balance impairments, sleep disturbances, and alterations in mood or behavior[22] (Box 20.3). Generally speaking, an athlete who has sustained a concussion may present with a Glasgow coma scale score of 13 to 15 and with only a brief, if any loss, of consciousness. Often, an athlete will present with symptoms, but imaging will not reveal any findings.[23]

However, because of the vast presentation of symptoms, it is necessary that the interdisciplinary team conduct a thorough examination and compare the current findings with the athlete's preseason baseline test results. The CDC's Heads Up program, with the initiative of increasing concussion awareness, provides resources for recognition of and recovery from concussion as well as recommendations for best practice. The CDC recommends that each athlete undergo both pre- and postseason baseline testing.[24] Baseline testing is inclusive of prior history of concussion with assessments of

---

BOX 20.3 Concussion Symptoms[24,25]

Patient-reported symptoms after concussion
- Headache
- Nausea
- Dizziness or imbalance
- Fatigue
- Sleep disturbance
- Visual difficulties (acuity and fatigue)
- Confusion
- Photosensitivity
- Anxiety and irritability
- Hearing difficulties or tinnitus
- Difficulty concentrating
- Noise sensitivity
- Atypical emotional response

length of recovery, balance, agility, and cognitive function (concentration and memory). Other medical conditions such as seizures, learning disabilities, anxiety, migraines, or depression should be noted as well. The ImPACT application test is a Food and Drug Administration (FDA)–cleared application that a healthcare provider may use to conduct the baseline screening; it involves the domains of verbal memory, visual memory, visual motor speed, and reaction time. It should be noted that the ImPACT Pediatric test has been validated for children aged 5 to 11 years.[25] Use of the ImPACT application requires licensing and training prior to administration.

Once an athlete has been properly examined and resultant concussive impairments have been identified, it is prudent for the physical therapy team to provide the patient and their parent or guardian, trainer, and coaches with education on the treatment recommendations. Interventions and the plan of care should take on an interdisciplinary approach and address the symptoms and impairments identified. Interventions should address patient education, activity intolerance, sensory integration, vestibular dysfunction, high-level balance and agility dysfunction, post-concussion headaches, photosensitivity, attention and dual-task performance deficits, and any identified musculoskeletal injuries.

RETURN TO PLAY

The CDC has recommended a six-step return to play progression. The athlete should be closely monitored for any symptoms prior to progressing to the next step in the process, and each step should take a minimum of 24 hours, thus allowing for approximately 1 week of recovery.[24] Immediately after sustaining a concussion, the athlete should rest for 2 to 3 days, after which light activity and moderate activity that does not worsen any symptoms may be resumed. The athlete should be assessed to determine whether any symptoms have worsened or new symptoms—such as altered consciousness or confusion, vomiting, or pupillary asymmetry have developed—prior to entering the stages to return to play. The six stages for return to play are detailed in (Table 20.5). Each stage has specific recommendations in terms of cardiovascular response to particular exercise and activity. Activities such as video gaming/virtual reality and driving and excessive cognitive load should be avoided in stages 1 through 3. Similarly, return to classroom activities must also be graded for return to the athlete's prior level of function. If return to play and return to classroom are occurring simultaneously, extra time within the stages may be warranted and continued until both domains are experienced without symptoms. Adjustments and accommodations may be necessary to

TABLE 20.5 **Return to Play Progression**		
Steps of Progression	**Functional Exercise of Each Step**	**Objective**
1) No Activity	Physical and cognitive rest	Rest and recovery
2) Light Aerobic Exercise	Walking, swimming, stationary cycling 60%–70% max heart rate. Avoidance of resistance training	Aerobic conditioning
3) Sport-Specific Exercises with Moderate Intensity	Moderate jogging, brief running, moderate-intensity stationary biking, moderate-intensity weightlifting (less time and/or less weight from their typical routine), non-contact activities	Add movement with head and body coordination
4) Heavy Noncontact Training Drill	Progression to complex multistep/task training drills—multiplanar movements	Improve aerobic capacity, coordination, and cognitive load
5) Full-Contact Practice	After medical clearance, return to normal training activities with control of factors	Coaching to assess functional skill set—regain confidence to return to play
6) Return to Play	Return to competition or game play	

From Centers for Disease Control and Prevention: *HEADS UP partners* (website): https://www.cdc.gov/headsup/partners/index.html. Accessed January 19, 2023.

facilitate a successful recovery. Accommodations may include wearing sunglasses for photosensitivity, use of ear plugs for sound sensitivity, extra time for tests and assignments, and access to a quiet area to allow for mitigation of sensory overload resulting from busy hallways and environments.

SUMMARY

As children and adolescents increase their participation in organized athletics, it is likely that more injuries will occur. The therapist must remember that children are not small adults and therefore require tailored interventions according to their physiologic and cognitive levels. Even within the realm of pediatrics, there are many physical, mental, and emotional differences between the age groups. A child cannot exercise in the same manner as an adolescent or adult because of physiologic and hormonal differences. Physiologic differences include heart size, volume of blood, and decreased stroke volume among others. Prepubertal hormonal differences do not allow the muscles to increase in size or strength. Children can participate in weightlifting and strengthening exercises; however, the strength gains are due more to neuromuscular improvements in coordination and muscle recruitment than to pure strength gains. Children should not begin strengthening exercises and weight training programs until they can fully understand and follow detailed instructions to prevent injuries.

Injuries that are common in children who participate in athletics are physeal (growth plates in the long bones) fractures, greenstick fractures, stress fractures, apophyseal (growth plates in the bone-tendon junctions) injuries, and muscle stress injuries resulting from bone growing at a more rapid rate than the attached muscles. In addition to musculoskeletal injuries, children and adolescents are susceptible to concussions, so careful attention must be paid to any postconcussive symptoms in an effort to facilitate appropriate return to play.

CASE STUDY: REVIEW THE FOLLOWING CASE OF A 16-YEAR-OLD MALE WHO SUSTAINED A CONCUSSION DURING A FOOTBALL GAME. THIS CASE FOLLOWS THE PROGRESSION OF THE PATIENT'S PRESENTATION TO RETURN TO PLAY

History and Systems Review

Referral for PT (outpatient setting): s/p concussion w/ Cervical Injury. Referred by ED to outpatient PT Concussion Clinic

First visit: 7 Days Post Injury

Funding source = Private Insurance

$20 copay/visit

Health Condition: 16 yo male who was playing football-tackled from behind and slammed forward onto his head/face. EMS summoned to the scene and transported him to ED w/ c-collar and backboard. Glasgow Coma Scale score of 15 at ED. Primary acute sx's: headache, nausea, dizziness, mild neck discomfort. No LOC or Amnesia surrounding event.

Head & Cervical Spine CT negative

ED Treatment: ondansetron (Zofran) 4 mg IV Push & d/c home w/ F/U in Concussion Clinic

Chief Complaint: (7 days post injury)

HA, Cervical Pain, Dizziness, Nausea, Diplopia, Hypersomnia, Photosensitivity

Medications/Supplements: Zofran and Percocet prescribed by ED – prn for up to 5 d. None thereafter.

Prior Medical History:

2–3 prior concussions last season (recovered <1 week)

(−) for personal Hx migraine, LD, ADHD, Motion Sickness

(+) Maternal Hx Migraine

Patient Perspective

Patient-Identified Problems/Goals:

- Reduce pain (HA, neck pain)
- Unable to work part-time (at hardware store)—needs to earn money for college
- Resume exercise/working out 5 d/week
- Play collegiate football

Participation Restrictions	Activity Limitations	Body Function/Structure Impairments
<ul><li>Limited ability to work (at hardware store) due to symptoms</li><li>Unable to play football on his current team</li><li>Limited socialization (driving, busy environments, etc.)</li><li>Can't exercise</li><li>Potential impact on ability to pay for college (stressor)</li><li>Able to play football in college?</li></ul>	<ul><li>Can't turn around, move head quickly, bend over without increase in symptoms—movements required at job and in school</li><li>Difficulty w/ reading, computer work</li><li>Difficulty driving and riding in car</li><li>Sleep disruption</li></ul>	**Post Concussion Symptom Scale:** (rated on 0–6 scale):

Post Concussion Symptom Scale: (rated on 0–6 scale):

Headache	6
Nausea	5
Vomiting	0
Balance Problems	3
Dizziness	5
Fatigue	2
Trouble falling asleep	0
Sleeping more than usual	6
Sleeping less than usual	0
Drowsiness	3
Sensitivity to light	6
Sensitivity to noise	3
Irritability	0
Sadness	4
Nervousness	2
Feeling more emotional	1
Numbness or tingling	0
Feeling slowed down	6
Feeling mentally foggy	6
Difficulty concentrating	5
Difficulty remembering	0
Visual problems	4
Total Symptom Score	67

- Constant Headache (4–8/10)
- Neck pain (2–7/10)
- Convergence: 8 cm

CASE STUDY: REVIEW THE FOLLOWING CASE OF A 16-YEAR-OLD MALE WHO SUSTAINED A CONCUSSION DURING A FOOTBALL GAME. THIS CASE FOLLOWS THE PROGRESSION OF THE PATIENT'S PRESENTATION TO RETURN TO PLAY—cont'd

Physical Therapist Perspective	**Contextual Factors**	**Personal Factors:** Highly motivated individual. Likes to be busy all the time; admits to feeling slightly depressed due to inactivity. Worried about resuming school and return to football. Patient has a 4.8 GPA on a 5.0 scale.
		Environment: Lives with parents and two siblings who are supportive. **Activity 1:** Reflection on patient history retrieved through case presentation. 1. **After reviewing the history of this case, what are the pertinent presenting factors? Provide support for your answers.** 2. **What type of recovery trajectory do you expect, given the information presented in the case history? What are the factors which help you arrive at this prediction?**
	Systems Review	**Cardiopulmonary system:** WNL **Integumentary system:** WNL **Neuromuscular system:** Impaired Neurocognitive Testing:

ImPACT® Clinical

Exam Type	Post-Injury 1	
Date Tested		
Last Concussion		
Exam Language	English	
Test Version	2.1	

Composite Scores		Percentile scores
Memory composite (verbal)	81	36%
Memory composite (visual)	58	13%
Visual motor speed composite	27.55	1%
Reaction time composite	0.84	1%
Impulse control composite	0	
Total Symptom Score	67	

Communication, affect, cognition, and learning style:

Intelligent, polite, somewhat subdued affect. Good eye contact and attention initially, but becomes overwhelmed easily; PT completed the evaluation in a quiet exam room with lighting dimmed

Musculoskeletal system: Normal except cervical/thoracic findings noted below

Continued

Impairments of Body Structure/Function

Activity 2: Interpretation of evaluation findings:
VOMS: (Vestibular Ocular Motor Screen)

	HA	Dizziness	Nausea	Fogginess	Total
Baseline	4	0	2	2	8
Smooth Pursuits	4	0	2	2	8
Horizontal Saccades	4	1	4	2	11
Vertical Saccades	4	1	4	2	11
Convergence	7	1	4	2	14
Horizontal VOR	6	7	4	2	19
Vertical VOR	6	7	5	2	20
Visual Motion Sensitivity	6	8	6	2	22
NPC (cm):	1) 40 cm	2) 38 cm	3) 36 cm	Average NPC: **38 cm**	

Additional Ocular Motor Exam:
- Pursuits—WNL
- Saccades—slowed
- Ocular Alignment—Exophoria w/ Cover Testing and Maddox Rod Testing
- Accommodation—WNL

Additional Vestibular Exam:
- Balance Screen: mCTSIB—WNL
- Head Impulse Test—WNL
- VOR Cancellation—WNL; subjectively w/ increased dizziness
- Gaze Holding—WNL with and without fixation
- Positional Testing—WNL
- Dynamic Visual Acuity Test—deferred

Cervical Exam:
- Cervical AROM: full and without increased pain in cervical spine
- Hypomobility in upper thoracic spine
- Cervical segmental mobility testing: Normal
- Alar/transverse ligament testing: negative
- PA pressure provocative for localized pain C6-T2
- + Right Utrap/levator tightness

Guiding questions to answer after reviewing examination findings:
1. What *general* interventions could be considered for management of this patient?
2. How would you prioritize these interventions at 1 week post injury?
3. What *physical therapy* interventions should be prioritized at this time?

CASE STUDY: REVIEW THE FOLLOWING CASE OF A 16-YEAR-OLD MALE WHO SUSTAINED A CONCUSSION DURING A FOOTBALL GAME. THIS CASE FOLLOWS THE PROGRESSION OF THE PATIENT'S PRESENTATION TO RETURN TO PLAY—cont'd

PT Perspective: Other Contributing Factors	**Activity 3:** Design an intervention. **Guiding questions for group discussion:** 1. What _general activity_ recommendations should be provided to this patient at this time? Consider: Work, reading, exercise, driving, sleep, socialization, computer, devices, etc. Provide rationale/evidence for these recommendations. **How long should these restrictions be maintained?** 2. Describe components of an initial physical therapy program. How would you implement this program (Frequency, duration, setting, etc.) 3. How would you progress this patient's physical therapy program? What outcome measures would you use to assess progression? 4. (When) should exertion activity be considered? How would you initiate the implementation of exertion activity? What assessments would you use to determine effectiveness and appropriateness?
Current Status	<u>Recent Achievements</u>: 5 weeks post injury At this point, symptoms and impairments have improved significantly; though he does have moderate symptoms intermittently. He has returned to his normal work schedule, tolerates busy environments with minimal increase in symptoms; and is performing light exercise (treadmill walking, stationary bike, light weight lifting) daily. When performing activities of higher intensity, he experiences dizziness and mild headaches. However, he reports ongoing "nervousness," "frustration" with not being able to exercise to his normal levels or participate in sports.

Evaluation/Diagnosis

20 yo male; 5 weeks s/p concussion with improving symptoms.
- Neck pain 0/10
- HA 0–5/10
- ABC 96%
- DHI 28/100
- Dizziness 0–7/10
- Convergence near point: 6 cm
- DGI 24/24; FGA 29/30
- VOR—performing VORx1 at 150 bpm with minimal symptoms

Prognosis/Goals

What additional goals would you suggest at this point?
Goals should reflect a progression toward full exertion and sport tolerance

Plan of Care:
1. Describe activities/interventions to achieve these goals.

Outcomes/Reassessment
1. Which of the above outcome measures would you use to report to the team if this patient is ready for discharge from physical therapy?
2. What criteria would be used to determine if this patient should be cleared to return to play?

CHAPTER DISCUSSION QUESTIONS

1. Why is a child's heart rate higher than an adult's during exercise?
2. How does strength improve in children without an increase in muscle mass?
3. Describe two skeletal injuries unique to children.
4. Describe Salter-Harris categories I and V of growth plate fractures.
5. What is Osgood-Schlatter disease? Who is more susceptible to getting this disease?
6. Describe general rehabilitation guidelines for childhood athletic injuries.
7. Why are foot stress fractures common in children?
8. Describe *Little Leaguer's elbow* injury.
9. Describe *Little Leaguer's shoulder* injury.
10. Describe aspects of the Major League Baseball Pitch Smart Program.
11. When can a child safely begin to participate in a strength-training program?
12. Identify and provide an example of an NMT program for injury prevention.

REFERENCES

1. Black LI, Terlizzi EP, Vahratian A. Organized sports participation among children aged 6–17 years: United States, 2020. *NCHS Data Brief.* 2022(441):1–8.
2. Safe Kids Worldwide: *Preventing sports-related injuries* (website): https://www.safekids.org/preventing-sports-related-injuries. Accessed February 3, 2023.
3. Daiki K, Gaynor P, Brett T, and others. The use of ratings of perceived exertion in children and adolescents: a scoping review. *Sports Med.* 2021;51(1):33–50.
4. Stricker PR, Faigenbaum AD, McCambridge TM. Council on Sports Medicine and Fitness: resistance training for children and adolescents. *Pediatrics.* 2020;145(6):e20201011.
5. Faigenbaum AD, Milliken LA, Loud RL, and others. Comparison of 1 and 2 days per week of strength training in children. *Res Q Exerc Sport.* 2022;73:416–424.
6. Faigenbaum AD, Milliken LA, Westcott WL. Maximal strength testing in healthy children. *J Strength Cond Res.* 2003;17:162–166.
7. Abbott A, Bird ML, Wild E, and others. Part I: epidemiology and risk factors for stress fractures in female athletes. *Phys Sportsmed.* 2019;48(1):17–24.
8. Stracciolini A, Casciano R, Friedman HL, and others. A closer look at overuse injuries in pediatric athlete. *Clin J Sport Med.* 2015;25:30–35.
9. Salter R, Harris W. Injuries involving epiphyseal plate. *J Bone Joint Surg.* 1963;45A:587.
10. Best R, Meister A, Huth J, and others. Surgical repair techniques, functional outcome, and return to sports after apophyseal avulsion fractures of the ischial tuberosity in adolescents. *Int Orthop.* 2021;45:1853–1861.
11. Chau MM, Klimstra MA, Wise KL, and others. Osteochondritis dissecans: current understanding of epidemiology, etiology, management, and outcomes. *J Bone Joint Surg Am.* 2021;103(12):1132–1151.
12. Gopinathan NR, Viswanathan VK, Crawford AH. Cervical spine evaluation in pediatric trauma: a review and an update of current concepts. *Indian J Orthop.* 2018;52(5):489–500.
13. Palazzo C, Sailhan F, Revel M. Scheuermann's disease: an update. *Joint Bone Spine.* 2014;81(3):209–214.
14. Patel DR, Joychan S, Govender M. Thoracolumbar back pain in adolescents. *J Pain Manag.* 2016;9(2):103–110.
15. Wu HH, Brown K, Flores M, and others. Diagnosis and management of spondylolysis and spondylolisthesis in children. *JBJS Rev.* 2022;10(3). doi: 10.2106/JBJS.RVW.21.00176.
16. Zaremski JL, Zeppieri G Jr, Tripp BL. Sport specialization and overuse injuries in adolescent throwing athletes: a narrative review. *J Athl Train.* 2019;54(10):1030–1039.
17. Saper MG, Pierpoint LA, Liu W, and others. Epidemiology of shoulder and elbow injuries among united states high school baseball players: school years 2005–2006 through 2014–2015. *Am J Sports Med.* 2018;46(1):37–43.
18. DeFroda S, McGlone P, Levins J, and others. Shoulder and elbow injuries in the adolescent throwing athlete. *R I Med J (2013).* 2020;103(7):21–29.
19. Pitch Smart USA: *Guidelines for youth and adolescent pitchers* (website): https://www.mlb.com/pitch-smart/pitching-guidelines. Accessed December 28, 2022.
20. Chéron C, Le Scanff C, Leboeuf-Yde C. Association between sports type and overuse injuries of extremities in children and adolescents: a systematic review. *Chiropr Man Therap.* 2016;24:41.
21. Ali M, Asghar N, Li A, and others. Incidence of concussion and recovery of neurocognitive dysfunction on ImPACT assessment among youth athletes with premorbid depression or anxiety taking antidepressants. *J Neurosurg Pediatr.* 2021;28(1):69–75.
22. Waltzman D, Sarmiento K. What the research says about concussion risk factors and prevention strategies for youth sports: a scoping review of six commonly played sports. *J Safety Res.* 2019;68:157–172.
23. Klein AP, Tetzlaff JE, Bonis JM, and others. Prevalence of potentially clinically significant magnetic resonance imaging findings in athletes with and without sport-related concussion. *J Neurotrauma.* 2019;36(11):1776–1785.
24. Centers for Disease Control and Prevention: *HEADS UP partners* (website): https://www.cdc.gov/headsup/partners/index.html. Accessed January 19, 2023.
25. Schatz P, Maerlender A. A two-factor theory for concussion assessment using ImPACT: memory and speed. *Arch Clin Neuropsychol.* 2013;28(8):791–797.

21

Prematurity Across the Settings

Kara Boynewicz, PhD, PT, DPT, ATC
Board-Certified Pediatric Clinical Specialist APBST

LEARNING OBJECTIVES

At the end of the chapter, the reader will be able to do the following:

1. Understand the perinatal complications that result in preterm birth and the implications for infants during a neonatal intensive care unit (NICU) stay.
2. Apply terminology used in the NICU environment.
3. Know the therapeutic interventions appropriate for babies in the NICU.

CHAPTER OUTLINE

KEY TERMS

Adjusted age
At-risk infant
Chronological age

Developmentally supportive care
Early intervention
Gestational age (GA)

Neonatology
Postconceptional age

Care of the neonate (the first 4 weeks of life) and provision of therapy services in the neonatal intensive care unit (NICU) require specialized knowledge and skills beyond basic physical therapy education and general pediatric practice.[1] Given the advanced knowledge and skill NICU practice requires, it is typically not considered an appropriate practice area for the physical therapist assistant (PTA).[2] However, infants discharged from the NICU often require continued therapy services in settings where PTAs do provide care (e.g., early intervention programs, family homes, preschools, and daycare centers). Providing comprehensive care for NICU graduates and their families requires the treating therapist to understand the family dynamics and stressors that accompany the birth of a premature or special needs infant, as well as knowledge of the infant's complex medical history (Box 21.1). This chapter will serve as an overview of therapeutic principles, commonly seen problems, interventions, equipment, and terminology associated with the NICU environment.

BOX 21.1   Commonly Used Abbreviations

Preparing to provide treatment for a NICU graduate will involve review of the medical record and/or NICU discharge summary. The list of abbreviations in Box 21.1 will help the PTA to discern some of the terminology.[1]

A's & B's	Apnea and bradycardia
AGA	Appropriate for gestational age
BAER	Brainstem auditory evoked responses
BPD	Bronchopulmonary dysplasia
bpm	Beats per minute (heart rate [HR])
BW	Birthweight
CHF	Congestive heart failure
CMV	Cytomegalovirus
CPAP	Continuous positive airway pressure (type of ventilation)
CS	Cesarean section delivery
CSF	Cerebrospinal fluid
GT	Gastric tube
Kcal	Kilocalories
MCA	Multiple congenital anomalies
NG	Nasogastric feeding tube (also known as *gavage*)
NJ	Nasojejunal feeding tube
NNS/NS	Nonnutritive suck, nutritive suck
PO	Per os ("by mouth"—usually indicates feeding taken from a nipple)
PROM	Premature rupture of membranes
PTL	Preterm labor
RDS	Respiratory distress syndrome
Sats	Oxygen saturation levels
SVD	Spontaneous vaginal delivery
TORCHS	Screening for toxoplasmosis fetalis, rubella, cytomegalovirus, herpes simplex, and syphilis
TPN	Total parenteral nutrition

OVERVIEW OF THE NICU

Neonatal intensive care nurseries have existed since the 1950s. With subsequent advances in technology and care, physicians were able to improve outcomes for the very-low-birthweight infant. With an increase in the number of surviving infants, the necessity of providing specialized care also grew. The complex needs of these very young infants necessitated involvement from multiple healthcare professionals. Physical therapists (PTs), occupational therapists (OTs), and speech-language pathologists began to expand their knowledge and scopes of practice to provide care for the premature and/or ill neonate, and these healthcare professionals are critical to the team.[3-5] Neonatology is now a technologically sophisticated area of pediatric medicine, and infants as premature as 23 weeks' gestation (17 weeks early) at birth have a 55% survival rate.[6]

The philosophies guiding NICU care have evolved over the decades. Theories guiding care in the late 1960s and early 1970s suggested that the preterm or ill infant in the NICU experienced a kind of sensory deprivation. Intervention at that time was guided by the belief that infants required supplemental sensory stimulation in an effort to mimic the intrauterine environment. However, further research indicated that these sick and preterm infants appeared to experience more stress from this imposed sensory stimulation; therefore, practice shifted to a model of reduced stimulation.[7]

The standard of care changed in NICUs with developmentally supportive care, which emerged in the 1980s after parents and medical staff noted a variety of negative physiologic, motor, state, and attentional responses. Optimal developmental care is based on minimizing this stress and increasing the infant's ability to self-organize through very careful monitoring of the infant's behavioral and physiologic cues. The rigorous minimizing of stress is shifting to controlled and conscious ways to give appropriate stimulation to preterm infants.[8,9]

Perspectives in care also recognize the family as the constant in the infant's life. Treatment is now directed toward facilitating parent-professional collaboration at all levels of care. One of the most important concepts of family-centered care recognizes the importance of an accessible healthcare system that is flexible, trauma informed, culturally competent, and responsive to family-identified needs.[10] This can be accomplished through the delivery of relationship-based individualized care geared to enhance the strengths of each infant and infant's family. This approach requires a high degree of interaction of family members with infants, as well as interpersonal and intrapersonal collaboration of families and professional caregivers.[11]

Classification of Newborn Infants

Newborn infants are typically classified by gestational age (GA) (number of weeks after conception). GA or estimated gestational age (EGA) is expressed in weeks. The terms *postconceptional age (PCA), adjusted age (AA),* and *chronological age (CA)* are also used. Classifications by GA are listed in Table 21.1.[12]

CA refers to the age of the child in days, weeks, or months from the time of birth. It is the actual amount of time since the child's birth. AA refers to the child's age after adjusting for prematurity. It is the age the child would be if they had been born at term, or the CA minus the weeks premature. For example, a child who is 16 weeks old (CA) but was 10 weeks premature has an AA of 6 weeks. Age is adjusted for prematurity until the child's second birthday. PCA is the CA plus the GA. Thus, a 4-week-old infant (CA) born at 28 weeks' gestation (GA) has a PCA of 32 weeks.

Infants are also classified by birthweight. Birth weights in the NICU environment are typically expressed in grams, as opposed to pounds and ounces. One pound is equal to 454 grams. The most common birthweight classifications are listed in Table 21.2.[12]

Newborns are further classified in terms of how adequate their weight is in relation to their PCA. The most common age-weight classifications are *appropriate for gestational age (AGA),* which encompasses the 10th through 90th percentiles; *small for gestational age (SGA),* for those infants who fall below the 10th percentile; and *large for gestational age (LGA),* for those who fall above the 90th percentile. *Intrauterine growth restriction (IUGR)* occurs when the development and maturation of the fetus are impeded or delayed by genetic factors, maternal disease, or fetal malnutrition caused by placental insufficiency.[12] Infants weighing less than the 10th percentile for GA or less than 2 standard deviations below the mean for GA are classified as IUGR.[2]

Apgar scores are an evaluation of an infant's physical condition, usually performed at 1 minute after birth and again at 5 minutes after birth. Scores are based on the sums of five factors that reflect an infant's ability to adjust to extrauterine life. The infant's heart rate (HR), respiratory effort, muscle tone, reflex irritability, and color are scored from a low value of 0 to a normal value of 2.[12] The five scores are combined, and the totals at 1 and 5 minutes are noted.

NICU Personnel

Neonatology is a technologically sophisticated area of pediatric medicine. The therapist working in the NICU is surrounded by a multitude of other professionals, all striving to meet one goal: optimizing the infant's potential for development.[3] All of these therapists will work in a highly collaborative manner with one another, as well as with the NICU personnel, with the neonatologist (physician) as the leader of the team. Each specialist is equipped with unique knowledge to enhance the quality of life for infants and their families.

According to American Academy of Pediatrics (AAP) guidelines, consultation with an allied healthcare professional (e.g., PT, occupational therapist (OT), speech-language pathologist) is suggested for NICUs with infants who have the greatest complex care needs.[5] In most NICUs, multiple therapy services personnel are employed, including PTs, OTs, and speech-language pathologists.[4,13] Speech-language pathologists are often consulted to address oral-motor and feeding/swallowing function.[14] Each infant will be cared for by a neonatal nurse with advanced training.

Other team members may include neonatal nurse practitioners (NNPs), who complete intensive training and are supervised by the neonatologist. They direct care

TABLE 21.1	Gestational Age Classifications
Classification	Age
Extremely preterm	<28 weeks
Very preterm	28–32 weeks
Moderate preterm	32–37 weeks
Term	37–42 weeks
Post-term	>42 weeks

TABLE 21.2	Birthweight Classifications
Classification	Weight
Extremely low birthweight (ELBW)	<1000 grams
Very low birthweight (VLBW)	1000–1500 grams
Low birthweight (LBW)	1500–2500 grams
Average birthweight	>2500 grams

for infants in the intermediate care setting/step-down nursery.[12] Also included in the NICU team is a respiratory therapist, who monitors ventilator equipment. A pharmacist is typically on staff and assigned exclusively to the NICU to assist doctors and nurses with the complex balance of multiple medications. A nutritionist assists doctors, nurses, and families in providing the appropriate number and type of calories to help these tiny patients grow. A lactation consultant is available to help mothers in pumping breast milk, and when the infant's health and development permit, bringing infants to their mothers to initiate breastfeeding. Social workers and parent liaisons are typically available to assist families with the emotional responses to their infant's complex care.

Common NICU Equipment

The NICU environment is filled with technology. Therapists working in the NICU require basic knowledge of the equipment for safe and effective delivery of service. Following is an introduction to some of the most commonly used equipment in the NICU.

- A *radiant warmer* is a bed with a mattress on an adjustable tabletop covered by a radiant heat source. This type of bed is used for the gravely ill or newly admitted neonate to allow open space for tubes and equipment and rapid access for personnel to assess and care for the infant.[12]
- A self-contained *isolette*, formerly known as an *incubator*, is an enclosed unit of transparent plexiglass; it provides a heated and humidified environment for temperature monitoring. Caregivers can gain access to the infant through portholes or by opening a door on the face of the unit. Many preterm infants remain in an isolette for the first several weeks until they can maintain appropriate body temperature.
- An *oxygen hood* is a plastic or plexiglass hood that typically covers the infant's head and provides a closed environment for controlled oxygen or humidification delivery.
- *Mechanical ventilators*: A *pressure ventilator* delivers positive-pressure ventilation. Pressures are limited, with the breath volume delivered dependent on the stiffness of the lungs. A *volume ventilator* provides positive-pressure ventilation, delivering the same tidal volume with each breath. A *negative-pressure ventilator* creates a relative negative pressure around the thorax and abdomen, thereby assisting ventilation without an endotracheal tube.[12]

- *Nasal and nasopharyngeal prongs* are used to provide continuous positive airway pressure (CPAP); the apparatus consists of nasal prongs of varying lengths and an adapter for pressure source tubing.
- *Monitor*: Usually one unit will display one or more vital signs on a digital display. Electrodes are placed on the infant's chest or abdomen and will typically display heart and respiration rates, as well as oxygen saturation. High and low limits are typically set, and an alarm will sound if the limits are exceeded. The following are recommended safe limits:
  - HR between 110 and 180 beats per minute (bpm). The ideal HR is between 120 and 160 bpm.[15] Factors that can cause fluctuations in HR are pain, seizures, medications, and reflux.
  - Respiration rate (RR) between 20 and 60 breaths per minute.[12] Factors that can cause fluctuations in RR include sepsis, reflux, apnea, medications, and anemia. Therapists working in the NICU should be aware that alarms may be set off when the infant is moving. Clinical observation of the infant's behavior and skin color will help to discern real from false alarms.[16]
- An *oxygen saturation monitor (pulse oximeter)* measures the amount of oxygen carried in the blood. Factors that can cause fluctuations in oxygen saturation include sepsis, hypoventilation, and lung oxygenation.[17] The target range for oxygen saturation for preterm infants should be 90% to 94%.[16] Lower saturation ranges (85%–89%) can set off an alarm and have been shown to reduce the risk of retinopathy of prematurity.[16]
- *Extracorporeal membrane oxygenation (ECMO)* is a lifesaving therapy for infants with severe neonatal respiratory failure who, despite intensive therapy, do not recover from hypoxemia or respiratory acidosis.[12] The procedure involves passing the infant's blood through a filter and supplementing it with oxygen outside the infant's body. Infants receiving ECMO are critically ill and are usually not candidates for therapy until they are stabilized and no longer receiving ECMO. Infants on ECMO are typically immobilized with their heads turned to one side.

REASONS FOR THERAPY REFERRAL

The goal of therapeutic intervention in the NICU is to optimize the infant's potential for development. NICU physicians and nurses recognize the valuable role therapists can play in optimizing outcomes for premature and ill newborns.[5] While referral criteria will vary between institutions, common reasons for referral include the following[18]:

- Cardiorespiratory issues with alterations in breathing patterns
- Decreased range of motion (ROM) or joint contractures
- Movement dysfunction, poor postural control, or asymmetric postures
- Known diagnosis or syndromes (e.g., spina bifida, Down syndrome)
- Altered neurobehavior, state control, and stress cues
- Disorganized feeding

Referrals are also frequently made to obtain a baseline evaluation for infants with questionable neurologic status.

COMMON MEDICAL DISORDERS

The majority of the many medical problems experienced by newborn infants are directly related to their premature birth and the immaturity of various systems. However, other problems can arise as a result of iatrogenic complications resulting from the medical management of life-threatening situations. Following is a list of the most prevalent neonatal medical problems, causes, and the effects on neonatal development.

Respiratory Disorders

Transient tachypnea of the newborn (TTN) occurs when an infant experiences minor respiratory difficulty soon after delivery.[19] This condition is characterized by fast breathing (>80 breaths per minute). Other clinical signs are nasal flaring, intercostal retractions, and cyanosis. For the majority of neonates, TTN generally resolves in 2 to 3 days. This condition is treated with oxygen, typically administered in an oxygen hood or via "blow by" (oxygen tubing placed near the infant's face).

Perinatal asphyxia occurs when a newborn does not breathe spontaneously. The asphyxia may develop before or during labor or occur immediately after delivery. Infants with perinatal asphyxia often experience neurologic problems. Associated conditions are hypoxic seizures or hypoxic ischemic encephalopathy (HIE).[20] Neurologic involvement may arise in infants that have experienced severe asphyxia.[20] Whole-body cooling can be initiated to help with the postinflammatory

process of HIE.[21] This consists of sedating the infants for 72 hours, lowering their body temperature, and then slowly warming them. This improvement in medical technology has greatly improved long-term developmental outcomes.[22]

Respiratory distress syndrome (RDS), also known as *hyaline membrane disease*, is a specific respiratory disorder common in premature infants and attributed to inadequate pulmonary surfactant.[23] It is caused by collapse of lung tissue due to lack of pulmonary surfactant and an overly flexible chest wall. As the air sacs collapse, the surface tension of the lungs increases, making ventilation very difficult. Medical management requires ventilatory support, typically via endotracheal intubation.

Bronchopulmonary dysplasia (BPD), or chronic lung disease (CLD), is the most common form of CLD among premature infants; it is a consequence of continued damage and abnormal healing of the lungs after a severe respiratory distress disorder.[24] Infants born at <32 weeks EGA who need supplemental oxygen after 36 weeks GA and infants born at ≥32 weeks GA who need additional oxygen after 28 days CA are defined as having BPD or CLD.

Apnea and bradycardia ("A's & B's") is another common problem in the NICU. Apnea is an absence of spontaneous respiration lasting longer than 20 seconds; it is commonly seen in premature infants.[25] Apnea is frequently accompanied by bradycardia, a slowing of the HR to less than 100 bpm. Apnea of the newborn frequently requires physical stimulation of the infant.[26] Bradycardia, if not directly related to apneic episodes, may be treated pharmacologically with caffeine. Some infants are discharged home with apnea monitors as well.

Cardiovascular/Cardiopulmonary Disorders

Patent ductus arteriosus (PDA) occurs when the fetal ductus arteriosus fails to close spontaneously at birth. When this happens, blood from the left side of the heart is able to pass to the right side, decreasing oxygenation and potentially causing cardiovascular overload. A PDA is more common in premature infants. The main diagnostic criterion is a characteristic heart murmur heard on auscultation and confirmed by an echocardiogram. Those PDAs that do not resolve spontaneously are treated pharmacologically or through surgical ligation.

Persistent pulmonary hypertension of the newborn (PPHN) is characterized by an increase in vascular tension in the lungs that causes a right-to-left shunt through the ductus arteriosus and foramen ovale; it generally resolves spontaneously. Infants with persistent PPHN are treated with medication or mechanical ventilation.[27]

Ventricular septal defect (VSD) is an abnormal opening in the septum separating the heart ventricles, permitting blood to flow from the left ventricle to the right ventricle and recirculate through the pulmonary artery and lungs, compromising peripheral oxygenation. It is the most common congenital heart defect and in many cases requires surgical correction.[28]

CNS Disorders

Intraventricular hemorrhage (IVH) describes bleeding into the ventricular system of the brain and occurs almost exclusively in premature infants.[12] Fifteen percent of infants with weights of less than 1500 grams and 80% of preterm infants weighing less than 1000 grams will have some degree of IVH.[29] Common symptoms include a bulging fontanel, sudden anemia, apnea, bradycardia, acidosis, high blood pressure, hydrocephalus, and changes in muscle tone and/or level of consciousness. The severity of IVH is classified according to the extent of the lesion as follows:

- Grade I: Subependymal, germinal matrix hemorrhage
- Grade II: Intraventricular bleeding without ventricular dilation
- Grade III: Intraventricular bleeding with ventricular dilation
- Grade IV: Intraventricular and intraparenchymal bleeding

The prognosis for infants with IVH is variable and depends on the severity of IVH, the presence or absence of other complications, and birthweight/GA.[30] Infants with grade I and grade II bleeds typically recuperate with little or no deficits; however, those with grade III and IV are at higher risk of developing cerebral palsy than those without IVH.[31] Infants with grade III and grade IV IVH are at increased risk for long-term neurologic impairments, cerebral palsy, and cognitive impairment.[32] Recent studies show that magnetic resonance imaging (MRI) is superior to cranial ultrasonography in detection, classification, and thereby in determining prognosis for infants with IVH.[33]

Periventricular leukomalacia (PVL) can occur as a severe form of IVH or as an independent diagnosis. This condition is characterized by ischemic white matter tissue surrounding the ventricles as a result of hypoxia associated with perinatal asphyxia. Diagnosis is established if paleness of the white matter is evident on cranial ultrasonography or a computed tomography (CT) scan. Infants with PVL are at exceptionally high risk for CNS damage and cerebral palsy.[34]

Miscellaneous Disorders

Retinopathy of prematurity (ROP) results from an alteration in the normal development of retinal blood capillaries. Found exclusively in premature infants, especially those with very low birthweights, ROP affects approximately 65% of infants with a birthweight of less than 1250 grams; 80% of those with a birthweight of less than 1000 grams will develop some degree of ROP.[35] The incidence of ROP is most consistently associated with early GA, low birthweight, and duration of mechanical ventilation. The following classification system is a simplified version of the International Classification of ROP[12]:

- Stage I: Thin demarcation line between the vascular and nonvascular regions of the retina
- Stage II: Demarcation line develops into a ridge that protrudes into the vitreous
- Stage III: Extraretinal fibrovascular proliferation occurs
- Stage IV: Fibrosis and scarring occur, with traction on the retina resulting in retinal detachment
- Plus disease: Occurs when vessels posterior to the ridge become dilated and tortuous

Routine ophthalmoscopic examinations are now performed in NICUs for all infants with a birthweight less than 1500 grams or GA less than 32 weeks and will continue into early childhood, until the retinas become fully mature. Laser surgery may be indicated if Stage IV ROP is detected to prevent permanent blindness.[36]

Necrotizing enterocolitis (NEC) is a serious disease in which the immature intestinal tissue, usually the intestinal wall, dies and sloughs off. Infants may develop intestinal hemorrhage, gangrene, submucosal gas, and in severe cases perforation of the intestine.[12] Typically seen in premature infants, NEC often first becomes evident around the third to tenth day of life as abdominal distention. Medical management can be complex, and surgical intervention is indicated when perforation of the intestines has occurred.[37] In severe cases a colostomy may be required. Oral or NG feeding will be suspended and reintroduced very gradually.

FRAMEWORK FOR THERAPY SERVICES

The framework for therapy services includes the model of the International Classification of Functioning, Disability and Health (ICF) to provide standard language. Common impairments with preterm infants include muscle tone, postural control, endurance with handling, ROM, and state regulation.[2] Common limitations in activity may include decreased tolerance with diapering and feeding, alterations in sleep-wake cycles, and changes in responsiveness to auditory and visual input.[18] Participation restrictions may include parent-infant interaction and growth. Personal factors include multiple comorbidities and temperament and attachment. Environmental factors include family support, lighting, and noise levels. Clinical care pathways have been developed to assist therapists working in the NICU to initiate the hands-on or hands-off examination and in knowing when appropriate interventions should be implemented.[38] In addition to the care pathways, neonatal competencies have been described for training and mentoring prior to initiating work in the NICU with medically fragile patients.[2,3]

INTERVENTION

Physical Therapy Assessment

The neonatal or infant screening includes the cardiovascular, pulmonary, integumentary, musculoskeletal, neurologic and neurobehavioral systems.[2] The examination includes the emergence/dominance of primitive reflexes, muscle tone, postural control, state regulation, neurologic reflexes, and ROM.[18] Standardized outcome measures appropriate for infants are available to PTs, OTs, and speech-language pathologists for assessing infants in the NICU. Some formal tools commonly used and modified are the following:

- Test of Infant Motor Performance (TIMP): Used to measure functional movement and postural control and can be used with infants as young as 34 weeks PCA through 4 months of life. The TIMP can discriminate among infants with varying risk for poor motor performance in early infancy, and it successfully shows change in motor performance over time.[39]
- NICU Neonatal Network Scale (NNNS): Used to provide a comprehensive assessment of both motor and sensory responses, neurologic integrity, and

behavioral function (i.e., neurobehavior) of healthy infants, preterm infants, and high risk infant.[40]
- Neurobehavioral Assessment of the Preterm Infant (NAPI): Used to assess neurobehavioral status of prematurely born infants, monitor effects of intervention, and document individual differences.[41]

Physical Therapy Intervention

Therapists working in the NICU assist families and NICU staff by providing education and coaching to enhance infant outcomes. Developmentally supportive care encompasses optimizing the infant's long-term outcomes and development and should be present in all interventions. The range of possible interventions includes fostering caregiver-infant interactions; positioning, feeding, and sensory stimulation or sensory/environmental modification; motor development intervention; splinting; and preparation for discharge.[42]

Fostering Parent Interaction/Caregiving

Increasing participation of the infant's potential is the primary goal of all NICU interventions. Therapists work as a part of a collaborative team to enhance the infant's outcome.[43] The birth of an infant with special needs or a premature birth creates profound stress on the family. Awaiting the birth of a baby is an emotionally charged time in the best of circumstances, but when problems occur, families experience emotional responses such as fear, apprehension, shock, guilt, anger, depression, frustration, helplessness, and denial. Such emotions will affect the family's perception of how their newborn is being cared for and how they are able to participate in that care.[44] Therapists working in the NICU and those working with NICU graduates must recognize these emotions and empower families to participate in providing care for their premature and ill infants.[45]

NEONATAL INTERVENTIONS

Providing information about the infant's condition and management

Recognizing, monitoring, and appropriately responding to the infant's cues, particularly stress indicators

Decreasing the infant's stress responses

Facilitating alertness and enhancing attentional stability

Optimizing the infant's interactive abilities through environmental modulation and appropriate timing of caregiving interventions, according to the infant's signals

Sensory/Environmental Modulation

Neonatal therapists must be able to accurately assess an infant's state or neurobehavioral readiness for intervention. Brazelton's state classification is the most commonly recognized indicator, with six defined states: deep sleep, light sleep, drowsy, quiet alert, active awake, and crying.[12] Current best practice in the NICU recognizes the quiet alert state as most appropriate for therapeutic intervention. Therapy sessions should be scheduled around periods of greater wakefulness to minimize disrupting the infant's rest. The physiologic responses and stress indicators that help caregivers and families recognize the presence of stress in an infant include gaze aversion, grimace, disorganized movements, finger/toe splays, changes in vital signs, spitting up, yawning, sneezing or hiccups, arching or extension, and crying.[46]

Interventions with evidence of sensory stimulation include kangaroo care, or skin-to-skin contact, with parents; music; language exposure; and multimodal interventions.[47] The Supporting and Enhancing NICU Sensory Experiences (SENSE) intervention promotes consistent, developmentally appropriate, responsive, sensory exposures, which include touch, music, and skin-to-skin contact.[48] This program includes parents administering the sensory input while in the NICU with kangaroo care, auditory stimulation, and touch.[49]

NEONATAL INTERVENTIONS

Careful observation to assess baseline level of stress and readiness for intervention

Gradual changes in lighting

Recognizing and inhibiting stress indicators

Gentle but firm stroking or deep pressure

Gentle vertical vestibular stimulation while holding the infant in an upright position

Unswaddling an infant who is swaddled

Presenting stimuli from one sensory modality at a time

Quiet talking or singing/humming

Infant massage

Positioning

Premature and very ill neonates have a number of positioning problems, which if not managed appropriately may lead to the development of postural abnormalities and a variety of developmental and movement problems.[50] The most common indicator for positioning intervention in the NICU is hypotonia. Hypotonia and hyperextension are common in premature infants, due in part to the lack of physiologic flexion and the immaturity of the nervous system.[51] When preterm infants are placed supine, they will typically assume a fully extended or hyperextended position as a result of the inability to move or flex against gravity. When placed prone, these infants will typically be unable to maintain prone flexion due to low tone and lack of strength and balance between flexors and extensors.

Common position-induced deformities include the following:

- Neck and trunk hyperextension with shoulder retraction and elevation
- "W" posturing of the upper extremities (shoulder abduction with external rotation and elbow flexion)
- "Frog-leg" positioning of the lower extremities (hip abduction and external rotation with knee flexion)

Care must also be taken to observe the infant's head shape. Head flattening, a common deformity, is the result of prolonged sidelying or supine positioning. The infant's skull assumes the shape of the surface on which it is lying, so infants positioned in sidelying positions for extended periods will have flattening of the sides of the skull.[52] Infants who are positioned supine for long periods will experience flattening on the posterior skull.[53]

Positioning is one of the least intrusive neonatal interventions and can be implemented even with the medically unstable infant. Even the gravely ill infant will require position changes. Infants born at less than 32 weeks' gestation are at high risk for disturbances in cerebral blood flow, especially in the first 3 days of life.[54] The infant's head, neck, and extremities should be positioned in midline when moving the infant to help prevent changes in their blood pressure and decrease the risk of IVH.[55]

Motor agitation or disorganized movements are commonly seen in infants in the NICU. Limiting this type of movement is desirable and can also be accomplished with appropriate positioning and containment/boundaries.[56] When placed prone, infants are said to sleep more, expend less energy and oxygen, breathe more slowly, and remain calmer.[12]

Handling and Motor Development Interventions

Handling interventions are aimed at preventing the development of atypical postural or movement patterns and facilitate efficient movements such as guiding infants to lifting their heads in prone, bring their hands to midline, and hold their heads in midline to enhance function.[9] Efforts are directed toward handling or positioning the infant to decrease neck and trunk hyperextension, shoulder retraction, and total body extension while facilitating active work in all of the flexor muscle groups. It has been shown that infants receiving handling in the NICU have improvements in their motor development.[57,58] As with all interventions, handling should be conducted in a gentle, graded manner with careful attention to the infant's responses.

Motor development interventions that have shown improvement in outcomes for infants in the NICU include handling and also postural control training, parent-directed training with individualized handling and motor stimulation of their infant, and parent-infant interaction.[9,59,60] This consists of placing infants in different positions, use of infant massage and therapeutic touch,[61] providing auditory and visual stimulation to elicit a response, and promotion of variable and self-directed movements.[9,61] The key for all interventions is including the family in care by means of education and coaching and having them provide the interventions to their infants.[62]

Feeding and Oral Motor Development

Therapists working in the NICU are often consulted to assist in the progression of oral-motor development and feeding. While feeding intervention is more often addressed by the OT or speech-language pathologist, in some settings PTs are also involved.

Preterm infants may have numerous issues surrounding feeding, including diminished reflexes, decreased muscle strength, and poor oral motor coordination.[63] These impact their ability to achieve compression on a pacifier, suck-swallow-breathe, and extract milk from a nipple.[64] Positioning, handling, use of pacifier, and state regulation strategies used by therapists contribute to infants' readiness to participate in oral feeding.[65] Infants may continue to experience feeding difficulties after discharge; therefore, a thorough understanding of the role of posture and regulation of physiologic state in facilitating efficient feeding is essential.

Splinting and Taping

Therapists are frequently consulted by NICU staff when an infant is believed to require splinting or taping of the upper or lower extremities.[14,66] Neonatal splinting should be considered in an effort to provide immobilization and support, to prevent contractures or for maintaining or increasing ROM for diagnosis such as talipes equinovarus.[67] Therapists must also take into very careful consideration the very fragile skin of newborns and premature infants. The role of the therapist is to fabricate the splint and educate the nursing staff and family about its use, wearing schedule, and precautions.[68]

Preparing for Discharge

While parents may look forward to the day they can finally bring their infant home, discharge from the NICU can also be a frightening and anxious time. Discharge planning should start on the day the infant is born, with milestones to help monitor the discharge process, and a discharge care path should be available for the therapist.[38] Milestones include transition to an open crib from an isolate and switch from use of a nasogastric tube to full oral feeding. The transition is further complicated for infants who go home still in need of medical supports such as oxygen or apnea monitors or for those who require continued in-home nursing care.[69] Therapists should spend time coaching and educating parents about the carry-over of therapeutic positioning and handling and the use of any equipment or splints that are recommended. The NICU team will likely also call on the services of a discharge planner or medical social worker to assist families in moving on to the next level of care. Referrals and recommendations for additional therapies through a home care agency or early intervention program are vital in helping families adjust to caring for the NICU graduate.[70]

NICU DEVELOPMENTAL FOLLOW-UP CLINIC

Infants born prematurely, those very sick at birth, those with a congenital or acquired diagnosis, or those needing oxygen support for an extended amount of time are still recovering when they go home.[71] NICU graduates can be considered at-risk infants as they may have difficulties with feeding, growing, breathing, and delays in development: their behaviors should be monitored closely because they are at risk for developmental delays.[72] This can be accomplished at a NICU follow-up clinic, comprised of an interdisciplinary team of health-care professionals who address the medical, nutritional, neurologic, developmental, and social needs of patients in a single location.[73] Families typically return to the hospital NICU follow-up clinic at regular intervals, where therapists take an active role in assessing the infant's progress and functional level or limitations and providing recommendations for continued therapy or access to early intervention services.[9] Some states have funded parents-as-teachers programs that send trained community workers or parenting peers into the homes of recently discharged infants. These individuals are trained to help parents acclimate their child to the home environment.

Early Intervention

Babies who have spent time in a NICU may be at risk for early medical or developmental challenges or delays, which are compounded if they have numerous medical complications.[74] The smaller they are at birth and the earlier they are born, the greater is the risk for developmental days, hence the term "at risk infant" is used. Identification of delays provides families with the resources needed and allows for referral for early intervention (Part C) services. A referral for physical therapy is commonly made to assist infants and their parents after discharge from the hospital. Common issues for infants in the first year of life include impairments in postural control and problem-solving in tummy time and delayed reaching skills.[75,76] Early therapy programs for NICU graduates have been shown to improve motor and cognitive development in infants.[77] Interventions focusing on family coaching, kicking activities, postural control, prone play, and parent-infant interaction have all been shown to improve outcomes.[78–81]

Early intervention is under Part C of the Individuals with Disabilities Education Act (IDEA) and provides services to children from birth to 3 years old.[82] Services provided by physical therapy in the early intervention setting focus to enhance the overall development of infants and toddlers, are family centered in the natural environment, embedded in the routines of the family, and follow the guiding documents of the Individualized Family Service Plan (IFSP).[82]

CASE STUDY OF A CHILD IN THE NICU

G.M. is a 33-week PCA infant girl referred for therapy services. G.M.'s primary NICU nurse reports G.M. is very floppy, has trouble moving her arms against gravity, and does not bring her hands together at midline. She tends to arch and is not able to lift her legs from the bed. She recently began to feed orally but has frequent A's & B's during and after feeding. The infant's history is significant for premature birth at 27 weeks EGA following a pregnancy complicated by breech positioning, premature rupture of membranes (PROM), and preterm labor (PTL). Delivery was by emergency cesarean section due to fetal heart rate deceleration. Birthweight was 1315 grams. G.M. required resuscitation and intubation and was then transferred to a Level III NICU 1 hour from home. Apgar scores were 1 and 8 at 1 and 5 minutes, respectively. Mechanical ventilation was initiated and continued for 7 days, at which time G.M. was transitioned to nasal CPAP. She is now receiving 1 liter of oxygen via nasal cannula.

Problems identified on review of the chart include grade III IVH, PDA treated with Indocin, and apnea. G.M.'s parents are often at her bedside, even though they must travel a great distance to be with her. She is their first child. The nurse reports they have frequent questions about her movements and facial expressions when they hold her. They are also concerned that she does not feed well and that her head is flat on the left side. They are very concerned about providing care for her after her discharge.

G.M. has been discharged home and has started receiving services through early intervention. She has an IFSP in place and has been receiving physical therapy services for 18 months. Answer the questions based on the following information.

ICF framework

Health Conditions: Prematurity 13 weeks. Status post ventilation.

Body Structure/Function: Hypotonia, oxygen dependent, plagiocephaly

Activity Implications: Infant movements against gravity; decreased feeds

Participation: Cannot participate in family routines

Environmental Factors: Needs medical support

Personal Factors: Two invested parents, but family is nervous, as GM is the first child

Movement System Analysis: Force production deficits in antigravity muscles

CHAPTER DISCUSSION QUESTIONS

1. What is G.M.'s newborn classification based on her gestational age and birthweight?
2. Review of the medical record indicates what complications during the pregnancy/delivery?
3. Further review revealed what other problems and risk factors that may impact outcomes?
4. After evaluating the infant in the NICU and meeting the parents, the PT provided information for all caregivers regarding positioning. What could the PT suggest to assist the family to enhance G.M.'s development with interventions?
5. Once in early intervention, what are some issues that are common to infants with G.M.'s medical condition and what interventions could be initiated?
6. What are some long-term complications that G.M. may encounter from her medical conditions resulting from her prematurity?

REFERENCES

1. Sweeney JK, Heriza CB, Blanchard Y. American Physical Therapy Association. Neonatal physical therapy. Part I: clinical competencies and neonatal intensive care unit clinical training models. *Pediatr Phys Ther.* 2009;21(4):296–307.
2. Sweeney JK, Heriza CB, Blanchard Y, et al. Neonatal physical therapy. Part II: practice frameworks and evidence-based practice guidelines. *Pediatr Phys Ther.* 2010;22(1):2–16.
3. Craig JW, Smith CR. Risk-adjusted/neuroprotective care services in the NICU: the elemental role of the neonatal therapist (OT, PT, SLP). *J Perinatol.* 2020;40:549–559.
4. Pineda RG, Lisle J, Ferrara L, et al. Neonatal therapy staffing in the United States and relationships to NICU type and location, level of acuity, and population factors. *Am J Perinatol.* 2021. Advance online publication. https://doi.org/10.1055/a-1678-0002.
5. American Academy of Pediatrics. *Guidelines for Perinatal Care/American Academy of Pediatrics (and) the American College of Obstetricians and Gynecologists.* 8th ed. Washington, DC: American Academy of Pediatrics; 2017.
6. Handley SC, Kumbhat N, Eggleston B, et al. Exposure to umbilical cord management approaches and death or neurodevelopmental impairment at 22–26 months' corrected age after extremely preterm birth. *Arch Dis Child Fetal Neonatal Ed.* 2023;108(3):224–231.
7. Als H. A synactive model of neonatal behavioral organization: framework for the assessment of neurobehavioral development in the premature infant and for the support of infants and parents in the neonatal intensive care environment. *Phys Occup Ther Pediatr.* 1986;6(3/4):3.
8. Pineda R, Smith J, Roussin J, et al. Randomized clinical trial investigating the effect of consistent, developmentally-appropriate, and evidence-based multisensory exposures in the NICU. *J Perinatol.* 2021;41(10):2449–2462.
9. Dusing SC, Tripathi T, Marcinowski EC, et al. Supporting play exploration and early developmental intervention versus usual care to enhance development outcomes during the transition from the neonatal intensive care unit to home: a pilot randomized controlled trial. *BMC Pediatr.* 2018;18(1):46.
10. Sanders MR, Hall SL. Trauma-informed care in the newborn intensive care unit: promoting safety, security and connectedness. *J Perinatol.* 2018;38(1):3–10.
11. Patel N, Ballantyne A, Bowker G, et al. Helping Us Grow Group (HUGG): family integrated care: changing the culture in the neonatal unit. *Arch Dis Child.* 2018;103(5):415–419.
12. Gardner S, Carter B, Enzman-Hines M, et al. *Handbook of Neonatal Intensive Care.* 9th ed. St Louis: Elsevier; 2021.
13. Rubio-Grillo MH. Performance of an occupational therapist in a neonatal intensive care unit. *Colomb Med (Cali).* 2019;50(1):30–39.
14. Ross K, Heiny E, Conner S, et al. Occupational therapy, physical therapy and speech-language pathology in the neonatal intensive care unit: patterns of therapy usage in a level IV NICU. *Res Dev Disabil.* 2017;64:108–117.
15. Alonzo CJ, Nagraj VP, Zschaebitz JV, et al. Heart rate ranges in premature neonates using high resolution physiologic data. *J Perinatol.* 2018;38(9):1242–1245.
16. Chandrasekharan P, Rawat M, Reynolds AM, et al. Apnea, bradycardia and desaturation spells in premature infants: impact of a protocol for the duration of "spell-free" observation on interprovider variability and readmission rates. *J Perinatol.* 2018;38(1):86–91.
17. Kumar N, Akangire G, Sullivan B, et al. Continuous vital sign analysis for predicting and preventing neonatal diseases in the twenty-first century: big data to the forefront. *Pediatr Res.* 2020;87(2):210–220.
18. Byrne E, Campbell SK. Physical therapy observation and assessment in the neonatal intensive care unit. *Phys Occup Ther Pediatr.* 2013;33(1):39–74.
19. Hermansen CL, Mahajan A. Newborn respiratory distress. *Am Fam Physician.* 2015;92(11):994–1002.
20. Mosalli R. Whole body cooling for infants with hypoxic-ischemic encephalopathy. *J Clin Neonatol.* 2012;1(2):101–106.

21. Harriman T, Bradshaw WT, Blake SM. The use of whole body cooling in the treatment of hypoxic-ischemic encephalopathy. *Neonatal Netw.* 2017;36(5):273–279.

22. Natarajan G, Pappas A, Shankaran S. Outcomes in childhood following therapeutic hypothermia for neonatal hypoxic-ischemic encephalopathy (HIE). *Semin Perinatol.* 2016;40(8):549–555.

23. Sweet DG, Carnielli V, Greisen G. European Consensus guidelines on the management of respiratory distress syndrome—2019 update. *Neonatology.* 2019;115(4):432–450.

24. Dumas HM, Fragala-Pinkham MA, et al. Cardiorespiratory response during physical therapist intervention for infants and young children with chronic respiratory insufficiency. *Pediatr Phys Ther.* 2013;25(2):178–185.

25. Zhao J, Gonzalez F, Mu D. Apnea of prematurity: from cause to treatment. *Eur J Pediatr.* 2011;170(9):1097–1105.

26. Eichenwald EC. Committee on Fetus and Newborn, American Academy of Pediatrics. Apnea of prematurity. *Pediatrics.* 2016;137(1):1–8.

27. Steinhorn RH. Evaluation and management of the cyanotic neonate. *Clin Pediatr Emerg Med.* 2008;9(3):169–175.

28. Hiremath G, Kamat D. Diagnostic considerations in infants and children with cyanosis. *Pediatr Ann.* 2015;44(2):76–80.

29. Ballabh P. Intraventricular hemorrhage in premature infants: mechanism of disease. *Pediatr Res.* 2010;67(1):1–8.

30. Chiriboga N, Cortez J, Pena-Ariet A, et al. Successful implementation of an intracranial hemorrhage (ICH) bundle in reducing severe ICH: a quality improvement project. *J Perinatol.* 2019;39(1):143–151.

31. Hollebrandse NL, Spittle AJ, Burnett AC, et al. School-age outcomes following intraventricular haemorrhage in infants born extremely preterm. *Arch Dis Child Fetal Neonatal Ed.* 2021;106:4–8.

32. Patra K. Severe intraventricular hemorrhage in a new decade: what do we tell parents? *J Perinatol.* 2014;34:167–168.

33. Wang Y, Song J, Zhang X, et al. The impact of different degrees of intraventricular hemorrhage on mortality and neurological outcomes in very preterm infants: a prospective cohort study. *Front Neurol.* 2022;13:853417.

34. Jiang H, Li X, Jin C. Early diagnosis of spastic cerebral palsy in infants with periventricular white matter injury using diffusion tensor imaging. *AJNR Am J Neuroradiol.* 2019;40(1):162–168.

35. Good WV, Hardy RJ, Dobson V, et al. The incidence and course of retinopathy of prematurity: findings from the early treatment for retinopathy of prematurity study. *Pediatrics.* 2005;116(1):15–23.

36. Bell EF, Hintz SR, Hansen NI, et al. Mortality, in-hospital morbidity, care practices, and 2-year out-comes for extremely preterm infants in the US, 2013–2018. *JAMA.* 2022;327(3):248–263.

37. Lin H, Mao S, Shi L, et al. Clinical characteristic comparison of low birth weight and very low birth weight preterm infants with neonatal necrotizing enterocolitis: a single tertiary center experience from eastern China. *Pediatr Surg Int.* 2018;34:1201–1207.

38. Campbell SK. Use of care paths to improve patient management. *Phys Occup Ther Pediatr.* 2013;33(1):27–38.

39. Campbell SK. Functional movement assessment with the Test of Infant Motor Performance. *J Perinatol.* 2021;41(10):2385–2394.

40. McGowan EC, Hofheimer JA, O'Shea TM, et al. Analysis of neonatal neurobehavior and developmental outcomes among preterm infants. *JAMA Netw Open.* 2022;5(7):e2222249.

41. Korner AF, Constantinou J, Dimiceli S, Brown BW Jr, Thom VA. Establishing the reliability and developmental validity of a neurobehavioral assessment for preterm infants: a methodological process. *Child Dev.* 1991;62(5):1200–1208.

42. Byrne E, Garber J. Physical therapy intervention in the neonatal intensive care unit. *Phys Occup Ther Pediatr.* 2013;33(1):75–110.

43. Barbosa VM. Teamwork in the neonatal intensive care unit. *Phys Occup Ther Pediatr.* 2013;33(1):5–26.

44. Cardin AD. Parents' perspectives: an expanded view of occupational and co-occupational performance in the neonatal intensive care unit. *Am J Occup Ther.* 2020;74(2):7402205030p1–7402205030p12.

45. Craig JW, Glick C, Phillips R, et al. Recommendations for involving the family in developmental care of the NICU baby. *J Perinatol.* 2015;35(suppl 1):S5–S8.

46. Milette I, Martel M-J, Ribeiro da Silva M, et al. Guidelines for the Institutional Implementation of developmental neuroprotective care in the neonatal intensive care unit. Part A: background and rationale. A Joint Position Statement From the CANN, CAPWHN, NANN, and COINN. *Can J Nur Res.* 2017;49(2):46–62.

47. Pineda R, Guth R, Herring A, et al. Enhancing sensory experiences for very preterm infants in the NICU: an integrative review. *J Perinatol.* 2017;37(4):323–332.

48. Pineda R, Raney M, Smith J. Supporting and enhancing NICU sensory experiences (SENSE): defining developmentally-appropriate sensory exposures for high-risk infants. *Early Hum Dev.* 2019;133:29–35.

49. Pineda R, Smith J, Roussin J. Randomized clinical trial investigating the effect of consistent, developmentally-appropriate, and evidence-based multisensory exposures in the NICU. *J Perinatol.* 2021;41(10):2449–2462.

50. Sweeney JK, Gutierrez T. Musculoskeletal implications of preterm infant positioning in the neonatal intensive care unit. *J Perinat Neonatal Nurs.* 2002;16(1):58.

51. Upadhyay J, Singh P, Digal KC, et al. Developmentally supportive positioning policy for preterm low birth weight infants in a tertiary care neonatal unit: a quality improvement initiative. *Indian Pediatr*. 2021;58(8):733–736.

52. McCarty DB, Peat JR, Malcolm WF, et al. Dolichocephaly in preterm infants: prevalence, risk factors, and early motor outcomes. *Am J Perinatol*. 2017;34(4):372–378.

53. Willis S, Hsiao R, Holland RA, et al. Measuring for nonsynostotic head deformities in pre-term infants during NICU management: a pilot study. *Early Hum Dev*. 2019;131:56–62.

54. Kumar P, Carroll KF, Prazad P, et al. Elevated supine midline head position for prevention of intraventricular hemorrhage in VLBW and ELBW infants: a retrospective multi-center study. *J Perinatol*. 2021;41(2):278–285.

55. Romantsik O, Calevo MG, Bruschettini M. Head midline position for preventing the occurrence or extension of germinal matrix-intraventricular haemorrhage in preterm infants. *Cochrane Database Syst Rev*. 2020;7(7):CD012362.

56. Madlinger-Lewis L, Reynolds L, Zarem C, Crapnell T, Inder T, Pineda R. The effects of alternative positioning on preterm infants in the neonatal intensive care unit: a randomized clinical trial. *Res Dev Disabil*. 2014;35(2):490–497.

57. Girolami G, Campbell SK. Efficacy of a neurodevelopmental treatment program to improve motor control of preterm infants. *Pediatr Phys Ther*. 1994;6:175–184.

58. Lee E-J. Effect of neuro-development treatment on motor development in preterm infants. *J Phys Ther Sci*. 2017;29:1095–1097.

59. Liu Y, Li ZF, Zhong YH, et al. Early combined rehabilitation intervention to improve the short-term prognosis of premature infants. *BMC Pediatr*. 2021;21(1):269.

60. Ustad T, Evensen KAI, Campbell SK, et al. Early parent-administered physical therapy for preterm infants: a randomized controlled trial. *Pediatrics*. 2016;138(2):e20160271.

61. Øberg GK, Girolami GL, Campbell SK, et al. Effects of dose on outcomes of a parent-administered exercise program in the neonatal intensive care unit. *Phys Ther*. 2020;100:741.

62. Khurana S, Kane AE, Brown SE, et al. Effect of neonatal therapy on the motor, cognitive, and behavioural development of infants born preterm: a systematic review. *Dev Med Child Neurol*. 2020;62(6):684–692.

63. Garber J. Oral-motor function and feeding intervention. *Phys Occup Ther Pediatr*. 2013;33(1):111–138.

64. Pineda R, Dewey K, Jacobsen A, et al. Non-nutritive sucking in the preterm infant. *Am J Perinatol*. 2019;36(3):268–276.

65. Griffith T, Rankin K, White-Traut R. The relationship between behavioral states and oral feeding efficiency in preterm infants. *Adv Neonatal Care*. 2017;17(1):E12–E19.

66. Borges Nery P, Snider L, Camelo JS Jr, et al. The role of rehabilitation specialists in Canadian NICUs: a 21st century perspective. *Phys Occup Ther Pediatr*. 2019;39(1):33–47.

67. Anderson LJ, Anderson JM. Hand splinting for infants in the intensive care and special care nurseries. *Am J Occup Ther*. 1988;42(4):222–226.

68. Trout SM, Whitaker AT. Management issues of congenital talipes equinovarus in the neonatal intensive care unit: a systematic review. *Foot Ankle Surg*. 2021;27(5):480–485.

69. Gupta M, Pursley DM, Smith VC. Preparing for discharge from the neonatal intensive care unit. *Pediatrics*. 2019;143(6):e20182915.

70. Smith VC, Love K, Goyer E. NICU discharge preparation and transition planning: guidelines and recommendations. *J Perinatol*. 2022;42(suppl 1):7–21.

71. Kang SR, Cho H. Research trends of follow-up care after neonatal intensive care unit graduation for children born preterm: a scoping review. *Int J Environ Res Public Health*. 2021;18(6):3268.

72. Orton JL, Olsen JE, Ong K, et al. NICU graduates: the role of the allied health team in follow-up. *Pediatr Ann*. 2018;47(4):e165–e171.

73. Voller SMB. Follow-up care for high-risk preterm infants. *Pediatr Ann*. 2018;47(4):e142–e146.

74. Hee Chung E, Chou J, Brown KA. Neurodevelopmental outcomes of preterm infants: a recent literature review. *Transl Pediatr*. 2020 Feb;9(Suppl 1):S3–S8. doi: 10.21037/tp.2019.09.10. PMID: 32206579; PMCID: PMC7082240.

75. Harbourne RT, Dusing SC, Lobo MA, et al. Sitting together and reaching to play (START-Play): protocol for a multisite randomized controlled efficacy trial on intervention for infants with neuromotor disorders. *Phys Ther*. 2018;98(6):494–502.

76. Dusing SC, Thacker LR, Galloway JC. Infant born preterm have delayed development of adaptive postural control in the first 5 months of life. *Infant Behav Dev*. 2016;44:49–58.

77. Spittle A, Orton J, Anderson PJ, et al. Early developmental intervention programmes provided post hospital discharge to prevent motor and cognitive impairment in preterm infants. *Cochrane Database Syst Rev*. 2015;2015(11):CD005495.

78. Dusing SC, Burnsed JC, Brown SE, et al. Efficacy of supporting play exploration and early development intervention in the first months of life for infants born very preterm: 3-arm randomized clinical trial protocol. *Phys Ther*. 2020;100(8):1343–1352.

79. Campbell SK, Cole W, Boynewicz K, et al. Behavior during tethered kicking in infants with periventricular brain injury. *Pediatr Phys Ther*. 2015;27(4):403–412.

80. Tripathi T, Dusing S, Pidcoe PE, Xu Y, Shall MS, Riddle DL. A motor learning paradigm combining technology and associative learning to assess prone motor learning in infants. *Phys Ther*. 2019;99(6):807–816.

81. Stuyvenberg CL, Brown SE, Inamdar K, et al. Targeted physical therapy combined with spasticity management changes motor development trajectory for a 2-year-old with cerebral palsy. *J Pers Med*. 2021;11(3):163.

82. Public L No. 108-446. Individuals with Disabilities Education Improvement Act of 2004 (website): https://www.govinfo.gov/app/details/PLAW-108publ446. Accessed September 30, 2022.

RESOURCES

When Your Baby's in the Neonatal Intensive Care Unit

www.kidshealth.org/parent/system/ill/nicu_caring.html
A Mothers Diary: How to Survive the Neonatal Intensive Care Unit, by Menetra Hathron

March of Dimes

Provides information on risk factors for a premature birth, common conditions treated in the NICU, terminology and equipment, prematurity, genetic disorders birth defects, and resources for families.
Cost: Free
http://www.marchofdimes.com

Seating and Wheeled Mobility

Roberta Kuchler O'Shea, PT, DPT, PhD

LEARNING OBJECTIVES

At the end of the chapter, the reader will be able to do the following:

1. Identify the three categories of seating components.
2. Identify the similarities and differences between manual and power mobility.
3. Advocate for appropriate seating and mobility equipment for a child.
4. Recognize laws that impact assistive technology.

CHAPTER OUTLINE

KEY TERMS

Assistive technology device
Assistive technology service

Contoured system
Custom-molded system

Planar system
Wheeled mobility

Assistive technology (AT) is an integral part of modern living and varies from low-level picture books to complex technologies that allow an individual with a disability to live independently. Availability of AT services and equipment spans the rehabilitation spectrum. In this chapter, seating and mobility will be the focus. (This text will not address the widespread availability of AT for computers, communication, home, and worksite modifications.) Prior to delving into descriptions of the equipment, it behooves one to understand the historical and legal developments of the AT field.

Attempts at integrating therapy goals into home and classroom settings have often included homemade adaptive equipment for positioning, mobility, and communication. An AT device is defined by legislation to include any item, piece of equipment, or product system that increases, maintains, or improves an individual's functional status.[1] In contrast an AT service is legally defined as any service—such as physical therapy, occupational therapy, or speech therapy—that directly assists someone with a disability in the selection, acquisition, or training of AT.[1] In recent years, AT has come to encompass a vast range of materials, designs, and applications. It is used to promote the development and acquisition of skills that a client lacks as a result of disease or injury. It can also provide compromises or adaptations in motor function when the attainment of certain skills is unrealistic or impossible.[2] Also referred to as *enabling technology*, AT can often generate new opportunities and open new doors for individuals with physical impairments or overall developmental delays.

Seating and wheeled mobility technologies are available to individuals with disabilities. Activity limitations—such as the inability to sit unsupported, the inability to walk or move from one place to another independently, the inability to effectively use the hands because of a weak or unstable trunk, or the inability to produce speech—are often primary reasons for recommending AT and AT services. Assistive technology that is correctly prescribed and used, especially in therapeutic positioning (adaptive seating), may help prevent secondary impairments such as skin breakdown, cardiopulmonary compromise due to scoliosis or slouched posture, and contractures or deformities due to inadequately supported body segments. Other potential benefits at this level are the reduction of tone or excessive muscle activity and a decrease in pathologic movements.

HISTORICAL OVERVIEW

In the past 3 decades, an explosion in the number and type of assistive devices has occurred. In 1972 the creation of several federally funded rehabilitation engineering centers focused efforts on research and development of new products, as well as on the delivery of services to the consumer.[3] This process brought together professionals from many fields: biomedical and rehabilitation engineering, physical therapy, occupational therapy, speech-language pathology, and special education. The Rehabilitation Engineering and Assistive Technology Society of North America (RESNA), an outgrowth of this shared interest, is an interdisciplinary association of professionals who bring applied technology to persons with disabilities.

Since 1975 many laws have been passed to ensure that the rights of people with disabilities are included in all education and work environments. These laws

include PL 101–476: Education of All Handicapped Children Act; 1986–2004 Amendments to the Individuals with Disabilities Educational Act (IDEA); PL 105–394: Technology-Related Assistance for Individuals with Disabilities Act of 1988 (TRAIDA [Tech Act]); PL 93–112: Rehabilitation Act; and PL 101–336: Americans with Disabilities Act (ADA). These laws have helped focus attention on and create a growing market for new technologies and products. Consumer demands for increased durability and performance have prompted manufacturers to apply technologies created by the aerospace, medical, and information industries to their own products. The field of AT represents a well-established cross-disciplinary specialty.

The 1988 federal legislation known as *TRAIDA*, or the Tech Act, defined ATs and services and recognized the importance of technology in the lives of individuals with disabilities.[2,4] The Assistive Technology Act of 1998 has extended funding to develop permanent comprehensive technology-related programs. All states and territories are eligible for 10 years, and states that have completed the 10 years are eligible for an additional 3 years of federal funding. IDEA funds programs that promote research and technology, and the 1998 Amendment states that AT devices and services be considered on all individualized educational plans (IEPs). In 2000, Quality Indicators for Assistive Technology Services became available to provide practitioners with a description of the essential elements of assessing, ordering, and implementing AT services under the auspices of IDEA.[5] It is the intent of these Indicators to assist therapists in providing appropriate and quality AT devices and services to children, especially young children. The Rehabilitation Act and the ADA protect individuals with disabilities against civil rights violations.

ASSISTIVE TECHNOLOGY TEAM

Team relationships entwine and define pediatric service provision. It is rare that an individual works in isolation with children without input from the families, other professionals, or the children themselves. AT implementation defines the importance and essence of team collaboration.

As in any rehabilitation team, the client/family must play an active role in the selection and procurement of the equipment. The makeup of the team and the setting in which it functions can vary greatly. For example, in many hospitals and rehabilitation centers with comprehensive technology service delivery programs, physicians (especially physiatrists and orthopedic surgeons) may be an integral part of the core team. In schools and residential centers, one or more of the client's primary therapists, along with an equipment supplier, may function as the core team.

A successful team recognizes that each of its members, even a minor player, contributes important information and perspective; communication must be multidirectional. The core team takes the responsibility for imparting information and training to the patient and caregivers to ensure proper use, maintenance, responsibility, and safety of the prescribed devices.

ASSISTIVE TECHNOLOGY FOR MOBILITY

A large portion of this chapter is dedicated to seating and mobility, as it is the most complex system of AT for the physical therapist (PT) and physical therapist assistant (PTA). However, there are several pieces of adaptive mobility equipment that merit discussion.

In order to gain independent mobility, a child may require an ambulation aid. These include canes, axillary crutches, Lofstrand crutches, forward walkers, reverse walkers, and gait trainers. Canes provide minimal balance support to a child. They offer effective assistance if the child has good static and dynamic balance. Canes give the child a stability boost. Some children prefer to use bilateral canes to gain stability. Many children prefer Lofstrand crutches over axillary crutches because they can use their hands for a task and allow the crutches to be suspended from the forearms, thus preventing the crutches from falling to the ground. There is some debate about the use of a forward walker versus a reverse walker. The forward walker may get away from the child as it rolls if the child is slow to pick up his or her feet. The reverse walker may pitch the child posteriorly and does not allow the child to ambulate in a typical alignment with the weight forward. Both seem to be successful in assisting children with ambulation and should be regarded equally. Gait trainers fully support the child and position the trunk in upright midline. It is also possible to position the lower and upper extremities as children use their legs to propel themselves in a walking/gait pattern. Toys that provide on-time mobility access are also important. Consider toy cars with adapted switches

or bumper cars with adaptive seating to allow a child to practice mobility and benefit from social, emotional, and cognitive growth.

SEATING SYSTEMS

The purpose of the seating system is to provide external postural sitting support for the child who has functional limitations due to impairments in musculoskeletal alignment, postural control, muscle tone, or strength. Seating is the interface between the child and the mobility device.[1] The goal is to enable the child to compensate for functional limitations and thereby maximize participation levels (Box 22.1). Letts states that to achieve stable sitting, biomechanical forces and moments in all planes must be balanced. "Good positioning" usually consists of an upright midline orientation of the entire body with a near-vertical alignment of the trunk and head. In children, the "90-90-90" rule is often used to maintain the hips, knees, and ankles at 90 degrees. However, this is not always feasible, typical, or appropriate for every child; and achieving a functional seated position must be assessed on an individual basis. It is important to note that as a child grows, it may not be reasonable (due to a longer leg length) to maintain the knees at 90 degrees. In this case, the decision to go with a different angled front rigging must be made. If the child has significant contractures of the lower extremities or trunk, it may not be possible to position them in 90 degrees of hip, knee, and ankle flexion. Kangas has seriously challenged the idea of static positioning, stating that it is unnatural

---

BOX 22.1   Potential Outcomes of Proper Seating and Positioning

Facilitation of optimal postural control to enable engagement in functional activities
Provision of an optimal balance between stability and mobility in the seated position
Maintenance of neutral skeletal alignment
Prevention of skeletal deformities
Maintenance of tissue integrity
Maintenance of a position of comfort
Decreased fatigue
Enhanced respiratory and circulatory function
Facilitation of caregiver activities

From Cook A, Polgar J. *Cook and Hussey's Assistive Technologies: Principles and Practice.* 3rd ed. St Louis: Mosby; 2008.

and impedes function. In the next section, studies that have examined the effectiveness of seating systems are reviewed, and considerations in prescribing seating systems are discussed.

Measuring the Client

It is imperative to record accurate body segment measurements when fitting a child for a seating system and mobility device. Final measurements should account for 2 or 3 years of potential growth. Figure 22.1 offers a template to assess body measurements. The measurements should be taken with the child seated.

Matching the Intervention to the Client's Level of Need

Postural support systems are typically classified into three levels: linear, generically contoured, and custom molded. The first and least intensive level of intervention is the linear (planar) system; it consists of a flat seat and back (Fig. 22.2). Children with good postural stability, sitting balance, and minimal external postural needs are the most appropriate candidates for this level of intervention. The seat and back are constructed of a solid base (plywood or plastic) covered by foam and upholstered with vinyl or knit fabric. Linear trunk or pelvic supports may be added. Many commercial variations are available, or they can be constructed in the clinic. This system is easily changed and adapted and is typically the least expensive for the client.

The second level of intervention is the generically contoured system, which provides external postural control by increasing the points of contact. The seat and back surfaces include generically contoured layers of foam, air, or fluid that can correspond to the curves of the body (Fig. 22.3). Contours also help distribute pressures more evenly. Contouring can range from simple to aggressive. Simple contouring can improve comfort and stability for many clients, and aggressive contouring may provide enough support for some clients with severe impairments. Table 22.1 lists the varieties of seating that can be fabricated in a clinic from solid bases with varying densities and configurations of foam, air, or fluid materials to create the contours. This level of system can accommodate for growth with modifications or adjustments to the positioning materials.

The third level of intervention is the custom-molded system. It provides an intimate fit by closely conforming to the shape of the client's body, thereby giving the most postural support. When carefully molded, it theoretically provides the greatest amount of pressure relief as well. The time and expense involved in the fabrication of these systems are considerable, and the molding process requires a great deal of skill. In the case of foam–in place technology, the final mold is created and fabricated on site and is ready for use immediately. In other cases, once the desired contoured mold is achieved, the shape is digitized and sent to a central fabrication center. A third option utilizes computer-aided design technology, which allows the clinician to bypass the construction of molds by mapping and digitizing body shape data directly using an instrumented simulator. The information is then transferred digitally to a computer-driven carving machine that produces the final custom-contoured cushion. These more aggressive contours may take the place of a trunk orthosis. It is important to note that custom-molded systems do not allow for growth and cannot be modified. Additionally, if a child is not positioned properly within the molded cushion, high-pressure spots can develop and result in trauma to the underlying soft tissues.

PRESCRIPTION AND APPLICATION OF SEATING SYSTEMS

The scope of this chapter and the rapidly evolving nature of technology preclude a thorough discussion of all options and features of postural support systems. Many excellent resources that describe these in more detail and provide problem-solving lists and charts exist.[1,6,8–10] In this section, attention is focused on some of the most salient points in the decision-making process (Fig. 22.4).

Seat Cushions

In most cases, the seat cushion is the most critical element of the seating system. The use of true linear seats is becoming rarer because most clinicians have found that a small amount of lateral contouring for even the highest-level sitter adds comfort and stability.[8,11] The benefit of adding contours to help relieve pressure problems is evidenced by the number of commercially available air- and fluid-filled pressure management cushions that have foam blocks and wedges to allow customization of cushion shape. Antithrust seats have a block of high-density foam placed just anterior to the ischial tuberosities; the foam block keeps the

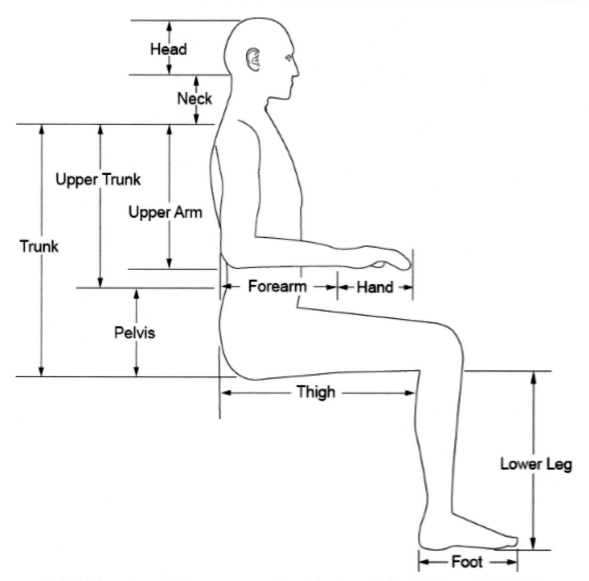

Fig. 22.1 Joint angle and body measurements taken during the evaluation. A_{sit} (right and left), behind hips/popliteal fossa; B (right and left), popliteal fossa/heel; D_{sit}, knee flexion angle; E, sitting surface/pelvic crest; F, sitting surface/axilla; G, sitting surface/shoulder; H, sitting surface/occiput; I, sitting surface/ crown of head; J, sitting surface/hanging elbow; K, width across trunk; L, depth of trunk; M, width across hips; N, heel/toe.

pelvis from sliding forward and equalizes pressure distribution along the thighs.[12] Antithrust design can be added to planar as well as contoured systems, but antithrust design is thought to work best with deep lateral contours of the pelvis and lateral thigh supports (adductor pads).

Seat placement within the wheelchair frame is an important consideration. A thick cushion or inappropriate mounting hardware can place the seat too high, compromising independent propulsion or resulting in loss of independent transfer. Poor seat placement can also change the center of gravity to an unsafe

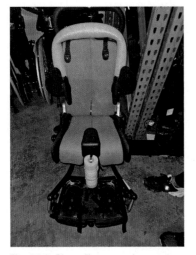

Fig. 22.2 Planar/linear seating system.

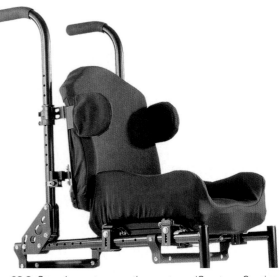

Fig. 22.3 Generic contour seating system. (Courtesy Sunrise Medical, Fresno, CA.)

position. Forward or backward placement, especially in very small children, can affect the knee angle required for foot placement on the footrests and can change the ease of wheeling by affecting access to the wheel rims or loading or unloading the front casters. For individuals who propel with their lower extremities, it is important to maintain a lower seat-to-floor height and a flat front edge of the seat cushion. Often, these individuals find it helpful to bevel the front edge

of the seat to allow full knee flexion without irritating the hamstrings.

Back Cushions

A back support with a gently curved surface can improve lateral trunk stability, posture, and comfort. Simple contouring and lateral support can often be achieved by

TABLE 22.1	**Various Types of Seating Fabrication Materials**	
Cushion Type	**Advantages**	**Disadvantages**
Foam	Inexpensive	Affected by light and air, which cause
	Lightweight	degradation of the foam
	Nothing leaks	Loses shape
Gel/viscous fluid	Good pressure relief	Heavy
	Easier than air to maintain	Chance of leakage
		May bottom out
Air without foam	Lightweight	Less stable
	Waterproof	Chance of puncture/damage
	Good pressure distribution over entire seated surface	High maintenance
	Adjustable via valves to relieve sores or provide postural support	
Thermoplastic elastomer/ urethane honeycomb	Lightweight	Can produce unwanted shear force if used without a cover
	Good support	
	No risk of leakage	
	Machine washable/dryable	
Custom-molded cushions	Designed to meet individual pressure and positioning needs	Expensive
		No ability to modify once fabricated

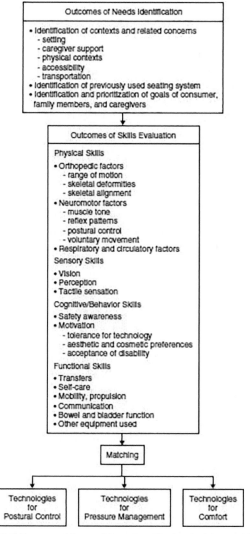

Outcomes of Needs Identification

- Identification of contexts and related concerns
  - setting
  - caregiver support
  - physical contexts
  - accessibility
  - transportation
- Identification of previously used seating system
- Identification and prioritization of goals of consumer, family members, and caregivers

Outcomes of Skills Evaluation

Physical Skills

- Orthopedic factors
  - range of motion
  - skeletal deformities
  - skeletal alignment
- Neuromotor factors
  - muscle tone
  - reflex patterns
  - postural control
  - voluntary movement
- Respiratory and circulatory factors

Sensory Skills

- Vision
- Perception
- Tactile sensation

Cognitive/Behavior Skills

- Safety awareness
- Motivation
  - tolerance for technology
  - aesthetic and cosmetic preferences
  - acceptance of disability

Functional Skills

- Transfers
- Self-care
- Mobility, propulsion
- Communication
- Bowel and bladder function
- Other equipment used

Matching

Technologies for Postural Control

Technologies for Pressure Management

Technologies for Comfort

Fig. 22.4 Framework for seating and positioning decision-making. (From Cook A, Polgar J. *Cook and Hussey's Assistive Technologies: Principles and Practice.* 3rd ed. St Louis: Mosby; 2008.)

shaping the back cushion. Many back cushions are available with accompanying customized support options. More aggressive contouring can be achieved using high-density foam blocks/wedges. A custom-molded back should be used for clients with severely fixed spinal deformities. Some children who need specific contact and support along the paraspinals but are still growing can benefit from a hybrid back cushion. This type of back cushion is custom molded and only contours along the paraspinal region and flattens laterally. Linear lateral trunk supports

are then added to the contoured back. This allows for growth and maintains significant proprioceptive input along the spine.

Sagittal plane alignment of the spine has traditionally been adjusted using lumbar rolls; however, control of sagittal curves begins with the pelvis and sacrum rather than the lumbar spine.[8,11]

Pelvic Stabilization

The most effective technique for pelvic stabilization control continues to remain largely a matter of clinical opinion and user preference.[8,11,12] A pelvic positioning device placed at a 45-degree angle at the seat-back junction is the most typical form of pelvic stabilization. For high-functioning individuals, placement of the belt across the anterior thighs, just in front of the hips, allows more natural active trunk and pelvic mobility.[8] The pelvic positioning belt can use a two-point or four-point attachment system. The four-point system allows for more comprehensive control of the pelvis and greater distribution of the pressures maintaining postural control. It is imperative that the pelvis be secured into the seating system properly so that the child cannot slide forward out of the seat.

Dynamic pelvic stabilization uses individually contoured pads that fit around the pelvis, with a pivot mechanism allowing anterior-posterior tilting of the pelvis without loss of stability.[13] Adjustments allow deformity accommodation, control of the amount and direction of tilting, and a dynamic force to return the pelvis to a neutral position. Anterior knee blocks, another form of pelvic stabilization, direct a long-axis force up the length of the femurs to counter sliding of the pelvis.[8,9]

Angles

There is no consensus about the effects of seat and spatial angles on alignment and function. Factors that must be considered in determining fixed angles include severity and nature of postural tone abnormalities, contractures and deformities, level of motor control for sitting, and design and purpose of the mobility base. Although the concept of upright 90-90-90 sitting is theoretically sound, it may not be a biomechanically possible option for many clients. Slight anterior wedging of the seat may improve head alignment or keep very young children from sliding. Opening the hip angle (tipping the front seat edge) may be necessary when hip extension contractures are present. Allowing the knees to flex brings the feet back under the seat and reduces the rotary force on the pelvis, thus minimizing the effect of tight hamstrings.

The anteriorly tipped seat has potential benefits for clients with hypo-extensible lower extremity musculature, but fair to good upper body control, who "sacral sit" on a flat surface. It is also used for the more severely involved child in a forward-lean position with a solid anterior chest support. Good pelvic stabilization must be achieved to prevent sliding. Unfortunately, when anteriorly tipped seating is used in wheelchairs, the client often lacks enough knee extension to keep the heels from interfering with caster movement.

In some cases, the seating system components can be instrumental in addressing the needs of clients with severe and abrupt extensor spasms.[14,15] Often, the severity of tone or spasms is exacerbated by the rigidity of a conventional system. These systems use hinges, pivot points, and springs to allow movement of the seat or back with the child and provide a gentle returning force. Some clients who use these systems have exhibited a decrease in the severity of spasms or fluctuating tone over a period of weeks, as well as improved comfort and ease of transfers.

Upholstery

Upholstery for seat and back cushions can be made out of a variety of materials. When choosing a covering, consideration must be given to whether the child is incontinent, whether the child is typically hot, and who will care for the coverings. Vinyl is a durable cushion covering; however, it can be hot and slippery and typically cannot be removed from the seating system. It also limits the ability of the foam underneath it to conform to the shape of the user. Synthetic knit fabrics with waterproof backing are also a popular choice of covering. They are less slippery, thus decreasing shear, and they can be removed for easy cleaning. Ideally, a child should have at least two sets of cushion covers so that one can be laundered while the other is in use.

Front Riggings

Front riggings, or leg supports, which are considered a component of the mobility base, are discussed here because of their direct influence on the entire seating system. Elevated leg rests are set farther forward of the seat than fixed leg rests and can contribute to forward

sliding on the seat or poor positioning of the feet for weight-bearing. They should never be ordered unless they are specifically required.

Choice of footrests on small pediatric chairs can be especially difficult because they may interfere with caster action. Footplates that extend backward under the seat are helpful when clients have tight hamstrings. Footplates can be positioned parallel to the floor or angled to match a client's foot/ankle deformity or their orthotic ankle angle. Shoe holders and foot straps maintain the feet in the desired location to assist with lower body stability and weight-bearing. For clients with deformities or limited joint movement, forcing the foot into neutral alignment on the footrest may impose undesirable stresses at the knees or hips.[8] Other clients who exhibit natural postural adjustments and placement of the feet during weight shifting and active movement should have their feet left free. If the child is learning to transfer independently, can already transfer independently, or is using a sit-to-stand transfer, the front riggings and footplates should be able to swing out of the way. An exception to this rule must be made for the client who uses tapered front riggings and fixed footplates for performance. These users will transfer out of their mobility base with the front riggings in a forward position.

Lateral and Medial Supports

Lateral trunk supports range from simple, flat, padded blocks to contoured, wraparound supports. Swivel or swing-away mounting hardware allows the wraparound supports to fit properly and enables the child to transfer into and out of the seating system easily.

Contoured seats usually provide the most effective lateral thigh and pelvic support, as well as good pressure relief. Square or rectangular pads such as lateral thigh supports can maintain position of the lower extremities and allow for growth. Medial thigh supports (abductor wedges or pommels) maintain hip alignment in neutral or slight abduction and should not function to stretch tight adductors or prevent forward sliding of the pelvis. Removable or swing-away pommels facilitate transfers and urinal or catheter use.

Anterior Supports

Anterior trunk supports maintain the spine erect and upright over the pelvis. Butterfly-shaped straps should not be used because they present extreme safety hazards. Instead, anterior support can be gained via an H or Y harness or anterior chest strap. An anterior chest support may be added to help secure the trunk within the seating system. Care must be taken to position the horizontal chest strap at the level between the mid rib-cage and the sternal notch so that the chest strap does not become a choking hazard if the child slides forward in the seating system. Padded axillary straps, sometimes known as *Bobath straps* or *backpack design straps,* also help maintain the trunk in an upright posture. They attach to the underside of the lateral thoracic support, are directed superiorly and medially over the front of the axilla, and attach at the top of the backrest, controlling shoulder protraction without crossing the chest. Trefler and Angelo reported no significant clinical differences in performance for children with cerebral palsy after completing a switch activation task while using different anterior chest supports. They concluded that style of anterior chest support should be based on client preference.

Headrest

Facilitating good head position can be one of the most difficult tasks. In the almost totally immobile client, the head is the one body part that is likely to move, and poor head positioning can make an otherwise effective postural support system fail. On the other hand, barium-swallow studies suggest that some clients with the most severe physical and cognitive impairments may need to adopt a forward-hanging head position to cope with increased oral secretions or reflux.[17] Correcting these clients' heads to a position that "looks good" may increase their risk of aspiration or choking.[18]

Support under the occiput provides better head support than a flat contact on the back of the head. Neck rings, two-step head supports, and contoured head supports are available in several options. Static and dynamic forehead straps position and maintain the head securely on the headrest. Collars with soft anterior chin support (which are not attached to the wheelchair) may be effective for clients who have constant neck flexion, regardless of seating angles. Care must be taken that the head support does not unduly block the child's peripheral visual fields or put undue stress on the cervical spine. Additionally, head supports can be the ideal mounting location for switches that control the AT or augmentative communication systems.

Upper Extremity Supports

Cutout trays are the most typical form of upper extremity support and can be designed for a multitude of special purposes. Posterior elbow blocks help reduce the tendency to retract the arms and maintain the upper extremities in a forward position. Clients with severe dystonia often prefer wrist or arm cuffs to reduce unwanted movement of one or both arms.

WHEELED MOBILITY

The purpose of the mobility base is dependent on the child's level of function. For some, the primary purpose will be independent mobility, and the therapist must determine how best to achieve this. For others, the purpose of the base is to provide a means of being transported by a companion, and this must be accomplished in a comfortable and efficient manner. In either case, the base serves the additional role of supporting the seating system. Selection of a mobility base requires consideration of the seating system it will support, the environments in which it will function, and the client's lifestyle (Box 22.2). Assessment for a new mobility base should ideally be done at the same time as assessment and simulation for the postural support system because much of the same information regarding the client and the environment must be gathered.

Many factors affect performance and mobility in users of manual wheelchairs, including human physiologic capacities such as strength and endurance, which are dependent on the user's diagnosis, age, sex, lifestyle, and build.[19] The position of the individual within the wheelchair, particularly in relation to the handrims or other propulsion methods, determines the mechanical advantage for the user to act on the chair. Wheelchair factors that affect mobility are rolling resistance, control,

---

BOX 22.2   Factors to Consider When Selecting a Wheelchair

Consumer profile: Disability, date of onset, prognosis, size, and weight

Consumer needs: Activities, contexts of use (e.g., accessibility, indoor/outdoor), preferences, transportation, reliability, durability, cost

Physical and sensory skills: Range of motion (ROM), motor control, strength, vision, perception

Functional skills: Transfers and ability to propel (manual or powered)

From Cook A, Polgar J. *Cook and Hussey's Assistive Technologies: Principles and Practice.* 3rd ed. St Louis: Mosby; 2008.

maneuverability, stability, and dynamic behavior. These depend on the quality and construction of the wheelchair and factors such as weight, rigidity of the frame, wheel alignment, mass distribution, and suspension. Wheelchair propulsion in children with spinal cord injury is similar to that in a neurologically matched group of adults.[17a] The adults wheeled faster, but the children spent a similar proportion of the wheeling cycle in propulsion, and the angular changes in the kinematics of the elbow and shoulder over time were the same for both groups. Therefore, applications intended to improve wheeling efficiency for adults may be appropriate for children as well.

The developmental consequences of impaired movement are another area of functional limitation and disability. The typical developing infant's experience with independent forward progression has a profound impact on perceptual, cognitive, emotional, and social processes.[21] For the immobile child, early provision of technology forms of mobility has the potential to minimize deficits in spatial, cognitive, affective, and social functions. Prone scooters, caster carts, and walkers are alternatives for some young children with functional upper extremities. For the child with more severe involvement, however, early power mobility offers the best choice and allows the child to increase his or her self-initiated movements during play.[19]

Studies indicate that children as young as 9 to 12 months can successfully learn independent power mobility within a few weeks.[23] Benefits attributed to the use of power mobility include increases in self-initiated behaviors, including change in location, rate of interaction with objects, and frequency of communication.[13,24] Others concluded that social participation of wheeled mobility users is a complex phenomenon.[18] However, the benefits frequently reported are increased peer interaction; increased interest in other forms of locomotion, including walking; increased family integration such as inclusion in outings; and decreased perception of helplessness by family members.[18] Field[25] concluded that the major issues affecting powered mobility performance are ability, technology features, environment, driving as an activity, and the interactions between these variables.

Training is always an important facet of ordering power mobility devices for children. Hasdai, Jessel, and Weiss[26] used simulator programs to provide training to clients aged 7 to 22 years. They determined that inexperienced drivers improved their overall driving performance after simulator training. The internet and virtual reality platforms have become training sites as well.

Selection of a Mobility Base

The goal in selecting a mobility base is to provide an appropriate means of efficiently getting from one location to another. It is inappropriate to require someone to rely on his or her everyday mobility for exercise. Prohibiting a child with marginal ambulation from using a manual wheelchair or prohibiting a child with marginal manual wheelchair skills from using a power wheelchair places both at risk for poor functional and academic performance due to excessive energy expenditure. A creative and structured fitness program is a more appropriate way of addressing strength and cardiovascular endurance goals.

It is generally agreed that positioning needs take precedence over the issuance of a mobility device. At the same time, the design of the seating system should maximize potential for independent function in the wheelchair whenever possible. This in turn influences chair modifications and the interface hardware needed. For example, if a 3-inch generically contoured foam cushion is necessary for pressure relief, but the client has short extremities (as in myelodysplasia), both independent transfers and wheeling will be more difficult. A possible solution is to order a chair frame with a lower seat height and without upholstery so that drop brackets can be used to lower the cushion between the seat rails. Variable seat-to-back angles allow adjustments of tilt and recline throughout the day. Tilt is useful for relief of pressure or relief of trunk or neck fatigue, and it provides a combination of active sitting and rest positions. When in a tilt system, the seat-to-back angle does not change. It is important to know that in order to get pressure relief under the Ischial Tuberosities, the client must be tilted approximately 45 degrees. Recline is useful for relief of fatigue, for hip or back pain, and for catheterizations or other hygiene procedures that must be performed in the chair. In a reclining seating system, the seat-to-back angle changes as the reclining position changes.

To assess driving skills and controller placement once the desired seating position has been obtained, some seating simulators can be mounted on a power base. A remote, attendant-held control can override the user's control, ensuring safety and appropriate feedback during assessment and training. The client should be offered test drives in a variety of bases, using appropriately simulated postural support wherever possible. Typically, children with adequate cognition of cause and effect can learn to drive well with practice.

The first step in selecting a mobility base is to determine what type of functional mobility is desired. Three general types of mobility bases are (1) companion chairs for dependent wheeling, (2) standard manual wheelchairs, and (3) power wheelchairs. Ideally, the selection should be based on the potential level of independent mobility, but other factors often come into play, including methods of transportation, type of housing, availability of training or supervision, and availability of funding.

The second step is choosing the style of the base. Within each type, there are several styles with different features and performance characteristics. Factors that influence this choice are the level and type of seating system required, the level of independence in other skills such as transfers and activities of daily living, the specific environments in which the chair will be used, the method of transportation, and the needs of caregivers.

Selection of size may influence both the style and type chosen and is based on client size, expected growth rate, growth capabilities of the chair itself, and the size and style of the seating system. Mobility bases designed specifically for pediatric clients are available in a variety of sizes and designs. Growth capabilities have been greatly improved as funding sources have demanded longer life from purchased items.

The final step is choosing the model and manufacturer of the chair. Often, the finer details of construction are important at this stage such as the proportions of the chair; angles; orientations; adjustability of parts such as footrests and armrests; and swing-away, detachment, or folding mechanisms. Other important influencing factors are performance characteristics, styling, comfort, rate of breakdown, availability of parts, service record, and cost. Regional preferences for various models and manufacturers are evident across North America.

Dependent Propulsion Wheelchairs

Dependent propulsion wheelchairs, transporter chairs, and dependent mobility bases are intended for individuals who will not need to access the wheels for independent mobility, including those with the most severe impairments and very young children (Fig. 22.5). In other cases, this type of chair may be used as backup transportation for a child who ambulates or uses a power wheelchair. Many styles of companion wheelchairs exist, and occasionally, manual wheelchairs are used as companion chairs. Companion chairs often include firm seats and backs and have a wide variety of positioning components as options. Alternatively, contoured or

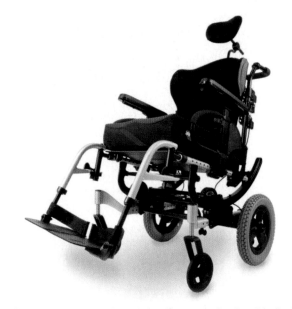

Fig. 22.5 A companion chair. (Courtesy Sunrise Medical, Fresno, CA.)

custom-molded seating systems can be fabricated and mounted on these frames. Some of these chairs can be used as vehicular transport seats and comply with federal safety standards. Others are designed for very young children and look and perform like a stroller.

When choosing a dependent mobility base, the primary caregiver must be considered a user as well. Attention should be given to his or her comfort and ease of use, including push handle height, rolling resistance, maneuverability, and ease of disassembly and transport. Parents of young children who are receiving their first mobility base and seating system may be very sensitive to the need for a wheelchair. Mobility bases that look like strollers are popular and are often much less threatening. Some funding sources deny stroller bases because of their limitations in growth and adaptability if the child's independent capabilities progress.

Manual tilt and recline features are incorporated into many companion chairs. A fixed angle of tilt or recline can be useful when designing the seating system for some clients. For others, the ability to vary the amount of tilt or recline throughout the day is critical for prevention of pressure sores, fatigue, and discomfort.

Manual Wheelchairs

The standard manual wheelchair has two large wheels, usually in back, for independent propulsion, and two

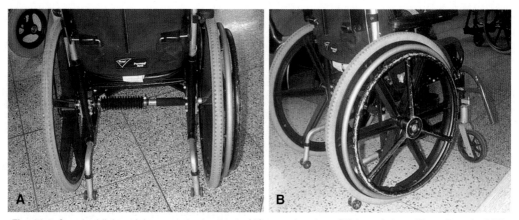

Fig. 22.6 Standard lightweight manual wheelchair. **(A)** posterior view; **(B)** lateral view. (From Campbell SK, Vander Linden DW, Palisano RJ. *Physical Therapy for Children*. 6th ed. Philadelphia PA: Elsevier; 2022.)

small swiveling casters in front (Fig. 22.6). Manual wheelchairs are often chosen as dependent mobility bases as well because of their ability to accept custom-designed seating systems, their ease of use, and their tilt and recline options. Lightweight and durable metals and fabrics, alternative wheel placement, improved frame proportions and designs, adjustability, and adaptability to custom seating have all helped streamline the manual wheelchair to improve its efficiency and control, ease of transfers, portability, and appearance. Lightweight chairs with the large wheels configured in front (the seating system is reversed) are much easier for young children to propel for short distances indoors. For the very active person, ultra-lightweight, high-performance chairs incorporate rigid frames and high-quality bearings for optimal performance. The serious athlete can find specialized designs dedicated to specific performance needs; these chairs barely resemble the traditional concept of a wheelchair.

One-arm-drive wheelchairs are designed for individuals with significant asymmetry of upper extremity strength and function that prevents bimanual propulsion. The classic style is the double-handrim on one side, with a linkage system to the other wheel. It is very important that a child has the opportunity to try this type of device before it is ordered and purchased to ensure it is a good match for the child's abilities and mobility patterns.

Power Mobility

Hays[17] described four functional categories of children using power mobility. The first group includes children who will never ambulate and who experience no independent mobility without the use of a power device. The second group includes children with inefficient mobility; that is, they ambulate or use a manual wheelchair but with unacceptable functional speed or endurance. The third group consists of children who have lost independent mobility through disease, brain injury, or spinal cord trauma. For this group, the developmental implications of independent mobility may be less important, but the acceptance of assisted mobility is a more significant issue. The fourth group includes children who require assisted mobility temporarily, either because they gain new ambulation skills through surgery or maturation or they recover lost function.

Advances in technology have brought independent power mobility to a greater number of individuals with severe disabilities than ever before. A wide variety of power bases and options are available, with more reliable and precise controls than ever before possible (Fig. 22.7).

The three main types of power wheelchairs are (1) the conventional design with integral seat and chassis (evolved from the traditional tubular manual wheelchair frame), (2) the powerbase or modular design with separate seat and chassis, and (3) scooters with either three- or four-wheeled platforms. Power chairs may be ordered with seats that tilt; backs that recline; and units that recline and tilt, take the user from sit to stand, include seat elevation, have leg rests that elevate, and headrests that adjust—all with the touch of a switch. Manufacturers have responded to an increased

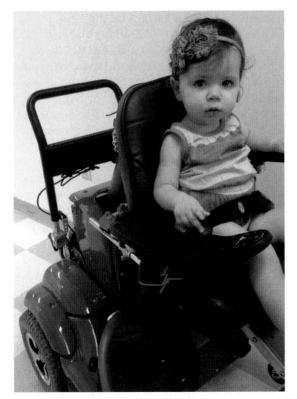

Fig. 22.7 Toddler sized power wheelchair. (From Campbell SK, Vander Linden DW, Palisano RJ. *Physical Therapy for Children.* 6th ed. Philadelphia PA: Elsevier; 2022.)

demand for pediatric power wheelchairs by producing wheelchairs that are lighter in weight, correctly proportioned for children, and have growth capabilities. Major advances in electronics have produced a greater variety of controls that are easier to access, more durable, and easier to adjust and customize. Power chairs are available in rear-wheel-, midwheel-, or front-wheel-drive options. The front-wheel and midwheel drives allow the user a tighter turning radius.

The style of power mobility base chosen will depend in part on the client's upper body control. Scooters are steered using a tiller that requires a significant amount of upper extremity active ROM and sitting balance. The control functions are usually mounted on the tiller and require a grip-type action of the thumb or fingers. Jones[19] described a range of scooters from "light duty mall crawlers to heavy-duty barnyard rut jumpers."[19] Scooters are easier to dismantle and transport in the trunk of a car and look least like a wheelchair. Although they remain popular among adults,

funding is not always an option because of their limited indoor mobility and poor vehicle tiedown capabilities. Manufacturers have responded by making them more rugged and suited to outdoor use. Whereas wheelchair bases are generally easy to adapt to a seating system, scooter-seating systems have little room for adjustability and adaptability.

The conventional and powerbase designs offer the greatest range of seating and control options. The entire seating unit can be removed from the pedestal mount of the modular base. Direct-drive motors of the powerbase improve power and control in turning. Front-wheel, midwheel, and rear-wheel drives offer different advantages and disadvantages in stability while driving and stopping, stability during recline or tilt, maneuverability in tight spaces, and ability to climb curbs. The type of drive system chosen for any given client must be as carefully considered as any other component of the wheelchair and seating system.

Power recline and power tilt capabilities offer excellent alternatives to individuals who need position changes throughout a long day of sitting. Power tilt and recline enable the user to perform different functions as needed because of pain, fatigue, or pressure concerns associated with sitting too long. The act of reclining, however, causes shearing of tissues due to the disproportionate movement between the client and the seating system. On returning to the upright position, most clients will have shifted position in the system, and the more complex the seating system, the more significant the effects. Power recliners are available in low-shear and zero-shear models to help address these problems. Power tilt-in-space models work well for the client who has severe hypertonia or contractures and cannot tolerate having the seat-to-back angle opened up or who, once having done so, cannot return to an upright position without significant sliding. Controls for powered wheelchairs are available in two basic types: proportional and digital. The former has a proportional relationship between movement of the joystick and speed of the chair or sharpness of turning, whereas the latter has an on/off relationship to chair movement. An example of a proportional control is a standard joystick found on many powered wheelchairs. It is customarily set up for hand access, mounted on either the right or left armrest. The joystick spindle moves in a 360-degree arc, allowing the user to achieve smooth, fluid turns.

The movement of the joystick controls the speed and the direction of the wheelchair. An alternative to the standard joystick is a joystick that is smaller and more compact. This feature allows a great deal of flexibility for joystick placement and requires specific mounting hardware to secure the control in the required location. Proportional joysticks are also available in short-throw models. The short throw model requires less movement and force for activation than the typical joystick. Joysticks are also available and are available in heavy-duty models that can withstand a great deal of force. Specialized joysticks that can be positioned for and activated using head control are available for some wheelchairs.

A digital control option may consist of four separate switches, with each switch controlling one direction—forward, reverse, left, and right. There are a variety of commercially available mechanical switches available for selection of the most appropriate switch for a child. Use of individual switches during assessment allows for evaluation of different configurations. For example, the switches may be separated and set up in arrays to evaluate head control, or each of the four switches may be positioned at different body sites. Digital controls tend to be less smooth while turning and changing between directions when compared with a proportional control because each direction is controlled by a separate switch with a separate electronic connection.

The recognition that age is no longer the determining factor in the successful use of powered mobility has helped define selection criteria. Children younger than 2 years have successfully used powered mobility independently as their primary means of mobility.[22] Furumasu, Tefft, and Guerette[20] developed an assessment to determine a child's readiness for powered mobility. This tool is based on Piagetian theories of development and evaluates the child on several learning domains. Furumasu, Tefft, and Guerette[20] also have developed a 6-hour protocol for instruction of young children. The protocol includes activities performed in increasingly more complex environments ranging from free play in an open gym to activities performed in community environments such as the mall or clinic.

An alternative perspective is that children may learn spatial relationships implicitly through training in a powered device.[21,27] Morgan provided a compelling argument for powered mobility for very young children based on the importance of mobility rather than "readiness for driving" skills. It was suggested that the child be allowed to explore movement in the device over a period of time, initially being restricted to a single direction in a small, safe environment. As the child's control over the powered device improves and verbal labels for what she or he is doing are provided, the concept of independent mobility will develop. Joystick- or switch-activated toys that are available at local toy stores make an excellent inexpensive alternative for power training of young children when the devices can be suitably adapted for seating and control.[27]

Simulators have proved to be successful training tools.[1] Inexperienced drivers following a simulator driving program improved their accuracy and performance. Whizz-Kidz in the United Kingdom provides a training program that includes basic, intermediate, and advanced training for manual and powered wheelchair users. The children are paired with a spotter and buddy to learn advanced skills that allow them to be safer and more independent in the community. Program information can be found at www.whizz-kidz.org.uk.

Virtual reality (VR) technology has enabled video gaming experiences to become wheelchair driver training experiences.[18,28] Bunning and colleauges investigated the effectiveness of wheelchair training using virtual environments.[28] All six participants demonstrated improved skills; however, they agreed that the VR wheelchair was more difficult to control than their own wheelchair. The authors recommended that a VR training environment is useful, although care must be taken not to make the environment overly complicated.[28] Criteria for safe driving include the ability to turn the chair on and off, follow a straight course, turn both left and right, back the chair up, maneuver around objects and persons, and stop quickly.[28]

The marginal driver is one of any age who may show borderline cognitive or physical skills or whose visual-perceptual skills interfere with driving ability. With supervision, these individuals may do well driving in a familiar setting, such as their school, but are not successful in novel or unpredictable community settings. The value of a powered wheelchair in increasing self-esteem and promoting independence in specific skills must be carefully weighed against the expense and amount of training and supervision required.

Several practical considerations are essential for the selection of powered mobility. Building accessibility and maneuvering space will affect where and how the device is used. Often, the powered wheelchair is stored and maintained at school, and a manual base is used at home. Care and maintenance of a powered wheelchair are more complex than for manual systems. Transportation is also a more complicated issue. Some school districts refuse to transport certain types of powered mobility devices such as scooters because they lack transportation-compliant tie-down brackets. The family may need a van for transporting the wheelchair, and a ramp or a lift may be required for loading and unloading because of the significant weight of the system. Responsibility for supervision, training, and routine wheelchair maintenance should be determined prior to ordering any system.

It is possible that many of these concepts could actually be taught through training in a power device. Kangas[29] provides a compelling argument for an experiential power mobility assessment for very young children that is based not on "readiness for driving" skills, but on the need for assistive mobility in any or all environments. She suggests that the child be allowed to explore movement in the device over a period of many sessions by first being restricted to a single turning direction in a small, safe environment. Only after the child has experienced going and stopping for the sake of being able to go again has he or she experienced mobility without regard for direction or purpose. This parallels the development of independent walking in toddlers. The child is never praised for "good driving" because this is meaningless. As the child's control over mobility expands and verbal labels for what is being accomplished are provided, the concepts described previously will develop. Power toys available at local toy stores make an excellent inexpensive alternative for power training of young children when the devices can be suitably adapted for seating and control.

TRANSPORTATION SAFETY

The US society is generally mobile and on the go. This includes children and adults who use wheeled mobility. In recent years RESNA and the American National Standards Institute (ANSI) have set federal standards for using wheelchairs within vehicle transportation. Best practice dictates that when at all possible, wheelchair users should transfer out of their wheelchair and into an age- or weight-appropriate vehicle seat with occupant restraint systems that meet all the federal safety standards. The wheelchair should be stored and secured within the vehicle to prevent it from becoming a harmful projectile.

If the wheelchair user cannot transfer, he or she should be seated in a wheelchair frame that meets ANSI/RESNA/WC19 standards. These wheelchairs have been frontal crash tested and have several advantageous features for use in vehicular transport. A WC19-compliant wheelchair should be used with a wheelchair tiedown and occupant restraint system (WTORS). Restraint systems that meet WTORS standards will be labeled as *SAE J2249*. Four tiedown straps are attached to strong places on the wheelchair frame, such as the welded frame joints. Attachment points should be as high as possible but below the seat surface. Rear tiedown straps should maintain a 30- to 45-degree angle with the vehicle floor. The wheelchair is secured to the floor of the vehicle at four identifiable crash-tested sites. It is imperative to face the wheelchair and occupant toward the front of the vehicle.

WC19 includes set standards for lateral stability of a wheelchair within a forward-moving vehicle because wheelchair users are often injured if the wheelchair tips after a quick stop or sharp turn in non-crash conditions. Effective May 2002, regulations included a wheelchair occupant crashworthy strap over the shoulder and pelvic belt that attaches to the side of the vehicle, across the user and is secured to the wheelchair frame. This configuration allows for restraint systems that fit more securely.

Wheelchair occupants should ride in an upright position with the back reclined less than 30 degrees. The headrest should be positioned to support the head and neck, and trays should be removed and secured. It must be noted that the pelvic positioning belt and the anterior chest support discussed previously are not considered occupant restraints for use in a motor vehicle.

EFFECTS OF MANAGED CARE ON ACQUISITION OF ASSISTIVE TECHNOLOGY

State-funded Medicaid programs, traditionally a major source of funding for children with disabilities, have contracted much of their coverage to private managed care insurance organizations, and in many cases, this has affected accessibility to durable medical equipment and specialized devices.[8,16] Denials for requested items may increase, either because a narrower interpretation is used in determining medical necessity or because nonstandard or customized items do not fit the billing codes. The time between the initial request and approval may be prolonged if the reviewers are less experienced in the needs of children with physical disabilities and require more explanation, making repeated requests and justification necessary. Choice of products may be affected because the amount that will be paid is often based on simpler adult equipment designs and does not cover the full cost of more expensive or more customized pediatric designs.

The capitation rate paid to medical equipment suppliers is often inadequate to cover actual expenses, thereby cutting profit margins and making it difficult to provide and service sophisticated or customized equipment. Medical and equipment needs of individuals with disabilities are much higher than many private companies anticipate. If a managed care company discontinues its contract for state Medicaid patients, this could leave those individuals with little or no choice of coverage and may require a change of provider. There is often a struggle with reconciling the variety of devices that are available for achieving independent function with the increasing restrictions in funding and availability. Therapists should feel comfortable writing additional support letters or letters of appeal for equipment that has been denied funding on first request. Additional information regarding the medical necessity of the device or components, stating the critical importance for the technology and the consequences that can result if the technology is not provided should be emphatically stated in the initial funding request and in all additional letters.

CASE STUDY OF A CHILD WITH SEATING AND MOBILITY DEVICES

Examination

History

General demographics: Anthony is an 11-year-old White male, and English is his primary language.

Social: Anthony attends 5th grade in an included classroom at his local public school. He is in Boy Scouts, on the school bowling team, and is involved in his church.

Growth and development: Anthony is left-hand dominant. He was born 8 weeks prematurely and contracted meningitis shortly after birth.

Living environment: Anthony lives with his two parents and his younger brother in an accessible single-family home. His father is a physical therapist.

History of current condition: Anthony needs a new seating and mobility system.

Functional status and activity level: Anthony requires minimum to moderate assistance with dressing and toileting. He can independently feed himself. He transfers with min-mod assist of 1. Anthony is independent in driving his power wheelchair indoors, within his community, and at school.

Medications: Anthony takes oral baclofen to decrease his spasticity.

History of current condition: Anthony received his first wheelchair at age 3 years. He initially used a linear seat and hybrid custom-molded back cushion with linear laterals on a power mobility system controlled by a joystick. It took him 6 months of driver training and practice to learn to drive the power chair independently.

Systems Review

Cardiopulmonary: There are no known pathologies or impairments.

Integumentary: There are no known pathologies or impairments. He has no history of pressure sores, and bilateral lower extremity scars are well healed.

Musculoskeletal: Bilateral de-rotation osteotomies 2 years ago.

Neuromuscular: See Tests and Measures.

Tests and Measures

Endurance: Anthony is able to perform all activities required of him without difficulty. He does not become short of breath or fatigued.

Anthropometric characteristics: Anthony is a slender adolescent of average height and weight for his age.

Arousal/attention/cognition: Within normal limits (WNL).

Assistive and adaptive devices: Anthony uses bilateral solid ankle ankle-foot orthoses (AFOs). He uses

CASE STUDY OF A CHILD WITH SEATING AND MOBILITY DEVICES—cont'd

utensil modifications so that he can independently feed himself. He uses a wheel-in shower with water sprayer and a raised toilet seat in the bathroom. He uses an adapted computer at school and home for educational purposes.

Community integration: Anthony is fully integrated into his community and school.

Cranial nerve integrity: Intact. Anthony wears glasses for visual acuity.

Environmental barriers: Anthony's school is a single-level structure with an accessible playground. He rides a wheelchair-accessible school bus to and from school. Anthony's home has recently been structurally modified to allow for wheelchair-accessible common areas (kitchen, living room, bathroom, den) and an accessible bedroom suite. An elevator was installed to allow Anthony access to the basement area. Both front and rear home entrances are wheelchair accessible.

Gait/locomotion/balance: Anthony has excellent sitting balance. He requires upper extremity support to maintain standing. Anthony can ambulate with both hands supported by another person but gains independent locomotion via his power wheelchair. Anthony uses a manual beach wheelchair (constructed of polyvinyl chloride tubing, mesh seat and back, and large inflated rubber wheels) when at the beach.

Integumentary integrity: All lower extremity scars are well healed.

Motor function: Anthony has spastic quadriplegia. He has increased spasticity in all four limbs that fluctuates with his activity level. He can roll and sit independently and transfer sit stand with min-mod assist of 1. When moving, he tends to be influenced by upper extremity flexion synergies and lower extremity extension synergies.

Gross motor function classification system level 4: Self-mobility with limitations. Child uses power mobility outdoors and in community.

Muscle performance: Modified Ashworth Spasticity Scale grade of 3; considerable increase in muscle tone, passive movement difficult.

Neuromotor development: Anthony's overall development is significantly influenced by his cerebral palsy, and he has a dominant startle reflex. He can volitionally move all extremities with effort. Anthony is left-handed and can easily move his left upper extremity and use his left hand to type and drive his power wheelchair. Anthony wears bilateral AFOs that fit him well. His current seating system and mobility devices no longer meet his needs. He has outgrown the customized seating system, and his mobility device is well worn and in need of repair. Anthony uses

an adaptive computer with a modified keyboard for his schoolwork.

Pain: Anthony has no complaints of pain.

Posture: Anthony is relatively symmetric when in his seating system. He tends to laterally flex to the left when sitting unsupported.

All ROM measurements are WNL except:

Left (Degrees)	Motion	Right (Degrees)
0	Ankle dorsiflexion	0
0	Ankle inversion	0
−5	Knee extension	−5
0	Hip extension	0
25	Hip abduction	20
0	Hip internal rotation	0
WNL	Wrist extension	0
WNL	Wrist pronation	To neutral
−10	Elbow extension	−10
100	Shoulder abduction	100
110	Shoulder flexion	110

Reflex integrity: Anthony has a positive Babinski sign bilaterally.

Self-care: Anthony requires minimal assistance for dressing and toileting. He can independently feed himself but requires assistance for food preparation. Anthony can independently manage his hygiene and oral care.

Evaluation
Prognosis
Anthony currently requires a new seating and mobility system. He needs a contoured seating system to maintain his musculoskeletal system in neutral and minimize deformities. He will continue to be independent and maintain good musculoskeletal alignment with a new system.

Direct Intervention
Coordination/Communication/Documentation
To obtain new seating and mobility equipment, Anthony will require a medical prescription, as well as a medical need form from his physician and therapists.

Following delivery of the new system, Anthony will receive training on maintenance and care of his seating and mobility system.

Prescription of Device
Seating system: Anthony's seating system should include a generically contoured seat with moderate pressure relief. Bilateral hip blocks and an adductor pommel will maintain

Continued

CASE STUDY OF A CHILD WITH SEATING AND MOBILITY DEVICES—cont'd

his lower extremity in neutral alignment. He will require a pelvic positioning device to maintain good positioning of his pelvis within the seating system. Anthony requires a low-maintenance pressure relief cushion. A fluid-filled cushion will provide appropriate pressure relief and sensory and kinesthetic feedback for his pelvis. A generically contoured back cushion with bilateral trunk lateral supports is recommended. The cushion contour should maintain Anthony's trunk in neutral alignment. Anthony requires a low-profile head support to protect against acceleration/deceleration injuries while in a motor vehicle.

Power mobility system: Anthony also requires a high-performance power mobility system that will integrate with his customized seating system. A mid-wheel-drive mobility system will allow him to achieve precise maneuverability at home, at school, and within the community. He should drive his system via a standard joystick input device placed on his left side. He will require 70-degree front riggings and footplates with shoe straps to maintain lower extremity positioning. Anthony's power chair also allows him to stand in the wheelchair. Using the power controller, Anthony transitions for sit to stand or stand to sit.

Re-examination
Anthony will need to be reassessed when the system is delivered. Anthony's seat/back may require slight modifications to ensure the most precise fit possible. Anthony should then be reassessed yearly.

Goals
1. Anthony will receive a new customized seating system to maintain good musculoskeletal alignment.
2. Anthony will receive a power wheelchair that interfaces with the recommended seating system, and the driver controls will be modified for his specifications.
3. Anthony will be independently mobile in his new seating and mobility system.

Analysis of Case Using the ICF Model
Body functions: Severe spastic quadriplegia, musculoskeletal malalignment and imbalances

Activity limitations: Requires a power wheelchair for mobility around home and community, requires assistance to complete motor tasks

Participation restrictions: Requires modified computer equipment at home and school, requires assistance to participate in most nonverbal activities

Environmental limitations: Requires accessible environments, requires assistance for activities of daily living, requires specialized transportation

Movement System: Anthony's hypertonia can be labeled as *fractionation deficit*. His weakness is labeled as *force production deficit*.

CHAPTER DISCUSSION QUESTIONS

1. What are the three categories of seating systems?
2. What are the two categories of wheeled mobility?
3. If a child can ambulate but requires assistance for balance, what are appropriate devices to consider to assist the child with ambulation at home and at school?
4. What kind of seating system and mobility system would be most appropriate for a child with diplegia who can ambulate but uses a wheelchair for long distances?
5. What is the difference between a midwheel-drive power wheelchair and a rear-wheel-drive power wheelchair?
6. What laws influenced the availability of AT for individuals with disabilities?
7. Why is the seating system an important component of a wheeled mobility or positioning system?
8. Your client is an 18-year-old girl with severe spastic quadriplegia. She attends a community college and lives at home. She has severe skeletal deformities, including scoliosis, hip dislocation, and leg-length discrepancy. Why would a custom-molded seating system and a midwheel-drive power chair be appropriate for her?
9. What is the difference between a tilt- in-space seating system and a reclining seating system? Give an example of when you would use each system.
10. If a child transitions from a manual mobility system to a power mobility system, what issues does the therapist need to be aware of?

REFERENCES

1. Sze S. A *Literature Review: an investigation of various types of assistive technology (AT),* https://files.eric.ed.gov/fulltext/ED490347.pdf. Accessed July 7, 2023.
2. Chambers D. Assistive technology supporting inclusive education: existing and emerging trends editor. In: Chambers D, ed. *Assistive Technology to Support Inclusive Education*: Emerald Publishing Limited; 2020.

https://www.emerald.com/insight/content/doi/10.1108/S1479-363620200000014001/full/html.

3. Hedman G. Overview of rehabilitation technology. In: *Rehabilitation Technology*. 1st ed. Milton Park, Abingdon-on-Thames, Oxfordshire: Routledge; 2020.

4. Langone J, Malone DM, Kinsley T. Technology solutions for young children with developmental concerns. *Infants Young Child*. 1999;4(11):65.

5. Long T, Tuscano K. *Handbook of Pediatric Physical Therapy*. 3rd ed. Philadelphia: Lippincott Williams & Wilkins; 2018.

6. Letts RM, ed. *Principles of Seating the Disabled*. Boca Raton, FL: CRC; 1991.

7. Kangas KM. Seating, positioning, and physical access. *DDSIS Newsletter*. 1991;14(2):4.

8. Bergen AF, Presperin J, Tallman T. *Positioning for Function: Wheelchairs and Other Assistive Technologies*. Valhalla, NY: Valhalla Rehabilitation; 1990.

9. Cook A, Polgar J, Encarnacao P. *Assistive Technologies: Principles and Practice*. 5th ed. St. Louis: Mosby; 2019.

10. O'Sullivan SB, Schmitz T. *Physical Rehabilitation: Assessment and Treatment*. 4th ed. Philadelphia: FA Davis; 2001.

11. Bergen AF. *Seating and Positioning Principles for the Neurologically Involved Client, Presented at the American Physical Therapy Association Combined Sections Meeting*, San Francisco; February 1992.

12. Siekman AR, Flanagan K. The anti-thrust seat: a wheelchair insert for individuals with abnormal reflex patterns or other specialized problems. In: *Proceedings of the 8th Annual Conference On Rehabilitation Engineering*. Washington, DC: RESNA; 1983.

13. Butler C. Effects of powered mobility on self-initiated behaviors of very young children with locomotor disability. *Dev Med Child Neurol*. 1986;28:325.

14. Evans MA, Nelson WB. A dynamic solution to seating clients with fluctuating tone. In: *Proceedings of the 19th Annual Conference on Rehabilitation Technology*. Arlington, VA: RESNA; 1996.

15. Orpwood R. A compliant seating system for a child with extensor spasms. In: *Proceedings of the 19th Annual Conference of Rehabilitation Engineering*. Arlington, VA: RESNA; 1996.

16. Trefler E, Angelo J. Comparison of anterior trunk supports for children with cerebral palsy. *Assist Technol*. 1997;9(1):15.

17. Hays RM. *Childhood Motor Impairments: Clinical Overview and Scope of the Problem. Presented at the Fourth International Seating Symposium*, Vancouver, BC; February 1988.

17a. Bednarczyk JH, Sanderson DJ. Kinematics of wheelchair propulsion in adults and children with spinal cord injury. *Arch Phys Med Rehabil*. 1994;75:1327.

18. O'Shea RK, Sposato B. Assistive technology. In: Campbell SK, ed. *Physical Therapy for Children*. 6th ed. Philadelphia: Elsevier; 2022.

19. Jones CK. In search of power for the pediatric client. *Phys Occup Ther Pediatr*. 1990;10(2):47.

20. Furumasu J. Considerations when working with the pediatric population. In: Lange ML, Minkel J, eds. *Seating and Wheeled Mobility: A Clinical Resource Guide*. Thorofare, NJ: Slack Inc; 2018.

21. Kermoian R. Locomotion experience and psychological development in infancy. In: Furumasu J, ed. *Pediatric Powered Mobility: Developmental Perspectives, Technical issues, Clinical Approaches*. Arlington, VA: RESNA; 1997.

22. Deitz J, Swinth Y, White O. Powered mobility and preschoolers with complex developmental delays. *Am J Occup Ther*. 2002;56(1):86.

23. Butler C, Okamoto GA, McKay TM. Powered mobility for very young disabled children. *Dev Med Child Neurol*. 1983;25:472.

24. Berry ET, McLaurin SE, Sparling JW. Parent/caregiver perspectives on the use of power wheelchairs. *Pediatr Phys Ther*. 1996;8(4):146.

25. Field D. Powered mobility: a literature review illustrating the importance of a multifaceted approach. *Assist Technol*. 1999;11(1):20.

26. Hasdai A, Jessel AS, Weiss PL. Use of a computer simulator for training children with disabilities in the operation of a powered wheelchair. *Am J Occup Ther*. 1998;52(3):215.

27. Morgan AM. Power mobility: optimizing driving. In: Lange ML, Minkel J, eds. *Seating and Wheeled Mobility: A Clinical Resource Guide*. Thorofare, NJ: Slack Inc; 2018.

28. Buning ME, Angelo JA, Schmeler MR. Occupational performance and the transition to power mobility: a pilot study. *Am J Occup Ther*. 2001;55(3):339.

29. Kangas KM. Clinical assessment and training strategies for the child's mastery of independent powered mobility editor. In: Furumasu J, ed. *Pediatric Powered Mobility: Developmental Perspectives, Technical Issues, Clinical Approaches*. Arlington, VA: RESNA; 1997.

RESOURCES

Rehabilitation Engineering and Assistive Technology Society of North America (RESNA)

RESNA
2001 K Street NW
3rd Floor North
Washington, DC 20006
PHONE: (202) 367-1121
FAX: (202) 367-212100
www.resna.org

Christopher and Dana Reeve Paralysis Resource Center

636 Morris Turnpike, Suite 3A

Short Hills, NJ 07078

1-800-539-7309

(Information on understanding paralysis and other conditions.)

American Academy of Cerebral Palsy and Developmental Medicine

555 East Wells, Suite 1100

Milwaukee, WI 53202

Phone: 414.918.3014

Fax: 414.276.2146

www.aacpdm.org

(Information on cerebral palsy and other developmental disorders.)

Orthoses for the Pediatric Patient

Roberta Kuchler O'Shea, PT, DPT, PhD, Matthew Okon, CPO/L
Maureen (Mo) Connelly Boyle, CPO/L, MPO

LEARNING OBJECTIVES

At the end of the chapter, the reader will be able to do the following:

1. Identify upper and lower extremity orthoses commonly used in the pediatric population.
2. Determine which planes of motion are controlled by orthoses.
3. Determine appropriate fit of an orthosis for a specific user.

CHAPTER OUTLINE

Orthoses can be used for a multitude of reasons. They help to control errant movement, offer stability to a weak or misaligned anatomic segment, and provide assistance in movement patterns. Orthoses can be fabricated from several materials including thermoplastics, metals, leather, and carbon fiber. It is important to work closely with an orthotist to determine the best material for the orthosis based on the patient's pathology and activity level. It is important to also consider the patient's growth potential or any expected changes in limb girth, patient weight,

or expected losses or gains in function. Typically, a physician will write the orthotic prescription in consultation with a rehabilitation team that includes a certified orthotist, the family, and the patient. The team may also include members from athletic training, physical therapy, and/or occupational therapy. It is important to remember that whenever motion is blocked by an orthosis, a compensatory movement will develop. This compensatory movement must be carefully balanced to ensure the orthosis is a benefit to the patient.

PATHOLOGIES THAT TYPICALLY REQUIRE ORTHOSIS INTERVENTION

Cerebral vascular accident (CVA)/stroke syndrome
Traumatic brain injury (TBI)
Cerebral palsy (CP)
Multiple sclerosis (MS)
Muscular dystrophy (MD)
Paraplegia
Tetra/quadriplegia
Spina bifida
Dystonia
Spinal muscular atrophy (SMA)
Hypotonia
Hypertonia

This text covers some of these pathologies in greater depth in other chapters. It is important to know that the orthotic intervention is used to correct the clinical signs and symptoms that result in musculoskeletal abnormalities.

THREE-POINT PRESSURE FOR CONTROL

The orthosis must use three points of contact/pressure when controlling motion. This gives the most optimal correction if a deformity is present. However, this may lead to concentrations of pressure at three points, if care is not taken to properly evaluate pressure-tolerant areas.

Planes of Movement Control

Sagittal: Divides body into left/right. Motions are flexion, extension, hyperextension, dorsiflexion, plantarflexion.

Frontal or Coronal: Divides body into anterior/posterior. Motions are abduction, adduction, elevation, depression, inversion, eversion.

Transverse: Divides body into superior/inferior. Movements are rotation, horizontal abduction, horizontal adduction.

THE ORTHOTIC EVALUATION

When assessing a client for an orthosis, the following should be considered:

Has the patient used an orthosis previously? If so, what type? Was the orthosis tolerated by the patient, and was the goal met?

What is the patient's current cognitive status and attitude toward wearing an orthosis?

If appropriate, is there family or caregiver support to assist the patient?

The orthotic assessment should include consideration of the following:
Condition of the extremity
Callouses
Scars
Abrasions or unhealed sores
Overall skin condition
Edema (static or fluctuating)
Sensation
Muscle tone
Hypertonia
Hypotonia
Dystonia
Fluctuating tone
Clonus
Range of motion of segment to be supported as well as joints above and below the segment
Dorsi/plantar flexion
Reduction of a varus or valgus deformity
Reduction of pronation or supination
Decisions to be addressed
What is patient's diagnosis?
What control is needed?
What assistance is needed?
What function should remain?

LOWER EXTREMITY ORTHOSES

Foot Orthosis

A foot orthosis is used for a patient who presents with collapse of the medial longitudinal arch, with no hindfoot involvement (Box 23.1). When the hindfoot presents with a coronal plane deformity such as excessive inversion or eversion, a University of California Berkeley Labs (UCBL) type of foot orthosis can be used (Fig. 23.1). A supramaleollar orthosis (SMO) is used when there is more severe involvement of the hindfoot, such as for patients who present with hypotonia (i.e., Down syndrome) (Fig. 23.2).

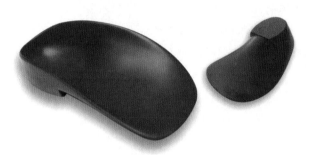

Fig. 23.1 Prefab UCB Style Pediatric Foot Orthosis. (© Nolaro24™ LLC, https://nolaro24.com/ls.html.)

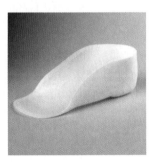

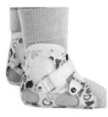

Fig. 23.2 Supramaleollar orthosis (SMO). (Reprinted with permission from SureStep.)

Ankle-Foot Orthosis

An ankle-foot orthosis (AFO) can be used to address both swing phase and stance phase abnormalities that are present in gait. It can be used to assist, resist, or stop motion in the sagittal, coronal, or transverse plane. In your evaluation, it is important to take into consideration the device design that will address the patient's functional needs with the least interruption of normal human locomotion (Fig. 23.3).

TYPES OF ANKLE-FOOT ORTHOSES

Flexible Ankle-Foot Orthosis

The flexible AFO, also known as a posterior leaf spring, addresses only swing-phase dorsiflexor weakness and allows for the least interference in gait during stance phase. The AFO will assist weak dorsiflexors to help reduce foot drop during swing phase but will not address any coronal plane abnormalities at the foot or ankle. The flexible AFO design will have little to no influence on the motion at the knee joint (Fig. 23.4).

Solid Ankle-Foot Orthosis

The solid AFO is designed to stop motion in all three planes at the ankle joint. This can be beneficial when working with a patient with reduced range of motion, spasticity, or paralysis/severe weakness. When designing an AFO, the orthotist/therapist needs to consider the patient's ankle angle, and a heel may be utilized on the AFO to effectively incline the patient's tibia during gait with the overall goal of restoring normal human locomotion. A solid AFO may also indirectly affect the knee in patients with knee buckling or hyperextension.

Articulated Ankle-Foot Orthosis

The articulated AFO allows for free motion into dorsiflexion and is typically designed with a plantarflexion stop. This allows the AFO to hold the foot at 90 degrees in swing phase, while allowing full motion of the ankle into dorsiflexion in the sagittal plane. The articulated AFO also provides coronal stability to improve hindfoot alignment in cases of hindfoot valgus or varus.

Ground Reaction Force Ankle-Foot Orthosis

The ground reaction force AFO is designed to maintain the knee in extension throughout stance phase via

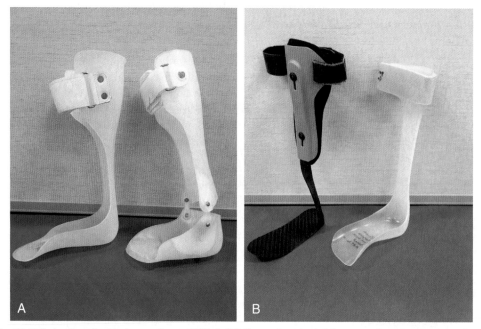

Fig. 23.3 Examples of ankle-foot orthoses (AFOs). **(A)** Pictured on the left is a custom-molded solid AFO and pictured on the right is a custom-molded hinged AFO. **(B)** Pictured on the left is a carbon fiber floor reaction AFO and pictured on the right is a custom-molded posterior leaf spring AFO. (From Chui K, Jorge M, Yen SC, and others. *Orthotics and Prosthetics in Rehabilitation*. 4th ed. Philadelphia: Elsevier; 2019.)

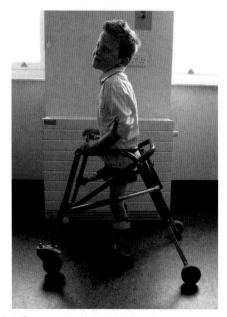

Fig. 23.4 Static ankle-foot orthosis. Child using a posterior walker, reported to promote upright posture and higher walking speeds than an anterior walker. (From Lissauer T, Clayden G. *Illustrated Textbook of Paediatrics*. 4th ed. St Louis: Elsevier; 2011.)

anterior pressure on the proximal tibia. This is seen in patients who present with crouch gait (i.e., spina bifida).

Carbon Ankle-Foot Orthosis

The custom carbon AFO utilizes energy-storing properties of the carbon fiber to encourage normalized gait patterns. The AFO is often designed with a posterior strut, which provides triplanar stability while still providing dynamic movement for the patient. These are prescribed for pediatric patients including those with hemiplegic cerebral palsy and spina bifida.

Knee Orthosis

The knee orthosis is prescribed for patients who require support exclusively to the knee joint. The knee orthosis is commonly prescribed to be worn by patients with sports-related injuries or during the postoperative period for patients who have undergone surgery to address ligamentous damage. Some patients will wear locked or unhinged knee orthoses at night to prevent or reduce contractures (Fig. 23.5).

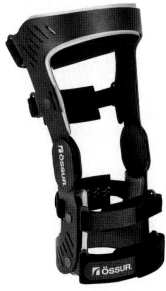

Fig. 23.5 Knee orthosis. Example of a knee brace that is used for nonsurgical treatment of anterior cruciate ligament (ACL) rupture or following surgery for ACL reconstruction. (© Ossur.)

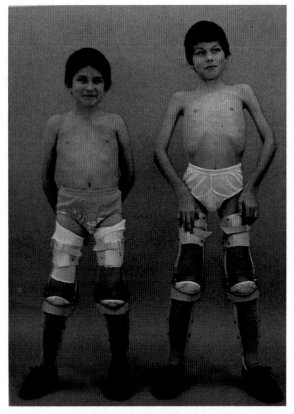

Fig. 23.6 Polypropylene knee-ankle-foot orthosis on two brothers (aged 12 years and 9 years) with Duchenne muscular dystrophy. They had continued ambulation in orthoses for 2 years and 6 months, respectively, after provision of orthoses. (From Dubowitz V. Deformities in Duchenne dystrophy. *Neuromuscul Disord.* 2010;20(4):282.)

Knee-Ankle-Foot Orthosis

The knee-ankle-foot orthosis (KAFO) extends from above the knee and distally to encompass the foot and fit inside of a shoe. The primary use of the orthosis is to provide increased control of the knee joint, such as in cases of excessive knee buckling or hyperextension when an AFO is not corrective enough (Fig. 23.6).

Hip-Knee-Ankle-Foot Orthosis

The hip-knee-ankle-foot orthosis (HKAFO) is an orthosis that extends further proximally than the KAFO to include a pelvic section. Typically, it is designed as a bilateral HKAFO that enables a patient to ambulate and is known as a reciprocating gait orthosis (RGO). RGOs can be utilized for patients with spina bifida (Fig. 23.7). RGOs are operated by unweighting one side to allow the linking mechanism to assist with hip flexion and progress the extremity forward. So, if the child leans backward on the right, the left lower extremity is assisted in hip flexion (Fig. 23.8).

Spinal Orthoses

In the pediatric population, spinal orthoses can be used to stabilize fractures, correct skeletal deformities, or support the trunk due to weakness or paralysis.

Often, these orthoses are fabricated from thermoplastic material and can have a bivalve design (anterior and posterior section) or a single opening at the anterior side of the orthosis.

Lumbosacral Orthosis

The lumbosacral orthosis (LSO) is utilized when support is required between the L2–L5 vertebrae. This design will act to limit flexion and extension of the lumbosacral spine. Often, the LSO is used for pediatric patients with sports injuries to the lower back or spondylolisthesis/spondylolysis of the lumbar vertebrae.

Thoracolumbosacral Orthosis

The thoracolumbosacral orthosis (TLSO) is used when patients require stability at the thoracic vertebrae up

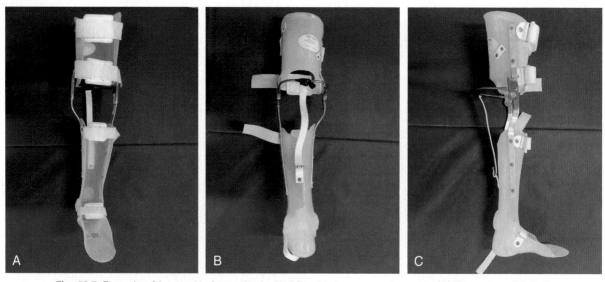

Fig. 23.7 Example of knee-ankle-foot orthosis (KAFO) with knee extension stop. **(A)** Front view; **(B)** Back view. **(C)** Side view. (From Chui K, Jorge M, Yen SC, et al. *Orthotics and Prosthetics in Rehabilitation.* 4th ed. Philadelphia: Elsevier; 2019.)

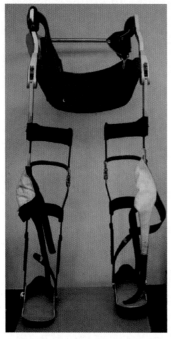

Fig. 23.8 Lateral view of a hip-knee-ankle-foot orthosis, prescribed for postoperative management after a complex total hip arthroplasty. Note the pelvic band, free hip joint, supportive thigh cuff, and free knee joint. The ankle-foot orthosis component is necessary for effective control of rotary forces through the femur and hip joint. (From Luqmani R, Robb J, Porter D, and others. *Textbook of Orthopaedics, Trauma, and Rheumatology.* 2nd ed. Edinburgh: Mosby; 2013.)

Fig. 23.9 Thoracolumbosacral Orthosis (TLSO) SureStep, with permission.

to T5. Often, children are fit with TLSOs to help correct scoliosis, to stabilize a traumatic spinal fracture, or to support the spine when the trunk musculature is severely weak as in cases of neuromuscular disorders. Patients wearing scoliosis TLSOs are prescribed a wear time by their physician; this must be at least 13 hours per day and can be as high as 23 hours per day to prevent progression of the scoliotic curve (Fig. 23.9).

Cervical Thoracic Orthosis

A cervical thoracic orthosis (CTO) provides support of the cervical spine with distal stabilization to the level of the xiphoid, including cervical flexion, extension, and rotation. This orthosis is used in the case of a spinal fracture or unstable cervical injury following trauma.

Cervical Orthosis

The cervical orthosis is used to provide stability to a patient's cervical spine by preventing excessive flexion, extension, and rotation. Pediatric patients may wear these following whiplash injuries or traumatic injury to the neck (Fig. 23.10).

Cranial Remolding Orthoses

A cranial remolding orthosis (CMO), also known as a cranial helmet or cranial band, gently prevents excessive growth in the direction that is most prominent, while leaving open spaces for the flattened areas of the baby's head to grow, forming a rounder, more even/symmetric shape.

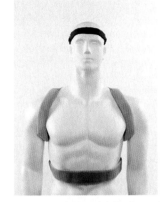

Fig. 23.10 Dynamic cervical orthosis from SureStep, with permission.

OTHER CONSIDERATIONS

Individuals who are wearing an orthosis must be educated regarding the correct donning and doffing of the orthosis. It is best to wear socks underneath lower extremity

---

CASES

Case 1

Allie is a 12-year-old dancer who has severe foot pain. She is also experiencing knee pain and occasional back pain. She is referred to physical therapy after an appointment with her primary doctor. She is also scheduled to see a sports medicine orthopedic doctor. The physical therapy assessment determines that Allie has significant pronation of both feet, which is resulting in a valgus foot position and valgus at her knees. It was recommended that she try over-the-counter shoe inserts that have a rigid arch with proper cushioning to maintain her midfoot alignment during her day-to-day activities. She will also wear taping support for her feet and ankles when she dances. Overpronation running shoes were recommended to help support her feet. Much to Allie's disappointment, it was recommended that she not wear flipflops without any foot support, as she cannot wear her orthoses in flipflops. She was also given an exercise program to help strengthen the intrinsic muscles of the feet and to help minimize lower extremity weakness found throughout the entire lower extremity chain.

ICF

Body structure and function: Weak foot intrinsic, weak hip abductors bilaterally, pain in lower extremities and occasional back pain.

Activity limitation: Can participate in dance classes and competitions without pain.

Participation limits: At risk for not making competitive dance teams.

Environmental: Needs to change preferred footwear to something more supportive. Add in exercise protocol to her daily routine.

Personal supports: Allie's family is very supportive and was able to purchase foot orthoses, taping supplies, and supportive sandals. Allie's dance coaches are also supportive and encouraging.

Movement System

Allie has force production deficits in the foot intrinsic musculature and hip musculature.

Case 2

Sebastian is a 6-year-old boy with diplegic cerebral palsy. He currently wears static AFOs that are about 18 months old. He is fully included in school and ambulates with a reverse walker. He is reporting that he is having difficulty squatting to retrieve objects from the floor. The team decided that Sebastian should try dynamic carbon AFOs with an SMO insert that will allow graded dorsiflexion and prevent plantarflexion. Sebastian receives weekly outpatient physical therapy to work on strength and coordination and balance

Continued

CASES—cont'd

activities. Sebastian also attends a weekly conductive education afterschool program 2 days a week to work on functional skills, better ambulation, and peer socialization.

ICF

Body structure and function: Tight heel cords but can get to 5 degrees dorsiflexion with passive range of motion (PROM) and mild tightness in bilateral hamstrings. Tends to walk on his toes when not wearing AFOs.

Activity limitations: Cannot squat to play with friends or retrieve objects easily from floor.

Participation limitations: Sebastian is involved with Scouts, buddy baseball, and golf. He enjoys playing with friends and visiting his grandparents' beach house. He wants to be a coach when he grows up.

Environmental supports: Sebastian attends an accessible school and rides the bus. At home, the bedrooms are upstairs, but with the use of the handrails, he can climb the five steps independently. He has a walker on his bedroom level and the main level of the house.

Personal factors: Sebastian is the youngest of six children adopted into his family. He has two dads (Mike and Erik) and many cousins, aunts, and uncles. Both sets of grandparents live close to Sebastian's family. All the children are in school full time, both dads work full time, and the grandparents help with afterschool routines.

Movement System

Sebastian has force production deficits in his bilateral quads and bilateral dorsiflexors. He also has fractionated movement deficits of the lower extremities.

Case 3

Katie is a 12-year-old with idiopathic thoracic scoliosis. Despite doing Schroth physical therapy exercises, she will require a TLSO to help minimize and prevent progression of the spinal curvature. Katies has a 35-degree curve in the thoracic spine with the convexity to the right. She has been fitted for a corrective TLSO called the Rigo-Cheneau style orthosis that has to be worn 16 to 18 hours per day. Katie continues to come to physical therapy for strengthening and stretching protocols. She has met other kids at physical therapy who wear different types of orthoses and enjoys talking to them.

ICF

Body structure and function: Thoracic scoliosis with convexity to the right.

Activity limitations: Katie cannot play sports this school year because of the orthosis-wearing schedule.

Participation: Katie continues to play in the school band and is involved in the 4H Club. Katie cannot ride her bike or motor scooter. She is very self-conscious about the orthosis, so she doesn't like to hang out with her friends like she used to. Because of the length of the orthosis, she is uncomfortable riding the bus, since the seats are fixed and the braces dig into her if she cannot slightly recline in her seat so she gets a ride to school from her parents.

Environmental: Katie lives in a semi-rural area with her mom, dad, two siblings, and her maternal grandparents. The family has a large dog named Oreo, three goats, and several chickens.

orthoses such as AFOs and to wear a thin T-shirt underneath a spinal orthosis such as a TLSO. Often, children with lower extremity orthoses will also need a larger or wider pair of shoes to accommodate the orthosis.

The patient's skin should be kept clean and dry and monitored for any redness or irritation. Because of the corrective pressure of orthoses, some redness is normal. However, if this does not dissipate after 20 minutes, the orthosis will need to be adjusted to relieve pressure in that area.

The orthoses should be regularly cleaned to prevent bacterial buildup. Thermoplastic designs may be wiped down with a damp cloth and soap or sprayed with rubbing alcohol for thorough cleaning.

The orthosis should be evaluated regularly for proper fit. Typical childhood skeletal growth and weight gain or loss will impact the fit of the orthosis.

REFERENCE

1. American Academy of Orthopedic Surgeons. *Atlas of Orthotics: Biomechanical Principles and Application.* 2nd ed. Maryland Heights, Missouri: CV Mosby Publishing; 1985.

Answers to Discussion Questions

CHAPTER 1

1. An increased likelihood of acquiring asthma, diabetes, morbid obesity, high lead levels, depression, or becoming a victim of violence; (a) suboptimal and infrequent health care; (b) exacerbation of chronic conditions; and (c) risky/unsafe living environments.

2. Some examples include offering park district programs that focus on overall wellness, health, and nutrition; neighborhood health centers that focus on entire family issues, including social and emotional status of the family; resources available to families to improve their quality of life; and before- and after-school programs that offer supportive and safe environments, relevant and age-appropriate health education and nutritional information, and extracurricular programs (sports, clubs, support groups).

3. Central nervous system, peripheral nervous system, visceromotor nervous system.

4. Cephalocaudal; proximal to distal; flexion to extension. Thus a young baby tends to develop head control and then trunk control, control of shoulders and hips prior to finger control, and works out of flexion, increasing the strength of the extensors before refining the strength of the flexors.

5. (a) Difficulty eating, difficulty maintaining head and eyes in midline; (b) difficulty with ADLs and IADLs (including feeding, dressing, washing), difficulty completing two-handed midline tasks, difficulty in crawling, cruising, and walking; (c) may develop scoliosis due to paraspinals over-firing unevenly, left compared to right.

6. Low tone, child appears floppy.

7. Hypertonia/hypotonia: difficulty sitting on classroom furniture and on floor, difficulty with walking, potential difficulty with language and communication. Athetosis: will need personal assistance and significant level of help in the classroom; child may have difficulty sitting in standard chairs at the table, participating in ambulation activities.

8. Central nervous system consists of the brain and spinal cord.

9. In the CNS the pathways and tracks tend to descend from the brain to their synapses in/near the spinal cord. The PNS information travels from the periphery to the spinal degree. The central nervous system may be referred to as *gray matter* and *white matter*. This nomenclature indicates which structures are myelinated and which are not. Myelinated structures are considered to be white matter, whereas nonmyelinated structures are considered to be gray matter. The peripheral nervous system consists of the nerves that connect the central nervous system and the peripheral muscles of the body. The peripheral nervous system has sensory fibers and innervates glands and skeletal, cardiac, and smooth muscles. The peripheral nervous system can regenerate after an injury, but the central nervous system cannot.

10. By the sixth week of gestation.

CHAPTER 2

1. Reliability determines if the tool is an accurate measure of what it claims to measure. An unreliable test cannot be used for clinical measurements.

2. No, a raw score is meaningless when comparing groups. The standardized score should be used to measure change over time.

3. Assessments can be used to screen for delays or abnormalities, provide a diagnosis, evaluate outcomes and progress, develop goals, collect data, and determine a prognosis. In the school setting the therapist uses assessment tools to help justify the number of minutes of services a child is receiving, especially if the number is uncharacteristically high.

4. The age-equivalent score is useful when assessing and describing developmentally delayed children who cannot achieve a developmental index score.

5. Test validity determines if the assessment tool accomplishes its intended purpose.

6. *Face validity* is the concept that the test strongly measures what it claims to measure. Thus is the face value of the assessment valid and true? *Content validity* requires that the assessment sample a reasonable range of target behaviors. Is the content of the assessment measuring what it claims to measure? *Concurrent validity* correlates the child's performance on an assessment to another valid assessment. Will the child achieve the same age level or developmental level on two different assessments given in the same time period? *Construct validity* requires that the test explain the child's achievement within a theoretical framework. *Predictive validity* describes how well the assessment tool predicts the child's performance at a future date.

7. The therapist may gain a richer understanding of the child.

8. Both assessment tools can be standardized. On the evaluation side, in a criterion-referenced exam, the child's performance is measured by the number of criteria the child has mastered on certain tasks. In the norm-referenced assessment tool, the child's performance is compared to standards set by a sample of children from the general population.

9. Two possible answers are:
The Pediatric Evaluation of Disability Inventory (PEDI) is a norm-referenced tool that assesses functional skills of children ages 6 months to 7.5 years. The PEDI measures capability and performance of functional activities in three content areas: self-care, ability, and social function. The Peabody Developmental Motor Scales, Second Edition (PDMS-2) uses a stratified sample relative to US census criteria. The PDMS-2 is designed to assess the gross and fine motor skills of children from birth through 6 years of age. Items are scored on a 3-point scale. Age equivalents, motor quotients, percentile rankings, and standard scores can be calculated for each child.

10. A therapist might choose to use a qualitative assessment style when studying student interactions at an inclusive fifth grade. The qualitative assessment will allow themes to develop over time, and the researcher will be able to record these themes and ask more questions. A researcher may use a quantitative measure when measuring motor quotients or assessing a child for eligibility purposes. In these cases, numbers are needed to determine the prognosis of the child.

CHAPTER 3

1. Work around/in the refrigerator on opening the door (child has to step and move as door opens); child can work on squat-to-stand activities by picking objects off floor and placing on refrigerator shelves or removing things from shelves; child can practice choice making by selecting things from the refrigerator; child can practice standing and weight shifting while playing wash the dishes/rinse the dishes at the sink.

2. Use snack time to work on squat to stand, sit to stand, or the reverse. Have the child play dress-up with oversized clothes and practice sitting or standing balance skills and sit-to-stand activities while donning or doffing clothes.

3. Children with more advanced skills can be seen as motor/language and/or cognitive models for children with less advanced skills. Typically developing peers receive exposure to children with delays or disorders.

4. Park district programs such as swimming, dancing, and gym.
Public library programs: Storytime can be used to practice time on task and attention to task. Early literacy will also help communication and cognition. The local YMCA or YWCA may offer motor activities that will help improve strength and coordination.

5. Children and adolescents ages 6 through 17 years should do 60 minutes (1 hour) or more of moderate-to-vigorous physical activity daily.

    • Aerobic: Most of the 60 minutes or more per day should be either moderate- or vigorous-intensity aerobic physical activity and should include vigorous-intensity physical activity on at least 3 days a week.

    • Muscle strengthening: As part of their 60 minutes or more of daily physical activity, children and adolescents should include muscle-strengthening physical activity on at least 3 days a week.

    • Bone strengthening: As part of their 60 minutes or more of daily physical activity, children and adolescents should include bone-strengthening physical activity on at least 3 days a week.

6. Resistance training, aerobic exercise, and motor learning are the top choices.

7. Group intervention, rhythmic intention, the conductor/teacher leading the group, and rhythmic intention.

8. Children with hemiplegia.

9. Physical therapy services held in the water environment. Aquatic therapy utilizes principles of water: viscosity, buoyancy, and hydrostatic pressure to provide resistance, unweight the body/joints, and improve mobility in reduced-gravity environment.

10. Use of mounting and riding a horse with certified hippotherapist trained to provide skilled rehabilitation. Hippotherapy has been shown to improve pelvis mobility and gait as the mobility of the horse's pelvis mimics the mechanics used for human kinematic in upright position.

11. Recognizes the influence of motor control and investigates the effects of postural control as a result of several interactions between complex neurologic and physiologic systems.

12. The main goal of PNF is to strengthen muscles within the functional movement patterns, including rotation. These movement patterns are known as *diagonals*. PNF is based on the developmental sequence and the sequential mastery of motor milestones. Spiral and diagonal movements are extremely important because these movements take strength, coordination, and control.

13. Strengthening programs do not cause a direct illness or injury to children.

14. Both have the potential to facilitate movement by increasing input or decreasing input to a region. Each requires some training to apply correctly.

CHAPTER 4

1. The family/caregiver knows and understands the needs of the child and family. If a goal or outcome is not important to the family, it will not be incorporated into the family's activities. If the activity is not part of a routine, then the child will have little time to practice and gain improvement toward mastering the goal/outcome. Additionally, the family/caregiver may be part of the few people who have seen the child across several environments and over a given time span; thus the family/caregiver can relay historical information that will be relevant to a current treatment plan.

2. With an interdisciplinary team: Goals are discipline specific, families may not be central to team functioning, team members implement their portion of the plan. Therapists on a transdisciplinary team will cross-treat and work on goals that may not necessarily be related to their specific discipline. They will also treat the child in a variety of environments so that the child has the opportunity to practice several skills in a variety of environments.

3. Medical: usually multidisciplinary or interdisciplinary. School: can be interdisciplinary or transdisciplinary. Early Intervention: transdisciplinary approach is often used.

4. Respectful listening: Pay attention and limit distractions, respond quickly to requests for information. Respectful speaking: Allow pauses in your speaking to allow for listener processing and so others can contribute, use a professional tone but limit professional jargon as much as possible, use an interpreter if needed to allow for accurate information transmission.

5. Related services assist the student to benefit from special education. Because of the related services provision in the law, physical therapy may be provided by and in the school, but this therapy must be educationally relevant and must support the child's IEP goals. The PTA can provide services and programming that work on the child's mobility within the school environment, including getting on and off the bus and in the playground area. The

PTA can also work within the classroom helping the child meet learning goals by providing classroom positioning, helping to arrange classroom furniture so the child can move within the space easily, or working on other modifications with the teacher to help the child learn and interact in the classroom setting.

CHAPTER 5

1. The collection of systems, including cardiovascular, pulmonary, endocrine, integumentary, nervous, and musculoskeletal, that interact to move the body or its component parts.
2. The movement system diagnoses for neuromuscular conditions allow pediatric physical therapists to examine, identify, and label movement-related dysfunction regardless of a child's health condition.
3. Initial conditions, preparation, initiation, execution, and termination.
4. Poor timing and sequencing of either intersegmental movements or postural responses (anticipatory and reactive) relative to balance demands.
5. Weakness is illustrated in the performance of tasks and in testing of body structures and functions.
6. The primary movement problem of infants and children with sensory selection and weighting deficit is difficulty with postural stability or orientation, or both, due to decreased ability to screen for and attend to information from the sensory system. Sensory seeking or sensory avoidance behaviors may be present. Whereas the primary movement problem of infants and children with sensory detection deficit is the inability to execute intersegmental movement due to a lack of joint position sense or multisensory failure affecting joint position sense, vision, and/or the vestibular system. SDD is a loss of joint position sense in one or more extremity.
7. Modifiers can be used to indicate an impairment that is not included in the description of a movement system diagnosis.

CHAPTER 6

1. Hallmark signs include reduced quality of movements, spasticity, muscle weakness, and ataxia. List the measurement tools that can be used in identifying children at risk for cerebral palsy: General

Movements Assessment (GMA), Harris Infant Neurological Examination (HINE), Test of Infant Motor Performance (TIMP).
2. Developmental pediatrician, neurologist, orthopedic surgeon, and a physiatrist. Other providers in the child's care may include an optometrist or developmental optometrist, physical therapist, occupational therapist, speech and language pathologist, developmental therapist, audiologist, dietician.
3. Intellectual disability, seizures, vision issues, hearing loss, orthopedic issues, dental problems, oral motor dysfunction, problems with spatial awareness, GERD.

CHAPTER 7

1. Motor vehicle accident, shaken baby syndrome, near drowning, sports injuries, tumors/neoplasm, child not restrained properly in a motor vehicle.
2. Typically classified with the Glasgow Coma Scale or the Ranchos Los Amigos Cognitive Recovery Scale.
3. Long-term impairments include decreased cognitive abilities; long- and short-term memory loss; and deficits in attention, reasoning, abstract thinking, judgment, problem-solving, and/or information processing. Child may also experience speech and language disorders, psychosocial behavioral issues, sensory deficits, perceptual motor disabilities, and decreased physical functioning.
4. Increase in scores reflects improved observable function in a particular area.
5. If a person receives a score of 3 in the subdomain of verbal response, this indicates that the person is verbal but may not be using appropriate words. However, sounds are consistently words and not just sounds or utterances.
6a. He should be classified as a level IV. At this stage, individuals are confused, agitated and alert, very active, aggressive, perform motor actions, but behavior is nonpurposeful; person will have an extremely short attention span.
6b. Limited ability to follow verbal and nonverbal direction, limited communication using yes/no inconsistently, limited wheeled mobility, limited ambulation. Strategies would include implementing a communication board with simple text and

color organization—morning activities in red, afternoon activities in green, evening activities in blue, for instance. Break down activities into smaller tasks, and order them with text or pictures so child can use as guide in completing activity. Use a smiley face with YES under it and a frown face with NO under it so that the child can point and indicate choice. Honor choice of yes or no, even if it seems inaccurate, to reinforce concepts. For example, if child indicates he does not want a snack, even though he really does, then deny snack at that time. Also, verbal commands need to be clear and concise. Limit commands to one to two steps, gradually building in complexity as child's understanding and memory improve. May need to get a chair lift or bilateral railings to assist child in getting to bedroom or perhaps relocate bedroom to a first-floor area temporarily.

CHAPTER 8

1. JRA is an autoimmune disease in which the body mistakenly identifies some of its own cells and tissues as foreign.
2.

	Pauciarticular	Polyarticular	Systemic
Subtypes	3	2	0
Joints involved	4 or fewer	5 or more	All and internal organs
Gender prevalence	5 times more in girls	3 times more in girls	0

3. Children with JRA often develop uveitis (iridocyclitis), which is inflammation of the iris and ciliary body.
4. Nonsteroidal antiinflammatory drugs (NSAIDs); disease-modifying antirheumatic drugs (DMARDs); biologic response modifier; and corticosteroids.
5. Pain relief, maintaining and gaining PROM and AROM, maintaining and increasing strength and endurance, improving the child's mobility and independent functioning.
6. Calcinosis, Raynaud phenomenon, esophageal dysmotility, sclerodactyly, and telangiectasias.
7. Localized scleroderma may display different types of skin involvement. Systemic juvenile scleroderma involves the internal organs and occurs less frequently in children than localized scleroderma.
8. Hard skin.

CHAPTER 9

1. Large birth weight, prolonged and difficult labor.
2. Reflux, larger size, intolerance for prone, use of car seat and exersaucer.
3. Muscular.
4. Attained full neck passive ROM, shows symmetrical movement and play in all positions, attained age-appropriate motor skills, no visible head tilt, parents aware of signs to monitor as Tommy grows and learns new motor skills. Come back for re-assessment 3–12 months after discharge or whenever those signs of asymmetry are noted.

CHAPTER 10

1. The most common clinical sign of DDH is limitation in hip abduction. On clinical examination, a "click" (Ortolani sign) is felt when upward pressure is applied at the level of the greater trochanter on the newborn or infant's flexed and abducted hip.
2. If no obvious clinical signs, then diagnosis is delayed until the child starts to ambulate.
3. Preoperative intervention may include lower extremity and trunk strengthening and parent/caregiver education. Positioning and handling techniques are an important aspect of the child's care both before and after surgery. Postoperatively the therapist reviews cast care (or traction/orthotic care) with the child's family/caregivers.

CHAPTER 11

1. CAVE: (C) cavus, a fixed plantar flexion deformity of the forefoot on the hind foot; (A) adductus, a fixed medial deviation deformity of the midfoot on the hindfoot; (V) varus, a fixed medial deviation deformity of the hind foot; (E) equinus, a fixed plantar flexion deformity of the ankle.
2. The baby's spine, upper extremities, and hips should be examined with both passive and active ranges of motion to detect any other abnormalities.
3. Genetics, orthopedics, PT.

4. In the provided case study, the child has some discomfort when WB on L LE and she can't run. These will add to her activity limitations.
5. Range of motion programing, strengthening programming especially on left. Be aware of potential secondary comorbidities, including scoliosis.
6. Goals should be age appropriate and focus on obtaining and mastering age-appropriate skills.
7. Swimming and water activities to help improve single leg stance on left, water will add buoyancy to help balance. Strengthening activities and ROM for left foot and lower extremity, SLS on left as tolerated on ground. Bilateral orthotics and serial casting of left to try to regain ankle motion.
8. Need to consider family's resources and access to ortho and pool. May need to use telehealth for monitoring if family can't make frequent appointments.
9. Gross Motor Function Measure, Peabody Developmental Motor Scales 2.

CHAPTER 12

1. Muscle atrophy, insufficient room within the uterus for normal fetal movement, central nervous system and spinal cord deformities, atypical development of tendons, bones, joints, or joint linings.
2. In one type of AMC the child presents with abducted and laterally rotated hips, flexed knees, clubfeet, medially rotated shoulders, extended elbows, and wrists in flexion with ulnar deviation. In the other type the child presents with flexed and dislocated hips, extended knees and clubfeet, medially rotated shoulders, flexed elbows, and flexed and ulnarly deviated wrists.
3. The members of the team typically include the child, family, orthopedic surgeon, and physical and occupational therapy.
4. Since muscle disuse and atrophy are hallmark characteristics of AMC, intensive therapy aims to get as much strength, endurance, and motor control as possible. Intensive therapy helps the child learn to move using different muscle groups than the child has used prior to therapy.
5. Work to achieve flexion in one UE and extension in the other UE.
6. Infant intervention will incorporate ways for the caregiver to hold the child and position the child when sleeping and feeding that will assist in gaining range, but also can occur as part of the typical family routine and interactions with the child.
7. Strengthening should be systemwide but focused on increasing and maintaining abdominal, hip, and knee strength.
8. When one hip is dislocated.
9. Kicking balls of varying weights; repetitive squat-to-stand activities, such as getting a sponge wet and then painting the wall with it; stepping activities/obstacle courses; jumping on a trampoline; riding a bike with adaptations if needed.
10. Swimming, horseback riding, and dance/movement classes.

CHAPTER 13

1. Cardiac involvement, cognitive delays, atlantoaxial instability.
2. Prone on elbows, supported sitting, support child over the shoulder.
3. Using sign language and verbal commands, limit immediate choice to two or three opportunities to choose from at a time, use pictures to help child understand the order of activities and which activities are going to occur.
4. Ascending and descending steps, jumping rope, swimming, rising up and down on tiptoes. The child may benefit from orthotics to help maintain foot position and balance.
5. Swimming, dance/movement class, bike riding, jumping on a mini trampoline.
6. Individual states' early intervention programs, National Association for Down Syndrome, local support groups, library, educational system.
7. Atlantoaxial instability, extreme joint laxity, hypotonia.
8. PTAs are an integral member of the therapy team and must help the child and family be involved members of the team as well. The PTA can help to motivate the child by making the exercises fun and functional. Therapeutic exercise should be embedded as much as possible into the child's daily routines.
9. Hypotonicity, ligament laxity, hearing loss, cardiac limitations.
10. She could roll the ball instead of kicking it. Susie could use a peer to kick the ball, and then she could run the bases.

CHAPTER 14

1. Headaches, irritability, lethargy, difficulty keeping eyes open, vomiting, seizures.
2. Bilateral AFOs and a reverse walker. This child may be able to progress to Lofstrand crutches.
3. Juan might consider using a walker or a manual wheelchair to conserve energy for the fieldtrip.
4. Washing dishes at the sink, organizing/rearranging the refrigerator contents, washing things that are up high so she needs to stretch to achieve.
5. Let him sit for 20 minutes and see if the redness diminishes, add padding to the lateral calcaneus area, contact Jackson's parents/guardian and suggest they make an appointment with the orthotist as soon as possible.
6. Latex-free supplies and equipment should be considered in the therapy gyms (e.g., equipment built from wood, metal, or other nonlatex materials).
7. Joe's program should include teaching him how to perform skin checks, strengthening exercises for the upper and lower extremities and trunk, and instruction in donning and doffing braces appropriately. He will need to practice the transfers in different settings: cafeteria, classroom, bathroom, etc. His program should also include activities to improve standing balance and weight shifting while using the braces. Joe's walker may be more cumbersome than he was used to. He will need to increase his awareness about where the walker is in relation to other people walking by and adjust his movements while using the walker.
8. She will require the use of a rental power wheelchair for school until she is able to resume using her manual wheelchair. Tess may be able to use forearm platform crutches, depending on her postsurgical instructions.

CHAPTER 15

1. Many autistic children have highly developed splinter skills. Individuals with autism often demonstrate poor eye contact when interacting with others; demonstrate marked impairment in facial expressions, body postures, and gestures; typically fail to form successful peer relationships; and exhibit limited or no joint attention. Odd or exaggerated responses to sensory stimuli are common in autistic children. Autistic children often rigidly adhere to routines or rituals with no apparent functional purpose.
2. The Children's Health Act of 2000, the New Freedom Initiative of 2001, and the Combating Autism Act of 2006.
3. Children with autism also frequently use stereotyped or repetitive language. They often may have standard rote responses to certain questions or situations, or may perseverate (uncontrollably repeat) a word or phrase.
4. Autistic children generally do not engage in spontaneous or imitative play. A child with autism often will demonstrate abnormally intense interest in unusually narrow areas of interest. Autistic children often rigidly adhere to routines or rituals with no apparent functional purpose.

CHAPTER 16

1. Identify the four criteria that must be met for a diagnosis of DCD:
   a. Motor skills and coordination are below what is expected for chronological age and experience.
   b. Motor difficulties are impacting daily living skills, school performance, leisure, and play.
   c. Symptoms begin in the developmental period.
   d. Symptoms cannot be explained by other intellectual, vision, neurologic, or motor impairments.
2. Weakness, poor balance, poor coordination, frequent falls, delayed developmental milestones.
3. Less physically active, sensorimotor delays, mental health issues, low self-esteem. They may be diagnosed with attention-deficit/hyperactivity disorder (ADHD), autism spectrum disorder (ASD), learning difficulties, sensory issues, speech difficulties.
4. Early diagnosis and intervention can improve developmental motor skills and improve success in the home, school, and community. It can prevent the secondary and long-term effects of developmental coordination disorder, which are obesity, low self-esteem, difficulties with academic achievement, and quality of life.
5. Balance and posture in sitting, sit to stand, standing, gait, and advanced motor skills (balance on one foot, jumping, hopping, running, skipping, catching and throwing a ball) should be observed. Coordination, fluidity of movement, and midrange control during

these activities. Sitting on a Swiss ball while doing another activity such as catching a smaller ball, reading, doing a puzzle, or tabletop activity.

CHAPTER 17

1. Children at this age are inquisitive and may pull scalding liquids onto themselves; children are also susceptible to abuse scald injuries secondary to their inability to escape the perpetrator or the situation.
2. First-degree burn: also known as *superficial burn*; painful but self-limiting; no scarring typically; due to overexposure to the sun.
   Second-degree burn: partial-thickness burns, including superficial or deep. Superficial partial-thickness includes damage to the epidermis; deep partial-thickness includes the epidermis and deep portion of the dermal layer; both cause increased sensitivity to pain and temperature in the area of the burn. Superficial partial-thickness burns appear red with large, thick-walled blisters; deep partial-thickness burns have a marbled, white edematous appearance with large, thick-walled blisters.
   Third-degree burn: known as *full-thickness burns*; total destruction of the epidermis and dermis and may include deeper tissues such as fascia, muscle, subcutaneous fat. Pain and temperature sensation is destroyed. Skin appears white, brown-black, charred, and leathery, and blistering does not typically occur.
3. Total burn surface area measures the percent of body tissue affected by the burn injury. There are three common methods used to measure TBSA: rule of nines, the palm of the child's hand, and the Lund-Browder chart.
4. They are both chemical burns. Acid burns produce coagulation necrosis, whereas alkalis cause liquidation necrosis (tissue is liquefied). Alkali burns tend to penetrate more deeply and are more dangerous.
5. Shock, edema, heterotrophic ossification, amputation, peripheral nerve involvement.
6. Tissue may form scar tissue secondary to the laying down of highly disorganized collagen; hypertrophic and keloid scarring may also occur. Itching may cause severe discomfort as the tissues heal.
7. Maintain range of motion, restore function.
8. Primarily for easy donning and doffing and for the cosmetic appearance of the mask.

CHAPTER 18

1. Hands, limbs, feet.
2. None.
3. Congenital and acquired.
4. Above knee = transfemoral; below elbow = transradial.
5. *Amelia* refers to the occasion where an entire bone/segment is missing; *hemimelias* refer to a longitudinal anomaly where all or part of one bone is missing; *phocomelia* refers to the congenital absence of the proximal section of the limb.
6. PFFD is a longitudinal deficiency where the femur is malformed and shortened. Typically the remaining femoral segment is held in flexion, abduction, and external rotation. This deformity is classified into four types: class A, B, C, or D. *Class A:* normal hip joint with intact and well-seated femoral head and acetabulum, shortened femoral segment with subtrochanteric varus angulation. *Class B:* femoral head present, acetabulum is adequate but defective, capital fragment within acetabulum. *Class C:* femoral head and acetabulum absent, short femoral fragment, no articulation between femur and acetabulum. *Class D:* femoral head and acetabulum absent, no relation between femur and acetabulum. Several surgical intervention strategies are available to the child with PFFD, depending on the length of the remaining limb.
7. A baby should be fitted with a passive prosthetic device before the age of 3 months.
8. Children will require an adaptation to allow them to achieve mobility. If the child has a transfemoral amputation, the child may be fitted with a device that will allow 4-point rocking and crawling. If the child has a transtibial amputation level, the child should be fitted for a prosthetic device when beginning to pull to stand.
9. This child requires a stable base of support. This child would benefit from a prosthesis with a single-axis knee hinge that manually and intentionally can be locked or unlocked. The knee is locked, usually via a webbing strap, in extension. The child ambulates with the knee locked in extension. The child should be encouraged to unlock the knee when returning to a sitting position.

10. Wear the prosthesis consistently. Pick up two objects and place them in their correct containers so that he can play with his toys.

CHAPTER 19

1. Physical activity, allergens, chemicals, smoke, respiratory coughs and colds.
2. Low-income children of color.
3. Child's asthma history, triggers and symptoms, ways to contact parent/guardian and healthcare provider, medications, physician and parent/guardian signatures, peak flow reading.
4. This device measures how well air is flowing into and out of a person's lungs. The person must be over 5 years old.
5. It is better to have a higher number/reading on the monitor.
6. Preventive medication is used to help decrease the inflammation of the airways or to decrease the triggers. Rescue medication helps to quickly open a person's airway during an asthma attack.
7. The person may take a dose of rescue medication prior to exercise. Modify routine if child has had a recent asthma attack.
8. Wheezing, shortness of breath, tightness of the chest, coughing, increased respiratory rate.
9. Stop exercising immediately.
10. High temperature, high barometric pressure, and the fall season were the most highly correlated factors associated with severity of symptoms.

CHAPTER 20

1. The child has a smaller heart size, which results in less stroke volume.
2. Strength improvements are due to improved coordination and neuromuscular recruitment.
3. Greenstick fractures and growth plate fractures.
4. Salter-Harris I: fracture along the entire growth plate without involving surrounding osteology. Salter-Harris V: compression fracture in the midsubstance or growth plate.
5. This is an avulsion of the bone where the patellar tendon attaches to the tibia. Children involved in jumping sports are most susceptible to Osgood-Schlatter disease.

6. Rehab programs should begin conservatively. Surgery is recommended rarely; more commonly rest is recommended. The rehabilitation program should consist of strengthening and flexibility, focusing on functional activities.
7. Stress fractures are not common in children. When they occur, they usually occur in the same spot in the foot. There are a large number of epiphyseal plates in a small area in the metatarsals, which is the most common site for stress fractures. These occur more often in females than males, especially during adolescence because of hormonal changes. Delayed menarche or amenorrhea increases the incidence of stress fractures.
8. Child experiences pain around the medial aspect of the elbow, possibly due to medial epicondylitis. Typically caused by overuse and most commonly seen in throwers.
9. This is caused by a proximal humeral growth plate fracture. This injury occurs primarily due to poor technique and underdeveloped musculature.
10. When the child is able to understand and follow detailed instructions on proper technique and progression.

CHAPTER 21

1. Extremely premature, very low birth weight.
2. PROM (premature rupture of membranes), PTL (preterm labor), fetal heart rate decelerations, cesarean section, VLBW, 1315 g.
3. Low Apgars, grade III IVH, PDA, first-time parents with long commute.
4. Speech-language pathologist, lactation consultant. She suggested prone swaddling as the best position for G.M. and suggested feeding time was the best time to attempt to interact with the baby. She provided parent education regarding reading baby's stress indicators, decreasing stress, and modifying the environment. She also recommended a gel pillow and frequent position changes to address concerns about head shape. She assured the family she would be available to answer questions and would provide a home program and referral to early intervention prior to discharge.
5. Interventions focusing on family coaching, kicking activities, postural control, prone play, and parent-infant interaction have all been shown to improve outcomes.

CHAPTER 22

1. Linear/planar, contoured, custom molded.
2. Power and manual.
3. It is best to consider the least amount of intervention, depending on the environment. At home the child may be able to cruise and take steps while holding on to furniture. At school the child may opt to use Lofstrand crutches to reduce fatigue and maintain balance. Some children prefer Lofstrand crutches to axillary crutches because the Lofstrand cuffs allow the child to maintain control of the Lofstrand and use the hands for motor skills. For instance, the child can push his tray through the cafeteria line with his hands while the Lofstrand crutch is kept from falling by the cuff. Depending on distances needed to travel and the child's speed and fatigue, it may be prudent to consider a walker for longer distances.
4. This child would benefit from a linear seating system that offered minimal pressure relief and positioning. The child would benefit from a lightweight manual wheelchair.
5. In a rear-wheel-drive chair, the steering and acceleration is generated in the rear wheels. This causes the sensation of the wheelchair user being pushed from behind. The midwheel-drive steering and acceleration is directly under the user's center of gravity. This gives the effect of the user moving as one with the chair. The midwheel drive chairs have a smaller turning radius, and they more closely mimic the turning performance of a typically developing child.
6. PL 101-476: Education of All Handicapped Children Act; 1986-2004 Amendments (IDEA); PL105-394: TRAIDA (Tech Act); PL 93-112: Rehabilitation Act; and PL 101-336: Americans with Disabilities Act.
7. The purpose of the seating system is to provide external postural support for the child in sitting when the child has functional limitations as a result of impairments in musculoskeletal alignment, postural control, muscle tone, or strength.
8. The custom-molded seating system will support her skeletal deformities well. A midwheel-drive power chair will allow her to maneuver more easily around campus, utilize public transportation easily, and it will integrate with the customized seating system.
9. A tilt-in-space system maintains the hip and knee angles as it tips on an axis. This system is recommended for individuals who need to tip back but have difficulty repositioning within the seating system. The reclining system allows flexion and extension of the lower extremities. This system is ideal for individuals who require frequent pressure-relief assistance and range of motion throughout the day.
10. The therapist should inquire about the ability of the child/family to transport and store the power system. The therapist should also inquire about accessibility issues at home/school/work. The therapist must also advise the child/family that they should complete a daily exercise regimen because caloric needs may drop significantly.

GLOSSARY

A

Acceleration dependent injury Related to the effects that occur when a force is applied to a movable head; may be either translational or rotational in nature.

Acquired limb deficiency Amputations caused by trauma, vascular disease, tumors, infections, or burn injuries.

Adjusted age (AA) Refers to the child's age after adjusting for prematurity. It is the age the child should be if they had been born full term, or the chronological age (CA) minus the weeks premature.

Age-equivalent score The mean chronological age represented by a certain developmental index score.

Amelia The occasion where an entire bone/segment is missing.

Amniotic band syndrome (ABS) The cause of several varying birth defects, including amputation of the arms, legs, and digits when the fetal parts are entrapped in a fibrous amniotic band in utero.

Asperger syndrome A neurobiological disorder in which children often demonstrate many autistic symptoms, including elevated sensitivities to certain sounds, tastes, textures, or light. Individuals with Asperger syndrome generally seem normal but often have difficulties with pragmatic language and can be overly literal or have problems with idiom and language use in a social context.

Assistive technology device (ATD) Defined by legislation to include any item, piece of equipment, or product system that increases, maintains, or improves an individual's functional status.

Assistive technology service Defined as any service, such as physical therapy, occupational therapy, or speech therapy, that directly assists someone with a disability in the selection and acquisition of an ATD or training in its use.

Asthma management plan A plan that includes the child's asthma history, triggers and symptoms, ways to contact the parent/guardian and healthcare provider, physician and parent/guardian signatures, the child's target peak flow reading, and a list of asthma medications. It

also includes the child's treatment plan for medications, based on symptoms and peak flow readings.

Atlantoaxial instability Is characterized by excessive movement at the junction between the atlas (C1) and axis (C2) and is due to either a bony or ligamentous abnormality.

Autism The most common of a series of related neurobiological disorders known collectively as *autism spectrum disorders* or *pervasive developmental disorders*.

Autism spectrum disorders Other forms of autism that include Rett syndrome, Asperger syndrome, childhood disintegrative disorder, and pervasive developmental disorder not otherwise specified.

Autoimmune disease One large group of diseases characterized by altered function of the immune system of the body, resulting in the production of antibodies against the body's own cells.

B

Blastocyte An undifferentiated embryonic cell.

C

Central nervous system One of the three systems the human nervous system is made of. It consists of the spinal cord, brainstem, and two cerebral hemispheres.

Cerebral palsy (CP) A permanent, nonprogressive neurologic disorder of motor function; describes a group of chronic conditions impairing control of posture and movement. CP appears in the first few years of life and generally does not worsen over time.

Chemical burn A burn injury that is divided primarily into two groups, acid and alkali. Acids produce coagulation necrosis by denaturing proteins upon tissue contact, and the development of this area of coagulation limits any extension of the injury. Alkalis cause a liquefaction necrosis, meaning the tissue is liquefied by contact with the alkali and then necroses as a result.

Child abuse Mistreatment of a child by a parent, guardian, or other caregiver.

Childhood disintegrative disorder A condition occurring in 3- and 4-year-olds

who have developed normally to age 2. Over several months, a child with this disorder will deteriorate in intellectual, social, and language functioning from previously normal behavior. An affected child shows a loss of communication skills, regression in nonverbal behaviors, and significant loss of previously acquired skills.

Chronological age (CA) Refers to the age of the child in days, weeks, or months from the time of birth.

Clubfoot deformity A birth defect in which the foot is turned inward, is stiff, and cannot be brought to a normal position.

Computerized tomography (CT) A medical imaging method that employs tomography, a process in which digital geometry processing is used to generate a three-dimensional image of the internal structures of an object from a large series of two-dimensional x-ray images taken around a single axis of rotation.

Conductive education An integrated system for children with cerebral palsy, spina bifida, and other motor disorders. Conductive education allows the child to learn to move within functional skills and is based on four primary principles: a conductor, the group setting, rhythmic intention, and a specific task series for each functional skill.

Congenital limb deficiency Amputations that occur in utero.

Contoured system One of three postural support systems that provides external postural control by increasing the points of contact, especially laterally. The seat and back surfaces are rounded by shaping layers of firm foam, air, or gel to correspond to the curves of the body.

Contrecoup injury The secondary reaction of the brain after initial force/injury.

Coup injury An injury in which the brain does not decelerate, rather it continues to move laterally until it is stopped by the lateral aspect of the skull.

Criterion-referenced measures Based on milestones of motor skills performed by typically developing clients; are more useful when developing a treatment plan or curriculum for a patient.

Custom-molded system One of three postural support systems and the third level of intervention that provides an intimate fit by closely conforming to the shape of the client's body, thereby giving the most postural support.

D

Developmentally supportive care Based on the belief that infants are vulnerable to sensory overload and overstimulation.

Diplegia A condition caused by cerebral palsy in which a child's functional problems occur primarily in the legs, with little or no involvement in the arms.

Disablement model (NAGI model) Widely used to describe a patient and the effect of injury or pathology on the patient's livelihood.

Down syndrome A genetic disorder caused by the presence of all or part of an extra chromosome 21.

E

Electrical burn Burn injuries are attributable to a variety of household mechanisms. Low-voltage injuries have very low morbidity and mortality. Both morbidity and mortality increase proportionally as voltage increases.

Embryonic stage Stage occurs during weeks 2 to 8 of gestation, in which rapid growth and development of the major body systems, including the respiratory, digestive, and nervous systems, occur.

Enablement model (ICF WHO model) The World Health Organization's model of enablement; describes how the patient's injury or pathology impacts activities and participation in society, based around the body structure and function, activity limitations and participation restrictions, and environmental factors.

Escharotomy Incisions through burns that may be necessary to reduce the pressures within the burns caused by the ever-increasing edema during the initial stages of burn progression. This is done to restore circulation when the tissue pressures compromise blood flow.

F

Fetal stage Constitutes the time 8 weeks postconception until birth. Rapid growth continues, organs and body systems become more refined. Fingernails, toenails, and eyelashes develop. The fetus actively moves within the uterus.

Full-thickness burn A third- or fourth-degree burn that involves the destruction of all the epidermal and dermal layers and extends down into the subcutaneous tissue.

G

Germinal stage Stage from fertilization until roughly 2 weeks gestational age in which the zygote implants into the uterine wall and divides.

Gestational age The age of a child expressed in number of weeks postconception.

Glasgow Coma Scale Aims to give a reliable, objective way of recording the conscious state of a person for initial and continuing assessment.

Gross Motor Functional Classification A classification system that categorizes children by degree of severity or functional capability. This system provides a qualitative, objective measure of prognosis of gross motor skills; a child can be classified at one of five levels, depending on the child's skill level.

Growth plate fracture A fracture in a long bone most commonly found near a joint; a common fracture among growing children.

H

Hemimelia Refers to a longitudinal anomaly where all or part of one bone is missing.

Hemiparesis A condition caused by cerebral palsy in which the child has weakness and poor motor control of one arm and one leg on the same side of the body.

Heterotopic ossificans The formation of real bone within soft tissue, which often causes pain, decreased range of motion, and swelling of the joint. This is a common risk for children who experience brain injury or spinal cord injury.

Homunculus A small anatomic model of the human form.

Hydrocephalus The enlargement of the ventricular system in the brain due to an increase in cerebrospinal fluid.

Hypertonia Increased rigidity, tension, and spasticity of the muscles caused by cerebral palsy; can sometimes lead to functional limitation, disability, or in severe cases reduced quality of life.

Hypertrophic scar Takes the form of a red, raised lump on the skin, but does not grow beyond the boundaries of the original wound; often improves in appearance after a few years.

Hypotonia Reduced tension or pressure.

I

Individualized educational plan (IEP) Describes the goals for the school year an educational team sets for children with delayed skills.

Individualized family service plan Establishes outcomes and related strategies, based on the caregiver's priorities, concerns, and professional assessments. The team, which includes the family and all evaluators, determines the amount of services to be provided and how best to meet the needs of the child in a natural environment.

Interdisciplinary A mix of practitioners from different disciplines who maintain their own professional roles and use a cooperative approach that is very interactive and centered on a common problem to solve.

Intracranial pressure The pressure exerted by the cranium on the brain tissue, cerebrospinal fluid, and the brain's circulating blood volume.

Iridocyclitis An inflammation of the iris and ciliary body.

J

Joint contractures A chronic loss of joint motion due to structural changes in non-bony tissue.

Joint inflammation A localized protective reaction of tissue in the joints to irritation, injury, or infection; characterized by pain, swelling, and sometimes loss of function.

K

Kinesio taping Used to support weakened muscles or prevent muscle overuse. Kinesio tape is flexible and has elastic properties that can strengthen a weakened muscle to prevent cramping or overcontraction.

L

Leukotaping Rigid strapping used to support a joint in a normal alignment. Muscle facilitation for appropriate firing can be achieved by laying the tape parallel to the muscle fibers.

Longitudinal deficiencies Unilateral or bilateral deficiency in which one of the bones in the segment is missing or malformed along the long axis of the segment.

M

Magnetic resonance imaging (MRI) Primarily used in medical imaging to visualize the structure and function of the body. It provides detailed images of the body in any plane.

Meningocele One of the levels of spina bifida in which the neural arches do not connect, and there is a sac covering the child's spinal column containing the herniation of the meninges. The spinal cord is not trapped, and these children often do not show any symptoms.

Micrognathia An abnormally small jaw.

Mosaicism Denotes the presence of two populations of cells with different genotypes in one individual who has developed from a single fertilized egg.

Multidisciplinary A mix of practitioners from multiple disciplines who work together in a common setting but without an interactive relationship.

Muscle atrophy Refers to a decrease in the size of skeletal muscle.

Myelomeningocele One of the levels of spina bifida in which the spinal cord and tissue protrude through the vertebral defect into an open area in the back. The spinal cord is malformed, and defects may extend below the level of the primary herniation. The defect can occur at any spinal level, but is often seen in the lumbosacral area.

N

Neonatology An area of pediatric medicine that seeks to optimize the infant's potential for development and measure the limits of viability for premature infants.

Neural tube defects Birth defects in the brain and spinal cord. The two most common neural tube defects are spina bifida and anencephaly.

Neurodevelopmental treatment Embraces knowledge of motor control and looks at the effects of postural control as a result of interactions between many neurologic and physiologic systems. Therapy that is meant for children with cerebral palsy or other motor disorders and enhances the individual's capacity to function.

Norm-referenced measures An assessment standardized on a normal population; allows standard scores, percentiles, and age-equivalent calculations to be made.

O

Osteochondritis dissecans An injury to the articular cartilage and the corresponding bone.

P

Partial-thickness burn A second-degree burn that penetrates more deeply; involves destruction of all the epidermal layers and extends into the dermis.

Pauciarticular JRA A pauciarticular (involving only a few joints) disease in which children test positive for antinuclear antibodies and have a high risk for iridocyclitis. Pauciarticular JRA can affect the spine, although possibly not until the late teens, and the children may test positive for the gene identified with adult ankylosing spondylitis.

Peak flow monitoring A monitoring system that employs a simple device that measures how well air is moving out of a patient's airways.

Percentage score Expresses the percent of items passed on a scale.

Percentile score *Percentile* means "per hundred." A percentile score gives an individual's ranking in a group. If a child scores in the 80th percentile on a test, the score is equal to or higher than the scores of 80% of the children who took the test.

Peripheral nervous system Connects nerves to the central nervous system; is built from sensory fibers that innervate glands and skeletal, cardiac, and smooth muscle.

Pervasive developmental disorder—not otherwise specified (PDD-NOS) A subthreshold condition in which the individual meets some but not all of the diagnostic criteria necessary for a diagnosis of autism. Children diagnosed with PDD-NOS demonstrate issues with socialization and behavior similar to but less severe than those evidenced by persons with autism; they have fewer if any language issues.

Phocomelia Refers to the congenital absence of the proximal section of the limb.

Planar system One of three postural support systems; it is the least intensive and consists of a flat seat and back.

Polyarticular JRA An arthritis in children that involves five or more large joints. Includes two subtypes. In the first subtype, children identified with a special kind of antibody in their blood known as *rheumatoid factor (RF)* often

have a more severe form of JRA. In the second subtype, children only experience joint involvement.

Postconceptual age (PCA) Child's chronological age (CA) plus the gestational age (GA). For example, a child with a CA of 4 weeks who was born at 28 weeks gestation has a PCA of 32 weeks.

Preventive medication One of two types of medication. Can be oral or inhaled; used to help decrease inflammation of the airways or to decrease the response to a trigger such as an allergen.

Primitive reflexes Any reflex normal in an infant, including grasp reflex, Moro reflex, and sucking reflex.

Proprioceptive neuromuscular facilitation Intervention for children with muscle imbalances to strengthen muscles within diagonal and rotational movement patterns. PNF is based on developmental sequence and the sequential mastery of motor milestones.

Prosthesis A device, either external or implanted, that substitutes for or supplements a missing or defective part of the body.

Q

Quadriparesis A condition caused by cerebral palsy in which some children have problems in all four extremities.

Qualitative assessment Assessment that interprets the phenomenon of performance, often in context of performance and presented as a descriptive narrative. This assessment will frequently be open ended, with no forced choice. Anecdotal observations and self-reports are examples of qualitative assessments.

Quantitative assessment Performance or achievement information or description made with objective, measurable data. Often this assessment is standardized and structured. Behavior occurrence as measured by behavioral objectives, task achievement, and specific values achieved (such as pounds lifted) is an example of a quantitative assessment.

R

Ranchos Los Amigos Levels of Cognitive Functioning Multilevel scale of cognitive recovery that ranges from 1 to 8; used for assessment of recovery, for communication between medical professionals and facilities, and to measure change and progress during the rehabilitation course.

Raw score Actual points earned on an assessment, or the number of items passed on a certain test.

Reliability Determines if the tool is an accurate measure of what it claims to measure.

Rescue medication One of two types of asthma medications, usually in the form of an inhaler (e.g., albuterol). This medication quickly helps to open the airways to help a person breathe easier.

Residual limb The part of the limb that remains after amputation.

Responsiveness The ability to detect minimally significant clinical change.

Retinal hemorrhage Hemorrhage inside the intraocular space caused by a sudden increase in venous pressure in the head. The rise in pressure is communicated by the optic nerve sheaths, causing blood to leak through damaged vessels; accompanied by retinal edema. Severe damage to the eyes may cause permanent, partial, or total blindness.

Rett syndrome An early-onset (prior to age 4) genetic condition associated with an abnormality on the X chromosome. Children develop normally through the first few months of life, then lose hand function and develop stereotyped hand movements that resemble hand wringing or hand washing around 5 months of age. Head growth slows, and social impairments similar to those in autism emerge.

Rigidity Significant resistance to movement.

Rotational injury Occurs when the brain remains stationary in a moving, rotating skull. Rotational injuries are related to shearing trauma and have been associated with diffuse axonal injuries.

Rule of nines A method of measuring the extent of a burn; divides the body surface into areas, each of which is considered to be 9% or a multiple of 9% of the total body surface area.

Scaled score Provides an estimate of the child's ability level along a continuum of items. Scores range from 0 to 100; 0 is low capacity, and 100 is highly capable.

Scheuermann disease A wedge-shaped fracture that has an overuse, postural cause.

Scleroderma Also known as *systemic sclerosis*, a connective tissue disease involving the skin, blood vessels, and immune system.

Secondary injury Occurs due to processes induced in response to the initial

trauma. Secondary injuries account for a significant portion of the overall damage that occurs with TBI.

Sensory integration Therapy that assists children by using controlled sensory input to help those with sensory processing difficulties. Three major components: normal sensory function, sensory integration dysfunction, and a programmatic guide for using sensory integration techniques.

Shaken baby syndrome A highly preventable disorder in which the brain is jolted back and forth inside the skull, creating first acceleration then deceleration movements inside the skull.

Spacer A large chamber fitted to an inhaler; useful in dispensing a dose of medication more effectively. Spacers increase the amount of medication that reaches the lungs instead of being deposited in the mouth and throat.

Spastic quadriplegia A condition caused by cerebral palsy in which a child experiences symptoms from both triplegia and diplegia.

Spasticity Pertaining to sudden, abnormal, involuntary muscular contraction consisting of a continued muscular contraction.

Spina bifida occulta Describes the condition where the neural arches do not connect, but there is no neural material located outside the spinal canal. This is the most common form of spina bifida, characteristically involving the lower lumbar spine. It is also the most benign, with typically no resultant neurologic effects or abnormalities.

Standard scores Describe deviations from the mean, or average, score for the group. Standard deviations are used to describe the divergence.

Standard tests Tests that include a set of tasks or questions that are intended to assess a particular type of behavior when presented under standardized conditions.

Strength training The use of resistance to muscular contraction to build the strength, anaerobic endurance, and size of skeletal muscles.

Superficial burn First-degree burns that are limited to the epidermis.

Systemic JRA Also known as *Still disease*, a type of JRA accompanied by high spiking fevers off and on for weeks and a rash on the chest and thighs. In addition

to joint involvement, internal organs such as the heart, liver, spleen, and lymph nodes can be affected.

Tethered cord syndrome Occurs when the spinal cord is fixed caudally because of pathology. The tethered spinal cord becomes stretched, distorted, and ischemic. The child with tethered cord may show atypical neurologic signs, including decreased strength, increased spasticity in the lower extremities, changing urologic patterns, back pain, or scoliosis.

Therapeutic taping Therapy for children with muscle weakness, joint instability, joint malalignment, and postural asymmetries; uses rigid or flexible taping to support and influence muscle groups.

TheraTogs An orthotic product that is designed to capture the benefits of taping without directly adhering to the skin.

Thermal burn Thermal burn injuries are the most likely to occur to infants and children; extremely common in young children and can occur from spilled food and beverages, including grease spills, hot tap water, clothes irons, curling irons, space heaters, and ovens/ranges.

Tone The normal tension found in muscles.

Total body surface area (TBSA) The amount of body surface over which a burn injury extends.

Transdisciplinary A team of practitioners from different disciplines in which members cross over professional boundaries and share roles and functions.

Translational injury An injury that causes a reaction to a force applied to the side of the skull with lateral movement of both the skull and the brain. This can cause significant brain damage.

Transverse amputation Occurs in the transverse plane of the extremity through the shaft of the involved bone.

Traumatic brain injury A traumatically induced physiologic disruption of brain functioning, resulting in partial or total impairments of one or more areas of functioning.

Triplegia A condition caused by cerebral palsy in which one arm and hand are virtually uninvolved, while all other limbs are involved.

Trisomy 21 One of the three types of chromosomal abnormalities that can lead to

Down syndrome. Trisomy 21 occurs in 95% of Down syndrome cases and results in an extra chromosome 21. Individuals with trisomy 21 have 47 chromosomes instead of the typical 46. Translocation occurs when the long arm of the extra chromosome 21 attaches to chromosome 14, 21, or 22.

V

Validity Determines if the assessment tool accomplishes its intended purpose.

W

Wheeled mobility Segment of the assistive technology available to individuals with disabilities.

Z

Zygote The result of fertilization, when the sperm and the ovum combine to form a new cell.

Note: Page numbers followed by '*f*' indicate figures, '*t*' indicate tables, and '*b*' indicate boxes.

A

Acceleration-dependent injury, 75
Achilles tenotomy, 115–122
Acquired amputations, 177
Acquired brain injury (ABI), 73
Acquired CP, 55
Acquired limb deficiency, 176
Age-equivalent score, 15
Ages and Stages Questionnaire, Second Edition (ASQ), 152
Alberta Infant Motor Scale (AIMS), 17*t*, 19, 63–64
Amelia, 176–177
American children, 6*b*
American Physical Therapy Association (APTA)
   Clinical Practice Guideline for Developmental Coordination Disorder, 160, 160*t*
   core values for PT and PTA, 36*b*, 36
   patient/client management model, 44*f*
   transforming society by optimizing movement, 42–43
Amniotic band syndrome (ABS), 177
Amputations
   lower extremity, 178*t*
   upper extremity, 178*t*
Ankle-foot orthosis (AFO), 188
   articulated, 249
   carbon, 249
   cervical, 249
   flexible, 249
   ground reaction force, 249
   hip-knee, 251
   knee, 250
   solid, 249
   spinal, 251
   thoracolumbosacral, 251
Antinuclear antibodies, 93
Aquatic therapy, 27*t*, 30
Arnold-Chiari malformation, type 2, 141*f*
Arthrogryposis multiplex congenita (AMC), 127*b*
   case study, 129*b*–130*b*
   causes of limited joint movement, 125
   clinical signs, 126*f*, 126–127, 127*b*
   definition, 125
   deformities of, 126–127
   incidence of dislocated hips, 127
   pathology, 125
   physical therapy assessment, 127
   physical therapy intervention, 127
     elbow flexion and extension, 127
     for infants, 127–128
     for preschool and school-age, 128
     serial casting to treat deformities, 127–128

Arthrogryposis multiplex congenita (AMC) *(Continued)*
     splinting and orthotic use, 127–128
     stretching and strengthening interventions, 127–128
     for toddler, 128
Articulated ankle-foot orthosis, 249
Assault/abusive head trauma (ABT), 73–74
Assessment
   goals and outcomes, 15–16
   norming sample, 14–15
   pediatric physical therapy, 17*t*
   purpose of, 14–15
   qualitative, 16
   quantitative, 16
   reliability, 16
   validity, 16
Assessment tools
   age-equivalent score, 15
   criterion-referenced, 16–18, 20
   norm-referenced, 16, 18–20
   in pediatric physical therapy, 20–21
   percentage score, 15
   percentile score, 15
   raw score, 15
   scaled score, 15
   standardized, 16
   standard scores, 15
   standard tests, 15
Asthma, 184
Asymmetric tonic neck reflex, 4
Ataxic CP, 56–57
Athetoid CP, 56–57
Athetoid tone, 10
Atypical development
   causes, 10
Atypical tone, 10
Autism, 148, 151*f*
   associated disorders in, 149
   case study, 153*b*–155*b*
   clinical signs
     hyper- or hyporeactivity, 151
     impairment in facial expression and body posture, 150
     limited or no joint attention, 150
     peer relationships, 150
     poor eye contact, 150
     restricted or repetitive behaviors, 150–151
     social communication and interaction skills, 149–150
   definition, 148
   intervention, 151–152
   pathology, 148
   physical therapy assessment, 152